Promotion of Physical Activity and Health in the School Setting

Antonio García-Hermoso
Editor

Promotion of Physical Activity and Health in the School Setting

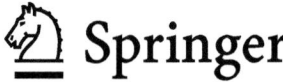

Editor
Antonio García-Hermoso
Navarrabiomed, Hospital Universitario de Navarra
Universidad Pública de Navarra (UPNA), IdiSNA
Pamplona, Navarra, Spain

ISBN 978-3-031-65594-4   ISBN 978-3-031-65595-1 (eBook)
https://doi.org/10.1007/978-3-031-65595-1

© The Editor(s) (if applicable) and The Author(s), under exclusive license to Springer Nature Switzerland AG 2024

This work is subject to copyright. All rights are solely and exclusively licensed by the Publisher, whether the whole or part of the material is concerned, specifically the rights of translation, reprinting, reuse of illustrations, recitation, broadcasting, reproduction on microfilms or in any other physical way, and transmission or information storage and retrieval, electronic adaptation, computer software, or by similar or dissimilar methodology now known or hereafter developed.

The use of general descriptive names, registered names, trademarks, service marks, etc. in this publication does not imply, even in the absence of a specific statement, that such names are exempt from the relevant protective laws and regulations and therefore free for general use.

The publisher, the authors and the editors are safe to assume that the advice and information in this book are believed to be true and accurate at the date of publication. Neither the publisher nor the authors or the editors give a warranty, expressed or implied, with respect to the material contained herein or for any errors or omissions that may have been made. The publisher remains neutral with regard to jurisdictional claims in published maps and institutional affiliations.

This Springer imprint is published by the registered company Springer Nature Switzerland AG
The registered company address is: Gewerbestrasse 11, 6330 Cham, Switzerland

If disposing of this product, please recycle the paper.

Preface

In the mission to provide children and young people the education and essential life skills they need, schools become pivotal arenas for promoting both cognitive development and physical well-being. Recognizing the inherent connection between physical activity and holistic health—encompassing physiological, physical, and mental dimensions—this book highlights the importance of integrating robust physical activity strategies within the school setting.

Children and adolescents, who spend a significant portion of their time within the school environment, present a unique opportunity to instill the values of regular physical activity. This emphasis not only aligns with preventive measures against pressing public health issues like childhood obesity and sedentary lifestyles but also acknowledges schools as influential spaces capable of shaping lifelong habits. Schools are the second most significant sphere of influence after the home, becoming a strategic hub for disseminating quality physical activity education on a large scale.

This book delineates the critical role schools play in promoting physical literacy and fostering an active school day for preschoolers, children, and adolescents. Beyond the evident health benefits, it investigates how school-based physical activity initiatives can positively impact academic learning and classroom behavior. The book provides an exhaustive account of the integration of physical activity strategies at various educational stages—from pre-primary to secondary school—incorporating updated evidence from successful investigations.

Furthermore, this collaborative effort from a diverse group of authors bridges the gap between theory and practice. By clarifying advances in both theory and research, the book not only showcases evidence-backed strategies but also serves as a practical guide for educators and policymakers. It outlines the complexities of planning, implementing, and evaluating school policies that foster a culture of physical activity. By incorporating these strategies, schools have the potential to cultivate an environment that not only reduces the risk of chronic diseases but also encourages a lasting appreciation for an active and healthy lifestyle. This collective effort strives to empower educators, professionals, and families alike in their commitment to the well-being and flourishing futures of the younger generation.

Pamplona, Navarra, Spain   Antonio García-Hermoso

Acknowledgments

I would like to express my sincere gratitude to Dr. Yasmin Ezzatvar for her invaluable support in designing all the figures in the book. Her dedication and expertise have significantly enriched this work, adding a visual dimension that complements and strengthens the content. Her collaboration has been essential for the completion of this book.

Contents

Part I Movement Guidelines and Recommendations

1. **Physical Activity and Sedentary Behavior in Children and Adolescents: Recommendations and Health Impacts** 3
   Yang Liu, Danqing Zhang, Youzhi Ke, Yiping Yan, Yangyang Shen, and Zhenghan Wang

2. **Twenty-Four-Hour Movement Behaviors for School-Aged Children and Adolescents** 41
   José Francisco López-Gil

Part II Assessment and Evaluation of Physical Health and Skills in School Settings

3. **Physical Literacy Assessment: A Conceptualization and Tools** 67
   Andreas Fröberg and Suzanne Lundvall

4. **Assessment of Physical Activity in Children and Adolescents** 89
   Jairo H. Migueles and Patricio Solis-Urra

5. **Health-Related Physical Fitness Assessment in School Settings** 107
   Kai Zhang, Cristina Cadenas-Sanchez, Brooklyn Fraser, and Justin J. Lang

6. **Motor Skill Assessment in Children and Adolescents** 133
   Nadia Cristina Valentini

Part III Physical Activity During School Hours

7. **Physical Activity and Health Through Physical Education** 167
   Adrià Muntaner-Mas

8	**Active Travel to and from School**	193
	Adilson Marques, Tiago Ribeiro, and Miguel Peralta	
9	**Physical Activity Opportunities During School Recess**	213
	Antonio García-Hermoso	
10	**Active Classrooms in School Curricula and Active Breaks**	233
	Abel Ruiz-Hermosa, David Sánchez-Oliva, and Mairena Sánchez-López	
11	**Multicomponent School-Based Physical Activity Programs**	251
	Collin A. Webster	
12	**School-Based Before-School Physical Activity Programs**	269
	Michalis Stylianou and James Woodforde	
13	**School-Based After-School Physical Activity and Sports Programs**	285
	Hyungsik Min, Donetta Cothran, and Pamela Hodges Kulinna	
14	**Integrating High-Intensity Interval Training (HIIT) into the School Setting: Benefits, Criticisms, and Recommendations**	303
	Angus A. Leahy, Jordan J. Smith, Narelle Eather, Nigel Harris, and David R. Lubans	
15	**How Can Muscle-Strengthening Activities Be Promoted in School Settings?**	327
	Ashley Cox	
16	**Inclusive Physical Activity Practices for Disabled Children and Adolescents**	359
	Thi Nancy Huynh, Justin Haegele, Maeghan E. James, and Kelly P. Arbour-Nicitopoulos	

Index 385

Contributors

Kelly P. Arbour-Nicitopoulos Faculty of Kinesiology and Physical Education, University of Toronto, Toronto, ON, Canada

Cristina Cadenas-Sanchez Department of Cardiology, Stanford University, Stanford, CA, USA

Veterans Affairs Palo Alto Health Care System, Palo Alto, CA, USA

Department of Physical Education and Sports, Faculty of Sports Science, Sport and Health University Research Institute (iMUDS), Granada, Spain

Donetta Cothran Department of Kinesiology, School of Public Health, Indiana University Bloomington, Bloomington, IN, USA

Ashley Cox Division of Musculoskeletal and Dermatological Sciences, Faculty of Biology, Medicine and Health, The University of Manchester, Manchester, UK

Narelle Eather Centre for Active Living and Learning, College of Human and Social Futures, University of Newcastle, Callaghan, NSW, Australia

Active Living Research Program, Hunter Medical Research Institute, New Lambton Heights, NSW, Australia

Brooklyn Fraser Menzies Institute for Medical Research, University of Tasmania, Hobart, TAS, Australia

Alliance for Research in Exercise, Nutrition and Activity (ARENA), University of South Australia, Adelaide, SA, Australia

Andreas Fröberg Department of Food and Nutrition, and Sport Science, University of Gothenburg, Gothenburg, Sweden

Antonio García-Hermoso Navarrabiomed, Hospital Universitario de Navarra, Universidad Pública de Navarra (UPNA), IdiSNA, Pamplona, Navarra, Spain

Justin Haegele Department of Human Movement Sciences, Old Dominion University, Norfolk, VA, USA

Nigel Harris Human Potential Centre, Auckland University of Technology, Auckland, New Zealand

Thi Nancy Huynh Faculty of Kinesiology and Physical Education, University of Toronto, Toronto, ON, Canada

Maeghan E. James Healthy Active Living and Obesity Research Group, Children's Hospital of Eastern Ontario Research Institute, Ottawa, ON, Canada

Department of Pediatrics, Faculty of Medicine, University of Ottawa, Ottawa, ON, Canada

Youzhi Ke Shanghai University of Sport, Shanghai, China

Pamela Hodges Kulinna Mary Lou Fulton Teachers College, Arizona State University, Tempe, AZ, USA

Justin J. Lang Alliance for Research in Exercise, Nutrition and Activity (ARENA), University of South Australia, Adelaide, SA, Australia

Centre for Surveillance and Applied Research, Public Health Agency of Canada, Ottawa, ON, Canada

School of Epidemiology and Public Health, Faculty of Medicine, University of Ottawa, Ottawa, ON, Canada

Angus A. Leahy Centre for Active Living and Learning, College of Human and Social Futures, University of Newcastle, Callaghan, NSW, Australia

Active Living Research Program, Hunter Medical Research Institute, New Lambton Heights, NSW, Australia

Yang Liu Shanghai University of Sport, Shanghai, China

José Francisco López-Gil One Health Research Group, Universidad de Las Américas, Quito, Ecuador

David R. Lubans Centre for Active Living and Learning, College of Human and Social Futures, University of Newcastle, Callaghan, NSW, Australia

Active Living Research Program, Hunter Medical Research Institute, New Lambton Heights, NSW, Australia

Faculty of Sport and Health Sciences, University of Jyväskylä, Jyväskylä, Finland

Suzanne Lundvall Department of Food and Nutrition, and Sport Science, University of Gothenburg, Gothenburg, Sweden

Adilson Marques CIPER, Faculty of Human Kinetics, University of Lisbon, Lisbon, Portugal

Jairo H. Migueles Department of Physical Education and Sports, Faculty of Sport Sciences, Sport and Health University Research Institute (iMUDS), University of Granada, Granada, Spain

Contributors

Hyungsik Min Mary Lou Fulton Teachers College, Arizona State University, Tempe, AZ, USA

Adrià Muntaner-Mas GICAFE "Physical Activity and Exercise Sciences Research Group", Faculty of Education, University of Balearic Islands, Palma, Spain

PROFITH "PROmoting FITness and Health Through Physical Activity" Research Group, Sport and Health University Research Institute (iMUDS), Department of Physical Education and Sports, Faculty of Sport Sciences, University of Granada, Granada, Spain

Miguel Peralta CIPER, Faculty of Human Kinetics, University of Lisbon, Lisbon, Portugal

Tiago Ribeiro CIPER, Faculty of Human Kinetics, University of Lisbon, Lisbon, Portugal

Abel Ruiz-Hermosa Faculty of Sport Sciences, Universidad de Extremadura, Cáceres, Spain

School of Education, Universidad de Castilla-La Mancha, Ciudad Real, Spain

Mairena Sánchez-López School of Education, Universidad de Castilla-La Mancha, Ciudad Real, Spain

David Sánchez-Oliva Faculty of Sport Sciences, Universidad de Extremadura, Cáceres, Spain

Yangyang Shen Shanghai University of Sport, Shanghai, China

Jordan J. Smith Centre for Active Living and Learning, College of Human and Social Futures, University of Newcastle, Callaghan, NSW, Australia

Active Living Research Program, Hunter Medical Research Institute, New Lambton Heights, NSW, Australia

Patricio Solis-Urra Department of Physical Education and Sports, Faculty of Sport Sciences, Sport and Health University Research Institute (iMUDS), University of Granada, Granada, Spain

Michalis Stylianou School of Human Movement and Nutrition Sciences, The University of Queensland, St. Lucia, QLD, Australia

Nadia Cristina Valentini Universidade Federal do Rio Grande do Sul, Porto Alegre, Brazil

Zhenghan Wang Shanghai University of Sport, Shanghai, China

Collin A. Webster Department of Kinesiology, Texas A&M University – Corpus Christi, Corpus Christi, TX, USA

James Woodforde School of Human Movement and Nutrition Sciences, The University of Queensland, St. Lucia, QLD, Australia

Yiping Yan Shanghai University of Sport, Shanghai, China

Danqing Zhang Shanghai University of Sport, Shanghai, China

Kai Zhang Healthy Active Living and Obesity Research Group, Children's Hospital of Eastern Ontario Research Institute, Ottawa, ON, Canada

School of Human Kinetics, University of Ottawa, Ottawa, ON, Canada

About the Editor

Antonio García-Hermoso, PhD, MSc, is a native of Plasencia, Spain, and a graduate of the University of Extremadura, Spain. Since 2019, Dr. García-Hermoso has been a member of the Navarrabiomed Research Center in Pamplona, Spain, where he serves as the head of the Physical Activity, Children, and Youth Unit. This unit is dedicated to analyzing the impact of exercise and physical activity on the physical and mental health of both ill and apparently healthy young people.

Dr. García-Hermoso has contributed to over 300 publications in peer-reviewed and PubMed-listed journals. He is a member of several international professional societies and serves on the editorial boards of *Translational Pediatrics* journal and the *Scandinavian Journal of Medicine and Science in Sports*.

Part I
Movement Guidelines and Recommendations

Chapter 1
Physical Activity and Sedentary Behavior in Children and Adolescents: Recommendations and Health Impacts

Yang Liu, Danqing Zhang, Youzhi Ke, Yiping Yan, Yangyang Shen, and Zhenghan Wang

1.1 Introduction

Physical activity (PA) is broadly defined as any bodily movement performed by skeletal muscles that leads to energy expenditure and can be quantified in kilocalories. Daily life PA encompasses occupational, sports, conditioning, household, and other activities. Within this spectrum, exercise represents a planned, structured, and repetitive subset of PA aimed at improving or maintaining physical fitness. Physical fitness consists of attributes that can be health- or skill-related, and the assessment of these attributes is possible through specific tests. These definitions, outlined by Caspersen [1] in 1985, serve as an internationalist framework for comparing studies that examine the relationship between PA, exercise, and physical fitness and health outcomes. Additionally, Pate et al. [2] proposed a model for classifying the Metabolic Equivalent of Task (MET) intensity of PA by categorizing patients into light (<3 METs), moderate (3–6 METs), or vigorous (>6 METs). This model provides a standardized approach for assessing the intensity levels of various physical activities.

On the other hand, sedentary behaviors, derived from the Latin word "sedere" (meaning "to sit"), are typically characterized by low energy expenditure, such as resting metabolic rate [3]. These behaviors include sitting during commuting, in the workplace, and in the domestic environment, as well as during leisure time [4]. Activities such as lying down, watching television, computer and game-console use, and other forms of screen-based entertainment, or sitting in an automobile, usually fall within the energy expenditure range of 1.0–1.5 metabolic equivalents of tasks (METs). Notably, one MET is defined as the energy cost of resting quietly, often expressed in terms of oxygen uptake as 3.5 mL·kg^{-1}·min^{-1} [5–7]. Sedentary

---

Y. Liu (✉) · D. Zhang · Y. Ke · Y. Yan · Y. Shen · Z. Wang
Shanghai University of Sport, Shanghai, China
e-mail: docliuyang@hotmail.com

behaviors involving both sitting and low levels of energy expenditure are highlighted [8]. The Sedentary Behavior Research Network defines sedentary behavior as any waking behavior characterized by an energy expenditure ≤1.5 METs while in a sitting or reclining posture.

1.2 Benefits of Physical Activity

The promotion of PA is a critical aspect of contemporary education and public health, impacting individuals' physiological, psychological, and social well-being [9]. Moreover, PA offers significant cardiovascular benefits, reducing mortality rates through activities such as swimming and aerobics [10, 11]. It also plays a crucial role in bone and muscle health, metabolic regulation, weight management, and mental health, combating issues such as depression and anxiety [12, 13]. Additionally, PA positively influences mood and stress relief, contributing to improved overall mental health [14, 15]. Socially, PA promotes interaction, teamwork, communication skills, and self-confidence. This synthesis supports the development of personalized intervention strategies in educational contexts [9].

1.2.1 Benefits of Physical Activity for Infants, Toddlers, and Preschoolers Under 5 Years of Age

Below are several benefits associated with regular PA practice in children under the age of 5.

1.2.1.1 Physical Development

Physical activity is a necessary condition for the healthy growth and development of young children, and the early childhood stage is a critical period for overweight and obesity. Between the ages of 0 and 2, the body's fat content rapidly increases. Starting at the age of 5–6, there is a second natural increase in body fat content. Early childhood body fat content is related to adult skin fold thickness and body mass index (BMI) and is a key factor in controlling the development of obesity [16]. PA in preschool children aged 3–6 years has a positive effect on one or more body composition-related indicators and can reduce the risk of obesity and overweight [17].

1.2.1.2 Bones and Muscles

To enhance bone health, young children should engage in activities that involve jumping and rolling. The distribution of osteoblasts on the surface of young children's bones is abundant. In the early stages of PA, muscle contraction generates tension and gravitational loads, which can stimulate osteoblasts, promote bone pathway development, and have long-term positive effects on adult bone pathway health. Engaging in early childhood gymnastics can have a positive impact on bone development and morphological outcomes in childhood [18]. Therefore, we should pay attention to the growth of young children's bones and muscles through the PA.

1.2.1.3 Psychological Development

Mental health, as a positive state of well-being, is the foundation for a good quality of life, especially for young children. There is a positive relationship between PA and mental health in young children [19]. The PA of young children not only enhance their cognitive abilities but also have a positive impact on their memory and learning.

1.2.1.4 Cognitive Ability

Young children are experiencing rapid physical and cognitive development, as well as habit formation and easy adjustment of lifestyle habits. Moreover, PA promotes cognitive development in young children [20]. Research has shown that engaging in positive games equivalent to moderate-to-vigorous PA (MVPA) can promote the development of young children's self-regulation abilities, thereby improving academic performance [21].

1.2.1.5 Memory and Learning

Studies have shown that PA interventions designed for preschool children can enhance working memory and motor competence [22]. Additionally, more time spent in MVPA are associated with better inhibitory control and working memory in this population [23].

1.2.1.6 Social Development

The socialization development of young children refers to the process in which they learn social rules, acquire social adaptability, master social skills, and form social relationships with others.

1.2.1.7 Team Collaboration and Social Skills

Social skills are an intrinsic factor in the mental health of young children [24]. During PA, young children inevitably interact and communicate with their peers, teachers, or family members. This kind of communication and exchange is used to express one's own wishes on the one hand, and on the other, one can understand the wishes of others and make corresponding responses, thus forming a role partnership. PA, especially organized sports, and structured sports games can help guide children to establish positive peer relationships. Research has shown that young children are more inclined to cooperate and develop common goals when engaging in outdoor PA, thereby generating companionship experiences among peers and cultivating empathy [25].

1.2.1.8 Personality and Willpower

Involving preschoolers in physically demanding activities that require self-control and perseverance may enhance their willpower and overall personality development because it provides them with opportunities to practice and strengthen these skills in a tangible and experiential manner [26]. By facing challenges and overcoming obstacles during such activities, preschoolers learn the value of persistence, discipline, and delayed gratification. This fosters the development of resilience and self-regulation, enabling them to better manage impulses and make constructive choices in various aspects of their lives [27].

1.2.2 Benefits of Physical Activity for Children

Physical activity has a positive and extensive impact on children, and the positive effects established during childhood persist into adolescence and even adulthood, playing a crucial role in child development. Below, we describe some of these benefits.

1.2.2.1 Physical Development

Children's active participation in PA contributes to healthy physical development, and the health benefits are reflected not only in cardiovascular and respiratory systems but also in strengthening skeletal muscles [28].

1.2.2.2 Cardiovascular and Respiratory Systems

Physical activity helps prevent cardiovascular disease (CVD) and improve cardiovascular health [29]. Research shows that the health benefits of moderate-to-high intensity PA are particularly significant [30], among which aerobic exercise is more effective [31]. Regular aerobic exercise, such as running, swimming, and playing football, can significantly improve the pumping efficiency of children's hearts, which delivers oxygen and nutrients throughout the body more efficiently, and the elasticity of the blood vessel walls and greater range of vasodilatation improve circulation and reduce the burden on the heart, thereby reducing the risk of cardiovascular disease [32, 33].

In addition, active PA helps improve the respiratory system [34], increase lung capacity, and improve respiratory system efficiency. Children are able to inhale oxygen more efficiently and deliver it to all parts of the body while expelling carbon dioxide more effectively.

1.2.2.3 Bones and Muscles

Physical activity during childhood has been shown to have a direct positive impact on musculoskeletal health [35]. Engaging in bone-strengthening activities during childhood can help reduce the risk of osteoporosis in adulthood, especially high-intensity PA [36]. Activities such as jumping, climbing, and resistance strength training stimulate the growth and proliferation of bones, increase bone density, and reduce the risk of fractures. Additionally, participating in a variety of muscle activities, such as pushing, pulling, and lifting heavy objects, is essential for the balanced development of a child's muscle groups. By targeting individual muscle groups, children are better able to build muscle strength, improve coordination, cope with various physical challenges in daily life, and thereby improve overall motor skills. This has a positive impact on the body's coordination and functionality [37].

1.2.2.4 Mental Health

Physical activity has a wide range of positive effects on cognitive development and mental health during childhood [38]. By participating in PA, children not only improve learning ability and memory but also help regulate their mood and reduce symptoms of anxiety and depression [39, 40]. The benefits of PA for mental health also extend to children with neurodevelopmental disorders [41].

1.2.2.5 Memory and Learning

The impact of children's PA on the brain is far from limited and directly involves specific brain areas, such as the hippocampus, for learning cognition and memory [42]. When engaging in PA, the hippocampus in the brain is activated to begin processing new information, learning, and memory. Exercise increases blood supply and promotes tighter connections between neurons. This neural activity improves children's learning and strengthens their attention, mental flexibility, and problem-solving skills [43]. Therefore, by participating in PA, children can be more active in learning, and their learning ability and memory can improve.

1.2.2.6 Behavioral Problems and Anxiety Symptoms

Childhood is a critical period for emotional and behavioral development, and nervous system regulation is also influenced by PA. Endogenous hormones released by exercise, such as dopamine and endorphins, have a positive regulatory effect on mood. These neurotransmitters help enhance children's emotional state and reduce symptoms of anxiety and depression [44]. In addition, by participating in group activities, children can establish more positive and healthy social relationships and improve their self-awareness and emotional regulation abilities [45]. Positive and healthy social relationships can reduce the incidence of problem behaviors in children and provide a healthy psychological support system. Overall, the learning and emotional benefits children gain from PA provide a strong foundation for their overall mental health.

1.2.2.7 Social Adaptation

Children actively develop friendships and foster teamwork through sports competitions and team activities. This not only provides opportunities to establish connections and make friends but also inspires responsibility, trust, and teamwork. These social sports experiences not only are positive at the moment but also, more importantly, continue to shape children's social skills over time [28].

1.2.2.8 Friendships and Teamwork

Children usually participate in sports competitions, games, or other activities with other children, and these experiences provide them with opportunities to bond with their peers and even make new friends. Additionally, when children participate in sports competitions or team activities, the team's collective honor and common goals can exercise their sense of responsibility, strengthen mutual trust, and deepen their sense of teamwork [46].

1.2.2.9 Self-Esteem and Social Skills Improved

The choice of PA provides children with a window to understand themselves. In addition to the acquisition of sports skills, children's sense of accomplishment, self-esteem, and self-confidence improve. By practicing with teammates, individuals learn to cooperate with others, share successes, cope with challenges together, form and maintain good interpersonal relationships, and acquire social skills [47]. In sports, there are broader possibilities for future development over time.

1.2.3 Benefits of Physical Activity for Adolescents

Adolescence is a critical developmental period during which individual lifestyle choices and behavioral patterns are formed, including decisions to engage in PA. The following section outlines the various health benefits of regular PA for encouraging everyone to actively participate.

1.2.3.1 Physical Health

Regular PA contributes to the physical health of adolescents in several ways. It helps improve cardiorespiratory fitness, build strong bones and muscles, control weight, and reduce the risk of developing various health conditions, such as heart disease, cancer, type 2 diabetes, high blood pressure, and obesity [48].

1.2.3.2 Growth and Development

Adolescence is the life stage between childhood and adulthood. It is a unique and important stage in the development of the full cycle of human life and a critical period for laying the foundation for health. Moderate PA promotes normal body metabolism, improves energy consumption efficiency, and helps individuals maintain a healthy and appropriate weight [49]. An increase in metabolic efficiency can increase nutrient absorption and utilization, ensure the acquisition of the materials and energy required by the body, and promote the growth and development of the body [50]. Moderate-to-vigorous intensity jumping and resistance exercise effectively stimulate bone proliferation and development, increase bone density, and enhance the stability of the skeletal system [51]. Moreover, the benefits of PA on skeletal muscles in adolescence can persist into early adulthood.

1.2.3.3 Prevention of Obesity and Chronic Diseases

As lifestyle changes lead to rising rates of obesity and chronic disease, one of the key measures taken to prevent these health problems is PA. Through exercise, adolescents can maintain a healthy weight, adjust insulin sensitivity, and reduce the risk of obesity and related diseases [52]. Moreover, PA can stimulate metabolic vitality and enhance the body's energy utilization efficiency. In addition, aerobic exercise, such as running and swimming, enhances the function of the cardiovascular system, maintains blood pressure stability, enhances cardiovascular system function, maintains blood pressure stability, reduces the risk of chronic diseases, and provides adolescents with an effective means to maintain cardiovascular health and prevent disease [53]. Therefore, active participation in PA not only supports adolescents' growth and development but also helps prevent potential health problems, foster healthy lifestyles, and promote lifelong healthy habits.

1.2.3.4 Mental Health

During adolescence, PA plays a multifaceted role in promoting mental health [38]. Regular PA not only helps regulate emotion and relieve academic stress but also improves emotional state through exercise of different intensities and types. Large-scale studies involving over 500,000 adolescents have shown that PA levels were positively associated with life satisfaction and inversely correlated with psychosomatic complaints in a dose-dependent manner [54]. Moreover, physical skills, self-esteem, and confidence improve [55]. As mentioned earlier, these benefits are also associated with adolescents with neurodevelopmental disorders [41].

1.2.3.5 Emotional Regulation and Stress Relief

Adolescence is often accompanied by mood swings and academic stress. PA improves mood by increasing the concentrations of dopamine, serotonin, and norepinephrine in the brain [56], high-intensity aerobic exercise is positively related to positive mood [57], and moderate-intensity anaerobic exercise can improve mood [58]. Regular exercise can relieve tension and anxiety and provide a positive and pleasant psychological experience. In addition, exercise can improve sleep quality [59], further relieve psychological stress, enable teenagers to better cope with challenges and stress, and maintain mental health.

1.2.3.6 Self-Esteem and Self-Confidence

By participating in various sports and PAs, adolescents can develop skills and improve self-awareness, thereby enhancing self-esteem and confidence [60]. Sports provide them with a platform to show their talent and achieve their goals, where they can gain a sense of accomplishment and enhance their confidence in their abilities. A healthy view of self-esteem is shaped to form, providing support when facing challenges later [61]. The formation of exercise habits, self-esteem, and self-confidence is conducive to building a strong and healthy psychology.

1.2.3.7 Social Adaptation

Regular PA plays a crucial role in fostering the social adaptation of adolescents in various ways. Studies indicate that PA significantly predicts social adaptation in adolescents, with higher levels of PA correlating with enhanced social adaptation skills. Moreover, engagement in sports and team activities not only cultivates leadership and teamwork skills but also fosters holistic and positive interpersonal relationships, laying a foundation for improved social integration [62].

1.2.3.8 Developing Leadership and Teamwork

Participation in sports and other team activities provides youth with unique opportunities to develop leadership skills and teamwork [63]. In a collective environment, we jointly pursue goals, assume responsibilities, and enhance cooperation and trust. The emphasis on cooperation in team sports enables them to learn effective communication, coordination, and problem-solving skills in teams. The team environment allows youth to practice leadership skills and teaches them how to guide and motivate team members. This experience has a profound effect on the development of positive social relationships among adolescents.

1.2.3.9 Promoting Positive Social Relations

Participating in school sports teams, clubs, or other team activities allows adolescents to cultivate deep friendships based on shared interests and promotes the development of positive social relationships [64]. PA not only provides emotional support to adolescents but also encourages the development of healthy interpersonal habits. Through interactions and shared experiences with teammates, adolescents form strong friendship bonds and acquire skills in conflict resolution, respect for others, and effective collaboration [65]. This socialization experience helps adolescents better integrate into society, establish positive relationships, and lay a solid foundation for their future social activities and relationships.

1.3 The Adverse Impact of Sedentary Behavior

Sedentary behavior is an important part of people's daily activity behavior and refers to the behavior of people who spend ≤1.5 METs while sitting, lying down, or leaning in the waking state [4]. Advances in technology and the popularity of smart devices have created environments that support people in becoming sedentary [66]; private car or public transportation has become the commonly chosen means of commuting; electronic devices such as television, computers, and cell phones have taken up a large portion of people's lives; and reductions in the frequency of active transportation and increases in screen time have greatly increased the proportion of sedentary behavior throughout the day, which is not beneficial to our physical and mental health.

Sedentary behavior is an independent health risk factor highly correlated with all-cause mortality and is one of the common causative factors for many noncommunicable diseases (NCDs) [67]. An increase in hours of sedentary behavior throughout the day corresponds to a decrease in hours dedicated to PA and/or sleep. Insufficient PA is one of the top four risk factors for death from NCDs [68], while sleep deprivation can also lead to attention deficit disorders, working memory deficits, negative moods, and many other problems [69]. Furthermore, longer periods of sedentary behavior itself can cause more physical and mental health problems.

In children and adolescents under 18 years old, the widely discussed topic of screen use reveals both positive outcomes (e.g., improved literacy with educational games) and negative outcomes (e.g., poorer body composition with general use). However, even adverse effects have a small effect size. Therefore, to enhance research, priority should be placed on nuanced measurements, focusing on content, context, and the environment [70]. Specifically, based on findings of Sanders et al. [70], the authors propose that guidelines should discourage excessive engagement with social media and the Internet, and explore modifying recommendations to encourage the use of educational apps and video games. However, these suggestions should be weighed against the minimal risks they pose to adiposity.

1.3.1 Effects of Sedentary Behavior on Infants, Toddlers, and Preschoolers Under 5 Years of Age

The health status of children and adolescents has garnered global attention in recent years, especially among preschool-aged individuals. The preschool stage is an important period for establishing a healthy lifestyle and an important focus for improving physical fitness and promoting healthy development, which is crucial for an individual's lifelong health. The Exercise Guidelines for Preschoolers [3–6] state that preschoolers should minimize sedentary behaviors every day, with screen time totaling no more than 60 min per day; the less, the better, and any sedentary behaviors should be limited to 60 min or less per session.

1.3.1.1 Physical Health

First, prolonged sedentary behavior leads to increased intake of snacks and decreased PA, leading to lower muscle strength in preschoolers, increasing the risk of childhood overweight and obesity [71, 72], while prolonged television viewing in preschoolers predicts higher levels of sweet teeth and BMI, and these types of suggestive advertisements for food may further exacerbate this association [73]. Additionally, sedentary behavior has been suggested to be a crucial factor contributing to reduced cardiorespiratory fitness [74]. Second, recent research has shown that basic motor skills are negatively correlated with sedentary behavior among preschoolers, that children who have higher levels of basic motor skills spend less time engaging in sedentary behavior, and that the development of basic motor skills in early childhood may lead to participation in a diverse PA program, thereby reducing the risk of obesity-related behaviors [75]. Locomotor skills are important fundamental movement skills for preschoolers, and developing locomotor skills may be an effective strategy for reducing sedentary behavior in young children [76]. Third, excessive screen time can increase snack intake and decrease PA, increasing the risk of overweight and obesity in children [77]; second, sedentary behavior can adversely affect strength and balance qualities in preschoolers.

1.3.1.2 Mental Health

It has been suggested that excessive screen time is associated with lower psychological well-being, including decreased curiosity, decreased self-control, distractibility, increased difficulty in making friends, and decreased emotional stability [77]. First, longer screen time in early childhood predicts a greater likelihood of peer rejection situations, such as being teased, beaten, or insulted by other students [73]. Second, prolonged screen time may also predict behavioral and emotional problems in children, including aggression, anxiety, depression, social isolation, decreased prosocial behaviors, and attention problems [78]. Symptoms of anxiety increase with increasing hours of sedentary behavior [79]. Studies highlight that increased screen exposure in preschoolers is correlated with lower social competence scores, higher scores for anger-aggressive behaviors, and anxiety withdrawal behaviors [71]. Third, the quality of sleep is also a marker of mental health, and good sleep quality can eliminate fatigue, protect the brain, restore physical strength, and regulate mental health. Sleep is crucial for preschoolers, and several studies have shown that the detection rate of sleep problems, such as shorter sleep duration, later bedtime, and more nighttime awakenings, increases with increasing duration of sedentary behavior in preschoolers. Sleep deprivation is an important risk factor for physical and mental problems in children. Finally, certain studies have indicated that sedentary behavior lasting more than 120 min per day may lead to lower self-esteem scores and reduced academic achievement in preschoolers [20].

Preschoolers who experience sleep deprivation have higher rates of anxiety and depression and are prone to aggressive behavior, irritability, and impulsivity [71].

Fourth, early exposure of young children to screening media, such as watching television, looking at cell phones, and playing video games, is detrimental to the development of cognitive flexibility, but not all sedentary behaviors, such as reading, on the other hand, promote cognitive functioning [70, 80].

1.3.1.3 Social Adaptation

Increased sedentary behavior decreases preschoolers' social and emotional skills, teamwork, and sharing awareness, which are necessary to support their social interactions with peers and adults. Screen-time behaviors often involve individuals leaning toward solitary activities, reducing opportunities for children to engage with the outside world, participate in play, and interact with peers. This reduction in interaction can easily lead to heightened irritability, aggressive behaviors, and social withdrawal, posing risks to preschoolers' socialization opportunities and the development of healthy social skills [81]; however, when preschoolers participate in video games with others, such as parents, brothers, sisters, or peers, there are more opportunities for interaction and communication, which can develop their social, teamwork, and emotional skills [82].

1.3.2 Effects of Sedentary Behavior on Children

Most studies have confirmed the minor impact of sedentary behavior on children's physical and mental health, as well as their social adaptation. Subsequently, we provide a detailed presentation of the various effects.

1.3.2.1 Physical Health

Sedentary behavior in children can give rise to various adverse effects on their physical health [70, 83]. First, there is an increased risk of cardiometabolic diseases, as sedentary behaviors are linked to such risks independently of PA levels. Additionally, sedentary behavior can contribute to obesity, thereby elevating the likelihood of associated health issues, including diabetes and cardiovascular diseases. Moreover, a sedentary lifestyle can result in reduced fitness, manifesting as decreased flexibility, muscular strength, and cardiorespiratory capacity. Prolonged sitting and sedentary behavior may also negatively impact bone density, potentially leading to decreased bone strength and an increased risk of fractures. Recent studies further highlight the negative association between sedentary behaviors and health outcomes in children, underscoring the detrimental effects of prolonged sitting and a lack of PA [84].

1.3.2.2 Mental Health

Notably, high levels of sedentary behavior correlate with increased depressive symptoms in children and adolescents [70, 85]. An inactive lifestyle is also associated with various mental health conditions, including anxiety symptoms, self-esteem, suicidal ideation, loneliness, stress, and psychological distress [83]. Prolonged periods of sedentary behavior can contribute to an increase in negative emotions, potentially impacting the mental well-being of children and adolescents [54, 86].

1.3.2.3 Social Adaptation

Sedentary behavior in children can detrimentally affect their social adaptation in various ways. Prolonged sedentary behavior, often associated with screen time, can diminish opportunities for social interaction and face-to-face communication with peers, which are crucial for developing social skills [87]. Additionally, it may influence the quality and quantity of social support, limiting the amount of time spent on social activities and building supportive relationships [87]. The association with negative emotions, such as stress and anxiety, further impacts social adaptation and the ability to engage in social activities. Moreover, children with high levels of sedentary behavior, particularly those experiencing obesity, may face an increased risk of bullying, significantly impacting their social adaptation and overall well-being [88].

1.3.3 Effects of Sedentary Behavior on Adolescents

Sedentary behavior in adolescents has been associated with various negative effects, including impacts on physical health and mental well-being. Some of the effects of sedentary behavior on adolescents are as follows:

1.3.3.1 Physical Health

Sedentary behavior in adolescents is significantly associated with markers of adiposity and cardiometabolic disease risk. Although evidence suggests an association between sedentary behavior and adiposity in youth, the causality and strength of this association are subjects of ongoing research and debate. Some studies propose that sedentary behavior, such as prolonged sitting and screen time, may contribute to adolescent obesity [89]. However, this relationship is influenced by various factors, including PA levels, dietary habits, and sleep patterns. Additionally, research indicates that, regardless of PA level, sedentary behaviors are linked to an elevated risk of cardiometabolic disease and all-cause mortality [83]. Specifically, sedentary behavior is associated with adverse effects on cardiometabolic health, including increased risk factors for cardiovascular disease and metabolic abnormalities [84].

1.3.3.2 Mental Health

Sedentary behavior in adolescents has been extensively studied, revealing noteworthy implications for mental health [90]. Prolonged periods of inactivity, especially when individuals are confined at home, have been associated with an increase in negative emotions. Furthermore, sedentary behavior can exert a detrimental influence on adolescents' motivation for PA, potentially resulting in reduced engagement in higher intensity exercises and diminished positive affect [91]. Importantly, research suggests that the interaction between sedentary time and mental health may compromise the positive effects of PA, thereby contributing to adverse mental health outcomes [90]. Finally, a recent review emphasizes that the use of social media may affect social comparison, social displacement, social stimulation, and self-determination [92].

1.3.3.3 Social Adaptation

Sedentary behavior in adolescents poses several challenges to social adaptation. Prolonged periods of sedentary behavior, often associated with screen time, may diminish opportunities for social interaction and face-to-face communication, impacting the development of interpersonal relationships [93]. Additionally, adolescents with higher sedentary behavior may exhibit less independence, heightened emotional reactivity, and difficulty regulating emotions, potentially affecting their social adaptation and relationships [94]. Furthermore, sedentary behavior may limit opportunities to develop and practice communication and social skills, potentially impairing adolescents' ability to communicate and interact effectively with their peers [93].

1.4 Recommended Levels of Physical Activity

Moderate PA, a key component of the World Health Organization's (WHO) health pillars, remains crucial amidst evolving lifestyle trends in children and adolescents. The international focus on promoting PA in this demographic population persists, with various strategies implemented in recent years. Recommendations play a vital role in guiding individuals in maintaining and enhancing physical health. At the school, societal, and scientific research levels, these recommendations influence educational methods, policy formulation, and academic research, contributing to the continuous development of theories and practices for the overall well-being of children and adolescents.

1.4.1 Principles of Implementing Recommended Physical Activity Levels

The principles guiding the implementation of recommended PA levels for children and adolescents are primarily derived from WHO guidelines and encompass principles of human rights, equity, evidence-based practice, and consistency with health goals [9, 95]. These studies emphasize the fundamental right to health, the necessity of addressing disparities, the reliance on robust scientific evidence, and the potential of PA to contribute to sustainable development goals and environmental sustainability. Implementation strategies should prioritize community engagement, consider diverse needs, and be built upon a solid evidence base.

1.4.2 Meeting Physical Activity Recommendations for Children and Adolescents

Several factors have been identified as correlates influencing compliance with recommended levels of PA in children and adolescents [96]. Access to facilities, particularly gymnasiums outside of school hours, is associated with greater adherence to MVPA recommendations for children [97]. Notably, significant between-country differences in daily MVPA compliance among children reflect both site characteristics and the importance of individual traits and local school contexts [97]. Additionally, age plays a role, with a tendency for adherence to PA to decline among adolescents as they become older [98]. Socioeconomic factors are found to influence PA levels according to demographic factors, with disparities associated with socioeconomic status impacting compliance with recommended activity levels [96, 99]. For children and adolescents with intellectual disabilities, various factors, including parental support, self-efficacy, and environmental influences, have been identified as correlates of PA compliance.

1.4.3 Overall Recommendations for Physical Activity

The WHO guidelines on PA and sedentary behavior provide evidence-based public health recommendations for children and adolescents in high-, middle-, and low-income countries [100], which provide a range of recommended amounts and intensities of PA. The guidelines consider that both moderate- and vigorous-intensity PA can promote health, can be undertaken by anyone at any skill level, and can be enjoyed by everyone. Various popular activities are recommended based on intensity, encompassing walking, cycling, wheeling, sports, active recreation, and play.

The guidelines emphasize the importance of gradually progressing and adopting collaborative approaches to PA. They underscore three key aspects: (a) necessity—highlighting the benefits of any PA; (b) modality—stressing that PA should be gradually increased in frequency, intensity, and duration; and (c) pathway—emphasizing the need for consultation with relevant professionals to determine the suitable type and intensity of activity.

1.4.4 Physical Activity Recommendations for Infants, Toddlers, and Preschoolers Under 5 Years of Age

Recommendations for PA in young children are contained in the WHO guidelines on PA, sedentary behavior, and sleep for children under 5 years of age [101], which are applicable to young children in high- and low-income or middle-income countries. The guidelines show that for children under 5 years of age to grow healthy, they must spend less time sitting with screens or confined to strollers and seats, get better quality sleep, and have more time for active play. From the perspective of school education, gamified activities imply that children's PA need to focus on fundamental motor skills and emphasize the teaching of basic PA skills to cultivate correct PA habits.

Currently, the WHO [101] and countries such as Canada [102, 103], England [104], and Australia [105] generally align with the key components of PA guidelines for children. Specifically, children under the age of one are recommended to accumulate 30 min of PA daily. The cumulative exercise time of children older than 1 year should be at least 180 min per day, which can be PA of all intensities. In addition, in terms of activity type, the types of actions recommended by the guide are also enjoyable games and help young children develop fundamental movement skills. It is important to note that in China [106] and according to the WHO [68], in addition to the recommended daily physical activity for young children, it is advised to engage in at least 120 min of outdoor activities daily to prevent myopia. Moreover, during adverse weather conditions like haze, high temperatures, or cold, it is recommended to appropriately reduce outdoor exercise time.

1.4.5 Physical Activity Recommendations for Children and Adolescents

The PA recommendations for children and adolescents vary by region but share the common goal of at least 60 min of daily activity. In North America [20, 107], the emphasis is on activities that strengthen muscles and bones, while in Asia, similar exercises are recommended with a focus on resistance and weightlifting in India [108] and strength training in Japan [109]. Oceania promotes intense aerobic activities along with muscle and bone strengthening [110, 111]. In Europe, there is an emphasis on a variety of activities, from vigorous aerobics to flexibility exercises in Denmark [112]. The WHO advocates for a combination of aerobic and strength activities [68]. These guidelines reflect the cultural diversity and unique health needs of each region, but all underscore the importance of an active lifestyle for overall youth health. However, it is noteworthy that there is a void in recommended PA guidelines for children and adolescents in Africa, but not for children under 5 years old [113]. Table 1.1 shows various examples of PA guidelines from different regions and countries.

Despite these recommendations, the global prevalence of compliance with PA guidelines among children and adolescents is low. According to the WHO, more than 80% of the world's adolescent population is insufficiently physically active, with significant differences in the prevalence of insufficient PA across genders, regions, and countries [95]. Other studies have reported similar findings, indicating that, globally, 81% of adolescents do not meet the recommended levels of PA [114, 115]. Additionally, the Active Healthy Kids Global Alliance (AHKGA) Global Matrix 4.0 Project, an initiative aimed at assessing, comparing, and contrasting the PA of children and adolescents in 57 countries worldwide, supports these findings. Overall, PA received the lowest global average grade (D) [116].

1.5 Overall Recommendations for Sedentary Behavior

The WHO released the Guidelines for PA and Sedentary Behavior, which propose that sedentary behavior has become a serious social, national, and general problem that endangers public health [68]. All age groups and specific population groups should actively limit sedentary behavior to promote comprehensive physical, mental, and social well-being. The most obvious and intuitive behavior associated with physical inactivity is the increasing use of electronic devices by children and adolescents, which leads to an increase in screen time and sedentary time. Sedentary time may include leisure play uninterrupted by electronic media. These play items/activities include puzzles, block drawings, painting, handicrafts, singing, music, etc. These projects, which are completed within static time, are important for children's development and beneficial for their cognitive development. Regardless of whether an individual's daily PA meets health recommendations, prolonged sedentary behavior has harmful effects on cardiovascular and metabolic health. Therefore, sedentary behavior is considered a risk factor for obesity and CVD and is distinguished from physical inactivity [4].

Table 1.1 Example of guideline recommendations for physical activity behavior from early childhood to adolescence across five continents and worldwide

Continent	Country	Source	Age (year)	Duration	Recommended specific physical activities
Africa	South Africa	South African 24-Hour Movement Guidelines for Birth to Five years [113]	0–1 years	≥30 min/day	Individuals should engage in various physical activities multiple times a day, including interactive floor play such as crawling. For immobile babies, at least 30 min of tummy time spread throughout waking hours, along with activities such as reaching and grasping, are recommended. When sitting, babies should participate in stimulating activities with a caregiver, such as playing with safe toys, engaging in baby conversations, singing, and storytelling.
			1–2 years	≥180 min/day	Individuals should engage in at least 180 min of diverse physical activities, including energetic play, throughout the day, with more being preferable.
			3–5 years	≥180 min/day	Preschoolers, typically aged 3–5 years, should engage in physical activities for a minimum of 180 min daily, with at least 60 min dedicated to energetic play that raises their heart rate, such as running, jumping, and dancing, spread throughout the day.
Americas	United States of America	Physical activity guidelines for Americans [107]	3–5 years	≥180 min/day	Adult caregivers of preschool-aged children should encourage active play that includes a variety of activity types.
			6–17 years	≥60 min/day	Children and adolescents should engage in muscle-strengthening activities at least 3 days per week.
	Canada	Canadian 24-hour movement guidelines for the early years (0–4 years) [117]	0–1 year	≥30 min/day	Being physically active several times in a variety of ways, particularly through interactive floor-based play; more is better.
			1–2 years	≥180 min/day	Engaging in a variety of physical activities at any intensity, including energetic play, throughout the day is beneficial—more is better.
			3–4 years	≥180 min/day	Time spent in a variety of physical activities spread throughout the day, including at least 60 min of energetic play, is beneficial—more is better.
		Canadian Children and Youth 24-Hour Physical Activity Guidelines [20]	5–17 years	≥60 min/day	At least 60 min of moderate-to-vigorous physical activity for a minimum of 3 days per week.

Asia	Saudi Arabia	The Public Authority Health of Saudi Arabia unveiled the Twenty-Four-Hour Movement Practice Guidelines [118]	1–2 years	≥180 min/day	Toddlers should engage in various physical activities totaling at least 3 h per day, including energetic and outdoor play, which can be spread throughout the day, with additional activities being beneficial.
			3–5 years	≥180 min/day	At least 3 h of various physical activities daily, including a minimum of 1 hour of energetic and outdoor play throughout the day. 1 hour or more of MVPA appropriately for their age.
			6–17 years	≥60 min/day	A minimum of 1 hour of MVPA per day, emphasizing aerobic activity. The interventions included vigorous physical activity, muscle strengthening, and bone strengthening activities performed at least 3 days per week within the daily 1-hour minimum. Participants participated in several hours of light PA per day.
	China	Physical Activity Guidelines for Chinese (2021) [106]	0–2 years	≥180 min/day	Engage in various forms of interactive activities with caregivers every day.
			3–5 years	≥180 min/day	Engage in at least 180 min of physical activity per day, including 60 min of energetic play, and encourage outdoor activity.
			6–17 years	≥60 min/day	Engage in muscle strengthening and bone strengthening exercises at least 3 days a week.
	India	Consensus Physical Activity Guidelines for Asian Indians [108]	5–17 years	≥60 min/day	Engage in resistance training and weightlifting exercises 2–3 days per week.
	Japan	Japanese national physical activity and health promotion guidelines [109]	3–6 years	≥60 min/day	Participate in a wide variety of physical activities using all parts of the body.
			7–18 years	≥60 min/day	Strength training should be performed 2–3 times/week for each major muscle group.
	Singapore	Singapore physical activity guidelines [119]	0–1 year	≥30 min/day	Encourage interactive floor-based activities for a minimum of 30-min a day.
			1–2 years	≥180 min/day	Spend at least 180 min engaging in a variety of physical activities of any intensity, spread throughout the day. Aim for daily outdoor play.
			3–6 years	≥180 min/day	Spend at least 180 min engaging in a variety of physical activities, with at least 60 min being moderate to vigorous-intensity activity, spread throughout the day.
			7–17 years	≥60 min/day	Engage in various high-intensity aerobic exercises, muscle-strengthening, and bone-strengthening activities for at least 3 days per week.

(continued)

Table 1.1 (continued)

Continent	Country	Source	Age (year)	Duration	Recommended specific physical activities
Oceania	Australia	A collaborative approach to adopting/adapting guidelines—The Australian 24-Hour Movement Guidelines for the early years (Birth to 5 years): an integration of physical activity, sedentary behavior, and sleep [105]	0–1 year	≥30 min/day	Being physically active several times in a variety of ways, particularly through interactive floor-based play, is beneficial; more is better. Currently, there are no available benchmarks; further research is required. For those not yet mobile, this includes at least 30 min of tummy time spread throughout the day while awake.
			1–2 years	≥180 min/day	At least 180 min spent in a variety of physical activities at any intensity, spread throughout the day; more is better. Including energetic play.
			3–5 years	≥180 min/day	At least 180 min spent in a variety of physical activities spread throughout the day, of which at least 60 min should be energetic play; more is better.
		Australian 24-hour movement guidelines for children (5–12 years) and young people (13–17 years): an integration of physical activity, sedentary behavior [111]	5–17 years	≥60 min/day	Engage in various high-intensity aerobic exercises, muscle-strengthening, and bone-strengthening activities for at least 3 days per week.
	New Zealand	Sit Less, Move More, Sleep Well Physical Activity Guidelines for Children and Young People [110]	5–17 years	≥60 min/day	Engage in physical activity at least 3 times per week.

Region	Country	Guideline	Age	Duration	Description
Europe	Ireland	Update of the National Physical Activity Guidelines for Ireland [120]	0–1 year	≥30 min/day	Be physically active several times a day in a variety of ways, particularly through interactive floor-based play; more is better. For those not yet mobile, this includes at least 30 min in prone position (tummy time) spread throughout the day while awake.
			1–2 years	≥180 min/day	Spend at least 3 h in a variety of types of physical activities at any intensity, including moderate- to vigorous-intensity physical activity, spread throughout the day; more is better.
			3–4 years	≥180 min/day	Spend at least 3 h in a variety of types of physical activities at any intensity, of which at least 1 h is moderate- to vigorous-intensity physical activity, spread throughout the day; more is better.
			5–17 years	≥60 min/day	Vigorous-intensity aerobic activities, as well as those that strengthen muscle and bone, should be incorporated at least 3 days a week.
	Denmark	Physical activity recommendations for children and adolescents [112]	0–1 year	N/M	Maximize floor-based tummy time for infants when they are Ensure that the infant is physically active in a variety of ways during the day. Ensure that the infant is able to move freely as much as possible.
			1–4 years	N/M	Ensure that the child is physically active in a variety of ways during the day. Ensure that the child can move freely as much as possible.
			5–17 years	≥60 min/day	If the 60-minute period is divided, each activity should last for at least 10 min. ENGAGE in physical activity of high intensity at least three times a week for at least 30 min to maintain or improve physical fitness and muscle strength. Activities should include those that increase bone strength and flexibility. Physical activity in addition to what is recommended will have further health benefits.
	United Kingdom	Chief Medical Officers' Physical Activity Guidelines [121]	5–18 years	≥60 min/day	One should engage in various types and intensities of physical activities throughout the week to develop motor skills, muscular fitness, and bone strength.
	Germany	National Recommendations for Physical Activity and Physical Activity Promotion [122]	0–3 years	N/M	Infants and toddlers should get as much physical activity as possible and be prevented as little as possible from following their natural instinct to move; a safe environment must be ensured
			4–6 years	≥180 min/day	Physical activity should amount to a total of 180 min/day and more, which can comprise instructed and non-instructed physical activity
			6–11 years	≥90 min/day	Children of primary school age should be moderately-to-vigorously physically active for 90 min or more each day. 60 min of that time can be spent on everyday activities, e.g., at least 12,000 steps/day
			12–18 years	≥60 min/day, with 60 min achievable through daily activities	One should engage in physical activities that promote muscle strength and endurance development 2–3 times per week.
	Switzerland	Updating national physical activity guidelines based on the global WHO guidelines: experiences and challenges from Switzerland [123]	0–1 year	≥30 min/day	Free activities several times per day.
			2–4 years	≥180 min/day	At least 180 min per day, regardless of intensity.
			5–17 years	≥60 min/day across the week	Vigorous intensity and muscle and bone strengthening PA at least 3 times/week. Do several times/week varied activities that strengthen bones, muscles and improve balance, coordination, and cardiovascular functions

(continued)

Table 1.1 (continued)

Continent	Country	Source	Age (year)	Duration	Recommended specific physical activities
	Worldwide	Guidelines on physical activity, sedentary behavior, and sleep for children under 5 years of age [101]	0–1 year	≥30 min/day	Be physically active several times a day in a variety of ways, particularly through interactive floor-based play; more is better. For those not yet mobile, this includes at least 30 min in prone position (tummy time) spread throughout the day while awake.
			1–2 years	≥180 min/day	Spend at least 180 min in a variety of types of physical activities at any intensity, including moderate-to vigorous-intensity physical activity, spread throughout the day; more is better.
			3–4 years	≥180 min/day	Spend at least 180 min in a variety of types of physical activities at any intensity, of which at least 60 min is moderate- to vigorous-intensity physical activity, spread throughout the day; more is better.
		WHO Guidelines on physical activity and sedentary behavior for children and adolescents, adults, and older adults [68]	5–17 years	≥60 min/day	One should engage in high-intensity aerobic activities and strength training exercises that promote muscle and bone development each week.

Min minutes, N/M not mentioned, MVPA moderate-to-vigorous physical activity, WHO World Health Organization

1.5.1 Sedentary Behavior Composition in Children and Adolescents

Spending time watching television is a prevalent sedentary behavior among youth, associated with metabolic risk factors and health issues [124]. Engaging in video games is another common sedentary activity that contributes to sedentary behavior in children and adolescents [115]. Using computers for non-academic purposes, such as browsing the Internet or playing games, is a significant sedentary behavior observed in young individuals [124, 125]. The use of smartphones and tablets for entertainment or communication purposes is also a common sedentary activity among children and adolescents. Additionally, sedentary behaviors like reading or studying while sitting for extended periods contribute to overall sedentary time in youth [115].

1.5.2 Recommendations for General Sedentary Behavior

The WHO guidelines on PA and sedentary behavior offer evidence-based public health recommendations tailored for children and adolescents across diverse income settings, encompassing high-income, middle-income, and low-income countries [68]. According to these guidelines, sedentary behavior for this demographic involves sitting or lying awake during low-energy consumption periods in various environments, including educational, family, community, and transportation settings. A key emphasis is placed on limiting sedentary time, particularly the duration spent on entertainment screens. The WHO's recommendations draw from established frameworks such as the Canadian 24-hour PA Guidelines for Children and Adolescents [117], the Australian 24-hour PA Guidelines for Children and Adolescents Aged 5–17, and the second edition of the US PA Guidelines [107].

While the WHO has proposed a recommended amount of PA for children and adolescents worldwide, the latest recommendation guidelines do not categorize specific age groups for children and adolescents and provide general recommendations only for reducing entertainment screen time. However, the PA and sedentary behavior guidelines introduced by countries such as Canada [117], Australia [111], and the United Kingdom [121] include detailed age groups for children and adolescents and provide comprehensive recommendations. These guidelines offer specific guidance tailored to different age ranges, ensuring that recommendations are appropriate and effective for promoting healthy behaviors among youth.

Specifically, in North America, both the United States [107] and Canada [20, 117] advocate for restricting recreational screen time to no more than 2 h per day. Similarly, Asian countries like Saudi Arabia [118], China [106], India [108], and Singapore [119] emphasize the need to limit screen time to varying degrees for children and youth. Oceania, represented by Australia [105] and New Zealand [110], echoes this sentiment by recommending less than 1 hour of screen time per day for young children. European nations like the United Kingdom [121], Germany [122], and Ireland [120] emphasize minimizing sedentary time overall, with varying guidelines on screen time limits. Switzerland [123] and Denmark [112] share a focus on reducing prolonged periods of inactivity, especially screen time, across different age groups. The WHO underscores the global importance of reducing sedentary behavior and limiting screen time for children aged 5–17 years [68] (Table 1.2).

1.5.2.1 Recommendations for Sedentary Behavior in Infants, Toddlers, and Preschoolers Under 5 Years

The WHO provides comprehensive guidelines for sedentary behavior in infants and young children. For infants under 1 year of age, prolonged sedentary positions, discouraged screen time and encouraged interactive activities such as reading, and storytelling are recommended. Similarly, for children aged 1–2, limiting sitting time to 1 hour at a stretch is advised, with a strong emphasis on minimal screen exposure. As children progress to ages 3–4, restrictions on sitting time continue, promoting alternative activities such as reading with caregivers. Caregivers should serve as positive role models by actively participating in physical activities with children and limiting their own screen time.

1.5.2.2 Recommendations for Sedentary Behavior in Children and Adolescents

The WHO advocates minimizing screen time for children and adolescents in its guidelines on PA and sedentary behavior [115]. This chapter includes examples of sedentary behavior guidelines from various countries and regions across five continents. Recommendations for managing sedentary behavior in children and adolescents universally highlight the importance of reducing screen usage time, generally suggesting a limit of no more than 2 h.

Table 1.2 Examples of recommended levels of sedentary behavior from early childhood to adolescence across five continents and worldwide

Region	Country	Source	Age	Recommendations of sedentary behavior
Africa	South Africa	South African 24-Hour Movement Guidelines for Birth to Five years [113]	0–1 year	It is advised that babies not be confined or strapped in for more than 1 hour at a time, whether in a pram, highchair, or on a caregiver's back or chest. Screen time (including televisions, cell phones, tablets, video games, and computers) is not recommended.
			1–2 years	When sitting, toddlers should participate in developmental activities such as reading, singing, playing games with blocks and puzzles, and storytelling with a caregiver. It is advised that toddlers not be confined or strapped in for more than 1 hour at a time, whether in a pram or highchair or on a caregiver's back or chest, and prolonged periods of sitting should be avoided. For toddlers younger than 2 years, screen time is not recommended. For those aged 2 years, screen time should be limited to no more than 1 hour, with less being preferable
			3–5 years	When sitting, preschoolers should participate in enriching activities such as reading, singing, puzzles, arts and crafts, and storytelling with caregivers and other children. It is recommended that preschoolers not be confined or strapped in for more than 1 hour at a time, and extended periods of sitting should be avoided. The screen time should be limited to no more than 1 h per day, with less being preferable.

(continued)

Table 1.2 (continued)

Region	Country	Source	Age	Recommendations of sedentary behavior
North America	United States of America	Early Childhood Obesity Prevention Policies [107]	0–5 years	Decrease sedentary behavior in young children. Child-care regulators and providers are encouraged to implement strategies to ensure that the amount of time that toddlers and preschoolers spend sitting or standing (such as occurs in car seats and highchairs) is limited. Limit young children's screen time. The report recommends that screen time (including television, cell phone use, and digital media involvement) be limited to, 2 h/d for children 2–5 years of age.
	Canada	Canadian 24-hour movement guidelines for the early years (0–4 years) [117]	0–1 year	Not being restrained for more than 1 hour at a time (e.g., in a stroller or highchair). Screen time is not recommended. When sedentary, engaging in pursuits such as reading and storytelling with a caregiver is encouraged.
			1–2 years	Not being restrained for more than 1 hour at a time (e.g., in a stroller or highchair) or sitting for extended periods. For those younger than 2 years, sedentary screen time is not recommended. For those aged 2 years, sedentary screen time should be no more than 1 h—less is better. When sedentary, engaging in pursuits such as reading and storytelling with a caregiver is encouraged.
			3–4 years	Not being restrained for more than 1 h at a time (e.g., in a stroller or car seat) or sitting for extended periods. Sedentary screen time should be no more than 1 h—less is better. When sedentary, engaging in pursuits such as reading and storytelling with a caregiver is encouraged.
		Canadian 24-hour movement guidelines for children and youth: An integration of physical activity, sedentary behavior, and sleep [20]	5–17 years	Limiting recreational screen time to no more than 2 h per day—lower levels are associated with additional health benefits. Limiting sedentary (motorized) transport, extended sitting time, and time spent indoors throughout the day.

Asia	China	Physical Activity Guidelines for Chinese (2021) [106]	0–2 years	Screen watching is not recommended.
			3–5 years	Sedentary behaviors should not exceed 1 hour each time. Screen time should be less than 1 hour per day.
			6–17 years	Sedentary behavior should not exceed 1 hour each time. Screen time should be less than 2 hours per day.
	India	Consensus physical activity guidelines for Asian Indians [108]	5–17 years	Leisure screen time limited to 2 h per day.
	Saudi Arabia	The Public Authority Health of Saudi Arabia unveiled the Twenty-Four-Hour Movement Practice Guidelines [118]	1–2 years	Avoiding restraint of toddlers for more than 1 h at a time in a stroller, car seat, or highchair, and discouraging prolonged sitting. Sedentary activities such as reading and storytelling should be encouraged when the child is not engaged in active play. Screen time for toddlers (1–2 years) is not recommended. For toddlers (2–3 years), sedentary screen time should be limited to no more than 1 h per day; less time is preferable.
			3–5 years	Preschoolers should be avoided for more than 1 h at a time in a stroller, car seat, or highchair. Be encouraged to engage in activities such as reading, storytelling, or coloring with a caregiver when sedentary. The sedentary screen time was limited to no more than 1 h per day for preschoolers; shorter durations were preferred.
			6–17 years	The recreational screen time should be limited to no more than 2 h per day, and prolonged sitting should be broken up whenever possible.
	Singapore	Singapore physical activity guidelines [119]	0–2 years	Limit the amount of time spent being sedentary, with recreational screen time not recommended. Instead, engage in imaginative play and storytelling activities.
			3–6 years	Limit the amount of time spent being sedentary, keeping recreational screen time to less than an hour a day
			7–17 years	Limit the amount of time spent being sedentary, particularly recreational screen time, by engaging in activities of any intensity, including those of light-intensity.

(continued)

Table 1.2 (continued)

Region	Country	Source	Age	Recommendations of sedentary behavior
Oceania	Australia	A collaborative approach to adopting/adapting guidelines—The Australian 24-Hour Movement Guidelines for the early years (Birth to 5 years): an integration of physical activity, sedentary behavior, and sleep [105]	0–1 year	Not being restrained for more than 1 h at a time (e.g., in a stroller, car seat or highchair). Screen time is not recommended. When sedentary, engaging in pursuits such as reading, singing, puzzles and storytelling with a caregiver is encouraged.
			1–2 years	Not being restrained for more than 1 h at a time (e.g., in a stroller, car seat or highchair) or sitting for extended periods. For those younger than 2 years, sedentary screen time is not recommended. For those aged 2 years, sedentary screen time should be no more than 1 h; less is better. When sedentary, engaging in pursuits such as reading, singing, puzzles and storytelling with a caregiver is encouraged;
			3–5 years	Not being restrained for more than 1 h at a time (e.g., in a stroller or car seat) or sitting for extended periods. Sedentary screen time should be no more than 1 h; less is better. When sedentary, engaging in pursuits such as reading, singing, puzzles and storytelling with a caregiver is encouraged.
	New Zealand	Sit Less, Move More, Sleep Well Physical Activity Guidelines for Children and Young People [110]	0–5 years	(a) Provide regular activity breaks to limit the amount of time a child spends sitting. (b) Discourage screen time for under two-year-olds and limit screen time to less than 1 hour every day for children aged 2 years or older—less is best. (c) Limit time in equipment that restricts free movement: All: From birth, encourage regular, unrestricted floor-based play (tummy time), on a safe surface. Be a role model: reduce your own screen use. Replace TV time with reading time, story time or doing jigsaw puzzles together. Avoid having the TV playing in the background. Remove the TV completely or limit having it on until the children have gone to bed. Do not have screens in (any) bedrooms. Set limited viewing times for all screens. Store DVDs, consoles, tablets, and electronic games out of sight. Break up long car journeys with regular stops (preferably at least once an hour), removing under five from their capsule/car seat at each stop. Encourage toddlers and preschoolers to walk instead of being in a pushchair.

Region	Country	Guideline	Age	Recommendation
Europe	The United Kingdom	Chief Medical Officers' Physical Activity Guidelines [121]	0–5 years	Break up inactivity.
			5–18 years	Children and young people should aim to minimize the amount of time spent being sedentary, and when physically possible should break up long periods of not moving with at least light physical activity.
	Germany	National Recommendations for Physical Activity and Physical Activity Promotion [122]	0–6 years	Avoidable sitting times should be reduced to a minimum. In addition to (motorized) transport, e.g., in a baby carrier or child seat, or periods spent inside unnecessarily, this relates in particular to reducing consumption of screen media to a minimum: Infants and toddlers: 0 min. Preschool children: as little as possible, maximum of 30 min/day.
			6–18 years	Primary school children: as little as possible, maximum of 60 min/day. Adolescents: as little as possible, maximum of 120 min/day.
	Ireland	Update of the National Physical Activity Guidelines for Ireland [120]	<1 years	Children should not be secured for more than 1 h at a time, whether in prams/strollers, highchairs, or strapped on a caregiver's back. Screen time is not recommended. When sedentary, engaging in reading and storytelling with a caregiver is encouraged.
			1–2 years	Children should not be secured for more than 1 h at a time, whether in prams/strollers, highchairs, or strapped on a caregiver's back, nor should they sit for extended periods of time. For 1-year-olds, sedentary screen time (such as watching TV or videos, playing computer games) is not recommended. For those aged 2 years, sedentary screen time should be no more than 1 h; less is better. When sedentary, engaging in reading and storytelling with a caregiver is encouraged.
			3–4 years	Children should not be secured in devices such as prams or strollers for more than 1 h at a time, nor should they sit for extended periods. Sedentary screen time should be limited to no more than 1 h; less is preferable. When sedentary, engaging in reading and storytelling with a caregiver is encouraged.
			5–17 years	Children and adolescents should limit the amount of time spent being sedentary, particularly the amount of recreational screen time
	Switzerland	Updating national physical activity guidelines based on the global WHO guidelines: experiences and challenges from Switzerland [123]	0–2 years	No screen time.
			3–4 years	Not more than 1 h/day
			5–17 years	Avoid prolonged periods of inactivity, especially screen time.
	Denmark	Physical activity recommendations for children and adolescents [112]	0–1 year	Avoid placing infants in baby bouncers, car seats and highchairs any longer than necessary.
			1–4 years	Avoid placing children in highchairs or strollers any longer than necessary. Screen time can adversely affect children's well-being. Although children may need or want sedentary activity on occasions it is important that they move as much as possible during the day.
			5–17 years	Limit the amount of screen time.

(continued)

Table 1.2 (continued)

Region	Country	Source	Age	Recommendations of sedentary behavior
Worldwide		Guidelines on physical activity, sedentary behavior, and sleep for children under 5 years of age [101]	0–1 year	Not be restrained for more than 1 h at a time (e.g., prams/strollers, highchairs, or strapped on a caregiver's back). Screen time is not recommended. When sedentary, engaging in reading and storytelling with a caregiver is encouraged.
			1–2 years	Not be restrained for more than 1 h at a time. This includes situations like being in prams/strollers, highchairs, or being strapped on a caregiver's back. Additionally, sitting for extended periods of time should be avoided. For 1-year-olds, it is not recommended to have sedentary screen time, such as watching TV or videos, or playing computer games. For children aged 2 years, sedentary screen time should be limited to no more than 1 h; less is preferable. When engaging in sedentary activities, it is encouraged to participate in reading and storytelling with a caregiver.
			3–4 years	Not be restrained for more than 1 h at a time, such as in prams/strollers, or sit for extended periods. Sedentary screen time should not exceed 1 h; less is preferable. When sedentary, it's encouraged to engage in reading and storytelling with a caregiver.
		WHO guidelines on physical activity and sedentary behavior for children and adolescents, adults, and older adults [68]	5–17 years	Reduce sedentary behavior time and limit screen time.

Min minutes, WHO World Health Organization

References

1. Caspersen CJ, Powell KE, Christenson GM. Physical activity, exercise, and physical fitness: definitions and distinctions for health-related research. Public Health Rep. 1985;100(2):126–31.
2. Pate RR. Physical activity and public health: a recommendation from the Centers for Disease Control and Prevention and the American College of Sports Medicine. JAMA. 1995;273(5):402.
3. Owen N, Healy GN, Matthews CE, Dunstan DW. Too much sitting: the population health science of sedentary behavior. Exerc Sport Sci Rev. 2010;38(3):105–13.
4. On behalf of SBRN Terminology Consensus Project Participants, Tremblay MS, Aubert S, Barnes JD, Saunders TJ, Carson V, et al. Sedentary Behavior Research Network (SBRN) – terminology consensus project process and outcome. Int J Behav Nutr Phys Act. 2017;14(1):75.
5. Tremblay MS, Colley RC, Saunders TJ, Healy GN, Owen N. Physiological and health implications of a sedentary lifestyle. Appl Physiol Nutr Metab. 2010;35(6):725–40.
6. Ainsworth BE, Haskell WL, Whitt MC, Irwin ML, Swartz AM, Strath SJ, et al. Compendium of physical activities: an update of activity codes and MET intensities. Med Sci Sports Exerc. 2000;32(Supplement):S498–516.
7. Pate RR, O'Neill JR, Lobelo F. The evolving definition of "Sedentary". Exerc Sport Sci Rev. 2008;36(4):173–8.
8. Owen N. Sedentary behavior: understanding and influencing adults' prolonged sitting time. Prev Med. 2012;55(6):535–9.
9. World Health Organization. Global action plan on physical activity 2018–2030: more active people for a healthier world [Internet]. Geneva: World Health Organization; 2018 [cited 2024 Feb 28]. 101 p. Available from: https://iris.who.int/handle/10665/272722.
10. Cheng W, Zhang Z, Cheng W, Yang C, Diao L, Liu W. Associations of leisure-time physical activity with cardiovascular mortality: a systematic review and meta-analysis of 44 prospective cohort studies. Eur J Prev Cardiolog. 2018;25(17):1864–72.
11. Oja P, Kelly P, Pedisic Z, Titze S, Bauman A, Foster C, et al. Associations of specific types of sports and exercise with all-cause and cardiovascular-disease mortality: a cohort study of 80 306 British adults. Br J Sports Med. 2017;51(10):812–7.
12. Nasstasia Y, Baker AL, Lewin TJ, Halpin SA, Hides L, Kelly BJ, et al. Differential treatment effects of an integrated motivational interviewing and exercise intervention on depressive symptom profiles and associated factors: a randomised controlled cross-over trial among youth with major depression. J Affect Disord. 2019;259:413–23.
13. Hillman CH, Buck SM, Themanson JR, Pontifex MB, Castelli DM. Aerobic fitness and cognitive development: event-related brain potential and task performance indices of executive control in preadolescent children. Dev Psychol. 2009;45(1):114–29.
14. Schnohr P, Kristensen TS, Prescott E, Scharling H. Stress and life dissatisfaction are inversely associated with jogging and other types of physical activity in leisure time—The Copenhagen City Heart Study. Scand Med Sci Sports. 2005;15(2):107–12.
15. Pasco JA, Jacka FN, Williams LJ, Brennan SL, Leslie E, Berk M. Don't worry, be active: positive affect and habitual physical activity. Aust N Z J Psychiatry. 2011;45(12):1047–52.
16. Dietz W. Critical periods in childhood for the development of obesity. Am J Clin Nutr. 1994;59(5):955–9.
17. Pate RR, Hillman CH, Janz KF, Katzmarzyk PT, Powell KE, Torres A, et al. Physical activity and health in children younger than 6 years: a systematic review. Med Sci Sports Exerc. 2019;51(6):1282–91.
18. Gruodyte-Raciene R, Erlandson MC, Jackowski SA, Baxter-Jones AD. Structural strength development at the proximal femur in 4- to 10-year-old precompetitive gymnasts: a 4-year longitudinal hip structural analysis study. J Bone Miner Res. 2013;28(12):2592–600.

19. Carson V, Lee EY, Hewitt L, Jennings C, Hunter S, Kuzik N, et al. Systematic review of the relationships between physical activity and health indicators in the early years (0-4 years). BMC Public Health. 2017;17(S5):854.
20. Carson V, Hunter S, Kuzik N, Gray CE, Poitras VJ, Chaput JP, et al. Systematic review of sedentary behaviour and health indicators in school-aged children and youth: an update. Appl Physiol Nutr Metab. 2016;41(6 (Suppl. 3)):S240–65.
21. Becker DR, McClelland MM, Loprinzi P, Trost SG. Physical activity, self-regulation, and early academic achievement in preschool children. Early Educ Dev. 2014;25(1):56–70.
22. Zhang JY, Shen QQ, Wang DL, Hou JM, Xia T, Qiu S, et al. Physical activity intervention promotes working memory and motor competence in preschool children. Front Public Health. 2022;10:984887.
23. Luo X, Herold F, Ludyga S, Gerber M, Kamijo K, Pontifex MB, et al. Association of physical activity and fitness with executive function among preschoolers. Int J Clin Health Psychol [Internet]. 2023 Oct 1 [cited 2024 Mar 4];23(4). Available from: https://www.elsevier.es/en-revista-international-journal-clinical-health-psychology-355-articulo-association-physical-activity-fitness-with-S1697260023000364.
24. Demir M, Jaafar J, Bilyk N, Mohd Ariff MR. Social skills, friendship and happiness: a cross-cultural investigation. J Soc Psychol. 2012;152(3):379–85.
25. Bento G, Dias G. The importance of outdoor play for young children's healthy development. Porto Biomed J. 2017;2(5):157–60.
26. Haimovitz K, Dweck CS, Walton GM. Preschoolers find ways to resist temptation after learning that willpower can be energizing. Dev Sci. 2020;23(3):e12905.
27. Compagnoni M, Sieber V, Job V. My brain needs a break: kindergarteners' willpower theories are related to behavioral self-regulation. Front Psychol. 2020;11:601724.
28. Kohl HW III, Cook HD. Educating the student body: taking physical activity and physical education to school [Internet]. Washington, D.C.: National Academies Press; 2013. [cited 2024 Feb 26]. Available from: http://www.nap.edu/catalog/18314
29. Pinckard K, Baskin KK, Stanford KI. Effects of exercise to improve cardiovascular health. Front Cardiovasc Med. 2019;6:69.
30. Li J, Siegrist J. Physical activity and risk of cardiovascular disease—a meta-analysis of prospective cohort studies. IJERPH. 2012;9(2):391–407.
31. Santos-Parker JR, LaRocca TJ, Seals DR. Aerobic exercise and other healthy lifestyle factors that influence vascular aging. Adv Physiol Educ. 2014;38(4):296–307.
32. Sattelmair J, Pertman J, Ding EL, Kohl HW, Haskell W, Lee IM. Dose response between physical activity and risk of coronary heart disease: a meta-analysis. Circulation. 2011;124(7):789–95.
33. Borges JP, Da Silva Verdoorn K. Cardiac ischemia/reperfusion injury: the beneficial effects of exercise. In: Xiao J, editor. Exercise for cardiovascular disease prevention and treatment [Internet]. Singapore: Springer Singapore; 2017 [cited 2024 Feb 26]. p. 155–79. (Advances in Experimental Medicine and Biology; vol. 999). Available from: http://link.springer.com/10.1007/978-981-10-4307-9_10.
34. Balbinot F, Claudino FCDA, Lucas PK, Martins APD, Wendland EM, Gerbase MW. Does regular exercise impact the lung function of healthy children and adolescents? A systematic review and meta-analysis. Pediatr Exerc Sci. 2023;35(3):186–94.
35. Janz KF, Letuchy EM, Eichenberger Gilmore JM, Burns TL, Torner JC, Willing MC, et al. Early physical activity provides sustained bone health benefits later in childhood. Med Sci Sports Exerc. 2010;42(6):1072–8.
36. Mitchell JA, Chesi A, Elci O, McCormack SE, Roy SM, Kalkwarf HJ, et al. Physical activity benefits the skeleton of children genetically predisposed to lower bone density in adulthood. J Bone Miner Res. 2016;31(8):1504–12.
37. Gunter KB, Almstedt HC, Janz KF. Physical activity in childhood may be the key to optimizing lifespan skeletal health. Exerc Sport Sci Rev. 2012;40(1):13–21.

38. Rodriguez-Ayllon M, Cadenas-Sánchez C, Estévez-López F, Muñoz NE, Mora-Gonzalez J, Migueles JH, et al. Role of physical activity and sedentary behavior in the mental health of preschoolers, children and adolescents: a systematic review and meta-analysis. Sports Med. 2019;49(9):1383–410.
39. Lubans D, Richards J, Hillman C, Faulkner G, Beauchamp M, Nilsson M, et al. Physical activity for cognitive and mental health in youth: a systematic review of mechanisms. Pediatrics. 2016;138(3):e20161642.
40. Rodriguez-Ayllon M, Neumann A, Hofman A, Voortman T, Lubans DR, Yang-Huang J, et al. Neurobiological, psychosocial, and behavioral mechanisms mediating associations between physical activity and psychiatric symptoms in youth in The Netherlands. JAMA Psychiatry. 2023;80(5):451.
41. Liu C, Liang X, Sit CHP. Physical activity and mental health in children and adolescents with neurodevelopmental disorders: a systematic review and meta-analysis. JAMA Pediatr [Internet]. 2024 [cited 2024 Feb 26]; Available from: https://jamanetwork.com/journals/jamapediatrics/fullarticle/2814312.
42. Bidzan-Bluma I, Lipowska M. Physical activity and cognitive functioning of children: a systematic review. IJERPH. 2018;15(4):800.
43. Slattery EJ, O'Callaghan E, Ryan P, Fortune DG, McAvinue LP. Popular interventions to enhance sustained attention in children and adolescents: a critical systematic review. Neurosci Biobehav Rev. 2022;137:104633.
44. Alizadeh PH. Possible role of exercise therapy on depression: effector neurotransmitters as key players. Behav Brain Res. 2024;459:114791.
45. Mah VK, Ford-Jones EL. Spotlight on middle childhood: Rejuvenating the "forgotten years". Paediatr Child Health. 2012;17(2):81–3.
46. Opstoel K, Chapelle L, Prins FJ, De Meester A, Haerens L, Van Tartwijk J, et al. Personal and social development in physical education and sports: a review study. Eur Phys Educ Rev. 2020;26(4):797–813.
47. Li J, Shao W. Influence of sports activities on prosocial behavior of children and adolescents: a systematic literature review. Int J Environ Res Public Health. 2022;19(11):6484.
48. Van Sluijs EMF, Ekelund U, Crochemore-Silva I, Guthold R, Ha A, Lubans D, et al. Physical activity behaviours in adolescence: current evidence and opportunities for intervention. Lancet. 2021;398(10298):429–42.
49. Cox CE. Role of physical activity for weight loss and weight maintenance. Diabetes Spectr. 2017;30(3):157–60.
50. Brooks GA, Butte NF, Rand WM, Flatt JP, Caballero B. Chronicle of the Institute of Medicine physical activity recommendation: how a physical activity recommendation came to be among dietary recommendations. Am J Clin Nutr. 2004;79(5):921S–30S.
51. Proia P, Amato A, Drid P, Korovljev D, Vasto S, Baldassano S. The impact of diet and physical activity on bone health in children and adolescents. Front Endocrinol. 2021;12:704647.
52. Short KR, Pratt LV, Teague AM. A single exercise session increases insulin sensitivity in normal weight and overweight/obese adolescents. Pediatr Diabetes. 2018;19(6):1050–7.
53. Pedersen BK, Saltin B. Exercise as medicine – evidence for prescribing exercise as therapy in 26 different chronic diseases. Scandinavian Med Sci Sports. 2015;25(S3):1–72.
54. Khan A, Lee EY, Rosenbaum S, Khan SR, Tremblay MS. Dose-dependent and joint associations between screen time, physical activity, and mental wellbeing in adolescents: an international observational study. Lancet Child Adolescent Health. 2021;5(10):729–38.
55. Booth JN, Ness AR, Joinson C, Tomporowski PD, Boyle JME, Leary SD, et al. Associations between physical activity and mental health and behaviour in early adolescence. Ment Health Phys Act. 2023;24:100497.
56. Stillman CM, Esteban-Cornejo I, Brown B, Bender CM, Erickson KI. Effects of exercise on brain and cognition across age groups and health states. Trends Neurosci. 2020;43(7):533–43.
57. Balchin R, Linde J, Blackhurst D, Rauch HL, Schönbächler G. Sweating away depression? The impact of intensive exercise on depression. J Affect Disord. 2016;200:218–21.

58. Sagelv EH, Hammer T, Hamsund T, Rognmo K, Pettersen SA, Pedersen S. High intensity long interval sets provides similar enjoyment as continuous moderate intensity exercise. The Tromsø Exercise Enjoyment Study. Front Psychol. 2019;10:1788.
59. Kline CE. The bidirectional relationship between exercise and sleep: implications for exercise adherence and sleep improvement. Am J Lifestyle Med. 2014;8(6):375–9.
60. Collins NM, Cromartie F, Davis S, Bae J. Effects of early sport participation on self-esteem and happiness. 2018 Jan 11; Available from: https://thesportjournal.org/article/effects-of-early-sport-participation-on-self-esteem-and-happiness/.
61. Liu Q, Jiang M, Li S, Yang Y. Social support, resilience, and self-esteem protect against common mental health problems in early adolescence: a nonrecursive analysis from a two-year longitudinal study. Medicine. 2021;100(4):e24334.
62. Li Y, Guo K. Research on the relationship between physical activity, sleep quality, psychological resilience, and social adaptation among Chinese college students: a cross-sectional study. Front Psychol. 2023;14:1104897.
63. Contreras-Osorio F, Ramirez-Campillo R, Cerda-Vega E, Campos-Jara R, Martínez-Salazar C, Reigal RE, et al. Effects of physical exercise on executive function in adults with depression: a systematic review and meta-analysis. IJERPH. 2022;19(22):15270.
64. Schaefer DR, Simpkins SD, Vest AE, Price CD. The contribution of extracurricular activities to adolescent friendships: new insights through social network analysis. Dev Psychol. 2011;47(4):1141–52.
65. Glick GC, Rose AJ. Prospective associations between friendship adjustment and social strategies: friendship as a context for building social skills. Dev Psychol. 2011;47(4):1117–32.
66. Wu J, Fu Y, Chen D, Zhang H, Xue E, Shao J, et al. Sedentary behavior patterns and the risk of non-communicable diseases and all-cause mortality: a systematic review and meta-analysis. Int J Nurs Stud. 2023;146:104563.
67. Patterson R, McNamara E, Tainio M, De Sá TH, Smith AD, Sharp SJ, et al. Sedentary behaviour and risk of all-cause, cardiovascular and cancer mortality, and incident type 2 diabetes: a systematic review and dose response meta-analysis. Eur J Epidemiol. 2018;33(9):811–29.
68. Bull FC, Al-Ansari SS, Biddle S, Borodulin K, Buman MP, Cardon G, et al. World Health Organization 2020 guidelines on physical activity and sedentary behaviour. Br J Sports Med. 2020;54(24):1451–62.
69. Krause AJ, Simon EB, Mander BA, Greer SM, Saletin JM, Goldstein-Piekarski AN, et al. The sleep-deprived human brain. Nat Rev Neurosci. 2017;18(7):404–18.
70. Sanders T, Noetel M, Parker P, Del Pozo CB, Biddle S, Ronto R, et al. An umbrella review of the benefits and risks associated with youths' interactions with electronic screens. Nat Hum Behav. 2023;8(1):82–99.
71. Barbosa SC, Coledam DHC, Stabelini Neto A, Elias RGM, Oliveira ARD. Ambiente escolar, comportamento sedentário e atividade física em pré-escolares. Rev Paul Pediatr. 2016;34(3):301–8.
72. Duncan MJ, Hall C, Eyre E, Barnett LM, James RS. Pre-schoolers fundamental movement skills predict BMI, physical activity, and sedentary behavior: a longitudinal study. Scandinavian Med Sci Sports. 2021;31(S1):8–14.
73. Pagani LS, Fitzpatrick C, Barnett TA, Dubow E. Prospective Associations between early childhood television exposure and academic, psychosocial, and physical well-being by middle childhood. Arch Pediatr Adolesc Med [Internet]. 2010 [cited 2024 Feb 26];164(5). Available from: http://archpedi.jamanetwork.com/article.aspx?doi=10.1001/archpediatrics.2010.50.
74. Kulinski JP, Khera A, Ayers CR, Das SR, De Lemos JA, Blair SN, et al. Association between cardiorespiratory fitness and accelerometer-derived physical activity and sedentary time in the general population. Mayo Clin Proc. 2014;89(8):1063–71.
75. Gu X. Fundamental motor skill, physical activity, and sedentary behavior in socioeconomically disadvantaged kindergartners. Psychol Health Med. 2016;21(7):871–81.
76. Laukkanen A, Pesola A, Havu M, Sääkslahti A, Finni T. Relationship between habitual physical activity and gross motor skills is multifaceted in 5- to 8-year-old children. Scandinavian

Med Sci Sports [Internet]. 2014 Apr [cited 2024 Feb 26];24(2). Available from: https://onlinelibrary.wiley.com/doi/10.1111/sms.12116.
77. Wong CW, Tsai A, Jonas JB, Ohno-Matsui K, Chen J, Ang M, et al. Digital screen time during the COVID-19 pandemic: risk for a further Myopia Boom? Am J Ophthalmol. 2021;223:333–7.
78. Parkes A, Sweeting H, Wight D, Henderson M. Do television and electronic games predict children's psychosocial adjustment? Longitudinal research using the UK Millennium Cohort Study. Arch Dis Child. 2013;98(5):341–8.
79. Gunnell KE, Flament MF, Buchholz A, Henderson KA, Obeid N, Schubert N, et al. Examining the bidirectional relationship between physical activity, screen time, and symptoms of anxiety and depression over time during adolescence. Prev Med. 2016;88:147–52.
80. McHarg G, Ribner AD, Devine RT, Hughes C, The NewFAMS Study Team. Infant screen exposure links to toddlers' inhibition, but not other EF constructs: a propensity score study. Infancy. 2020;25(2):205–22.
81. Hinkley T, Brown H, Carson V, Teychenne M. Cross sectional associations of screen time and outdoor play with social skills in preschool children. Martinuzzi A, editor. PLoS One. 2018;13(4):e0193700.
82. Hinkley T, Timperio A, Salmon J, Hesketh K. Does preschool physical activity and electronic media use predict later social and emotional skills at 6 to 8 years? A cohort study. J Phys Act Health. 2017;14(4):308–16.
83. Tremblay MS, LeBlanc AG, Kho ME, Saunders TJ, Larouche R, Colley RC, et al. Systematic review of sedentary behaviour and health indicators in school-aged children and youth. Int J Behav Nutr Phys Act. 2011;8(1):98.
84. Saunders TJ, Chaput JP, Tremblay MS. Sedentary behaviour as an emerging risk factor for Cardiometabolic diseases in children and youth. Can J Diabetes. 2014;38(1):53–61.
85. Lee E, Kim Y. Effect of university students' sedentary behavior on stress, anxiety, and depression. Perspect Psychiatr Care. 2019;55(2):164–9.
86. García-Hermoso A, Hormazábal-Aguayo I, Fernández-Vergara O, Olivares PR, Oriol-Granado X. Physical activity, screen time and subjective well-being among children. Int J Clin Health Psychol. 2020;20(2):126–34.
87. Zou L, Wang T, Herold F, Ludyga S, Liu W, Zhang Y, et al. Associations between sedentary behavior and negative emotions in adolescents during home confinement: mediating role of social support and sleep quality. Int J Clin Health Psychol. 2023;23(1):100337.
88. García-Hermoso A, Hormazabal-Aguayo I, Oriol-Granado X, Fernández-Vergara O, Del Pozo CB. Bullying victimization, physical inactivity and sedentary behavior among children and adolescents: a meta-analysis. Int J Behav Nutr Phys Act. 2020;17(1):114.
89. Biddle SJH, García Bengoechea E, Wiesner G. Sedentary behaviour and adiposity in youth: a systematic review of reviews and analysis of causality. Int J Behav Nutr Phys Act. 2017;14(1):43.
90. Hoare E, Milton K, Foster C, Allender S. The associations between sedentary behaviour and mental health among adolescents: a systematic review. Int J Behav Nutr Phys Act. 2016;13(1):108.
91. Kracht CL, Beyl RA, Maher JP, Katzmarzyk PT, Staiano AE. Adolescents' sedentary time, affect, and contextual factors: an ecological momentary assessment study. Int J Behav Nutr Phys Act. 2021;18(1):53.
92. Perlmutter E, Dwyer B, Torous J. Social media and youth mental health: assessing the impact through current and novel digital phenotyping methods. Curr Treat Options Psych [Internet]. 2024 [cited 2024 Mar 6]; Available from: https://doi.org/10.1007/s40501-024-00312-1.
93. Zakiyatul Fuadah D, Siswoaribowo A, Diniaty E. Sedentary lifestyle with social interaction in adolescent. JANH. 2021;3(2):71–6.
94. Werneck AO, Collings PJ, Barboza LL, Stubbs B, Silva DR. Associations of sedentary behaviors and physical activity with social isolation in 100,839 school students: the Brazilian Scholar Health Survey. Gen Hosp Psychiatry. 2019;59:7–13.

95. World Health Organization (WHO). Global status report on physical activity 2022: country profiles [Internet]. [cited 2024 Feb 28]. Available from: https://www.who.int/publications/i/item/9789240064119.
96. Sterdt E, Liersch S, Walter U. Correlates of physical activity of children and adolescents: a systematic review of reviews. Health Educ J. 2014;73(1):72–89.
97. Gomes TN, Katzmarzyk PT, Hedeker D, Fogelholm M, Standage M, Onywera V, et al. Correlates of compliance with recommended levels of physical activity in children. Sci Rep. 2017;7(1):16507.
98. Shao T, Zhou X. Correlates of physical activity habits in adolescents: a systematic review. Front Physiol. 2023;14:1131195.
99. Butcher K, Sallis JF, Mayer JA, Woodruff S. Correlates of physical activity guideline compliance for adolescents in 100 U.S. cities. J Adolesc Health. 2008;42(4):360–8.
100. World Health Organization (WHO). WHO guidelines on physical activity and sedentary behaviour. Geneva: World Health Organization; 2020.
101. World Health Organization. Guidelines on physical activity, sedentary behaviour and sleep for children under 5 years of age [Internet]. Geneva: World Health Organization; 2019. [cited 2024 Feb 28]. 33 p. Available from: https://iris.who.int/handle/10665/311664
102. Tremblay MS, Chaput JP, Adamo KB, Aubert S, Barnes JD, Choquette L, et al. Canadian 24-hour movement guidelines for the early years (0–4 years): an integration of physical activity, sedentary behaviour, and sleep. BMC Public Health. 2017;17(S5):874.
103. Tremblay MS, LeBlanc AG, Carson V, Choquette L, Connor Gorber S, Dillman C, et al. Canadian physical activity guidelines for the early years (aged 0–4 years). Appl Physiol Nutr Metab. 2012;37(2):345–56.
104. Get Ireland active: promoting physical activity in Ireland. Dublin: Health Service Executive; 2009.
105. Okely AD, Ghersi D, Hesketh KD, Santos R, Loughran SP, Cliff DP, et al. A collaborative approach to adopting/adapting guidelines - the Australian 24-hour movement guidelines for the early years (birth to 5 years): an integration of physical activity, sedentary behavior, and sleep. BMC Public Health. 2017;17(S5):869.
106. Composing and Editorial Board of Physical Activity Guidelines for Chinese. Physical activity guidelines for Chinese (2021). Biomed Environ Sci. 2022;35(1):1–3.
107. Piercy KL, Troiano RP, Ballard RM, Carlson SA, Fulton JE, Galuska DA, et al. The physical activity guidelines for Americans. JAMA. 2018;320(19):2020.
108. Misra A, Nigam P, Hills AP, Chadha DS, Sharma V, Deepak KK, et al. Consensus physical activity guidelines for Asian Indians. Diabetes Technol Ther. 2012;14(1):83–98.
109. Ohta T, Tabata I, Mochizuki Y. Japanese national physical activity and health promotion guidelines. J Aging Phys Act. 1999;7(3):231–46.
110. Ministry of Health. Sit less, move more, sleep well physical activity guidelines for children and young people [Internet]. 2017 [cited 2024 Mar 5]. Available from: https://www.tewhatuora.govt.nz/assets/Our-health-system/Preventative-Health/physical-activity-guidelines-for-children-and-young-people-may17.pdf.
111. Care AGD of H and A. Australian Government Department of Health and Aged Care. Australian Government Department of Health and Aged Care; 2021 [cited 2024 Mar 4]. Australian 24-hour movement guidelines for children (5 to 12 years) and young people (13 to 17 years): an integration of physical activity, sedentary behaviour, and sleep. Available from: https://www.health.gov.au/resources/publications/australian-24-hour-movement-guidelines-for-children-5-to-12-years-and-young-people-13-to-17-years-an-integration-of-physical-activity-sedentary-behaviour-and-sleep?language=en.
112. The Danish Health Authority. Health promotion package – Physical activity [Internet]. Copenhagen, Denmark; 2018. Available from: https://www.sundhedsstyrelsen.dk/-/media/English/Publications/2020/Forebyggelsepakke-fysisk-aktivitet-(Engelsk)/Health-promotion-package-on-physical-activity.ashx?sc_lang=en&hash=F3BB1EEB328D772F7DD3A4DF4E9B6866.

113. Laureus Sport for Good Foundation. South African 24-hour movement guidelines for birth to five years: an integration of physical activity, sitting behaviour, screen time and Sleep Cape Town [Internet]. South Africa: Sports Science Institute of South Africa; 2018. Available from: https://www.laureus.co.za/wp-content/uploads/2018/11/EYMG-2-pager-ONLINE.pdf.
114. Garcia-Hermoso A, López-Gil JF, Ramírez-Vélez R, Alonso-Martínez AM, Izquierdo M, Ezzatvar Y. Adherence to aerobic and muscle-strengthening activities guidelines: a systematic review and meta-analysis of 3.3 million participants across 32 countries. Br J Sports Med. 2023;57(4):225–9.
115. Chaput JP, Willumsen J, Bull F, Chou R, Ekelund U, Firth J, et al. 2020 WHO guidelines on physical activity and sedentary behaviour for children and adolescents aged 5–17 years: summary of the evidence. Int J Behav Nutr Phys Act. 2020;17(1):141.
116. Tremblay MS, Barnes JD, Demchenko I, Gonzalez SA, Brazo-Sayavera J, Kalinowski J, et al. Active Healthy Kids Global Alliance Global Matrix 4.0—a resource for physical activity researchers. J Phys Act Health. 2022;19(11):693–9.
117. Tremblay MS, Carson V, Chaput JP, Connor Gorber S, Dinh T, Duggan M, et al. Canadian 24-hour movement guidelines for children and youth: an integration of physical activity, sedentary behaviour, and sleep. Appl Physiol Nutr Metab. 2016;41(6 (Suppl. 3)):S311–27.
118. Public Health Authority. Twenty-four-hour movement practice guidelines for Saudi Arabia. An integration of physical activity, sedentary behavior, and sleep duration [Internet]. Saudi Arabia: Public Health Authority; 2017. Available from: https://faculty.ksu.edu.sa/sites/default/files/24hr_s_movement_practice_guidelines_for_saudi_arabia_1619026105.pdf.
119. Health Promotion Board, Singapore. Singapore physical activity guidelines, 2022; Available from: https://www.healthhub.sg/sites/assets/Assets/Programs/pa-lit/pdfs/Singapore_Physical_Activity_Guidelines.pdf.
120. Murtagh E, Power D, Foster CH Murphy M, Healy S, Hayes G, et al. Update of the National Physical Activity guidelines for Ireland-final research report. 2024 [cited 2024 Mar 5]; Available from: https://repository.rcsi.com/articles/report/Update_of_the_National_Physical_Activity_Guidelines_for_Ireland_-_Final_Research_Report/24762942.
121. Department of Health & Social Care. UK Chief Medical Officers' physical activity guidelines, 2019 Sep 7; Available from: https://assets.publishing.service.gov.uk/media/5d839543ed915d52428dc134/uk-chief-medical-officers-physical-activity-guidelines.pdf.
122. Rütten A, Pfeifer K. National Recommendations for Physical Activity and Physical Activity Promotion [Internet]. 2016 [cited 2024 Mar 4]. Available from: https://open.fau.de/server/api/core/bitstreams/9f5d8dba-b112-4721-9026-667c740f15ac/content.
123. Kahlmeier S, Frei A, Kriemler S, Nigg CR, Radtke T, Manike K, et al. Updating national physical activity guidelines based on the global WHO guidelines: experiences and challenges from Switzerland. Curr Issues Sport Sci. 2023;8(1):014.
124. Sisson SB, Church TS, Martin CK, Tudor-Locke C, Smith SR, Bouchard C, et al. Profiles of sedentary behavior in children and adolescents: the U.S. National Health and Nutrition Examination Survey, 2001–2006. Int J Pediatr Obes. 2009;4(4):353–9.
125. Dias PJP, Domingos IP, Ferreira MG, Muraro AP, Sichieri R, Gonçalves-Silva RMV. Prevalence and factors associated with sedentary behavior in adolescents. Rev Saude Publica. 2014;48(2):266–74.

Chapter 2
Twenty-Four-Hour Movement Behaviors for School-Aged Children and Adolescents

José Francisco López-Gil

2.1 Introduction

There is convincing evidence that suggests a strong correlation between various health indicators in the youth population and their physical activity (PA), sleep duration, and sedentary behaviors, such as screen time [1–3]. In this sense, the 24-hour movement guidelines for young people emphasize the need to shift their focus from individual behaviors to incorporating all movement-related behaviors throughout the day [4]. According to these guidelines, preschoolers (3–4 years) are recommended to engage in a minimum of 180 min of PA, with at least 60 min being considered moderate to vigorous PA (MVPA), limiting sedentary screen time to less than 1 h, and ensuring 10–13 h of good-quality sleep [5, 6]. Furthermore, children and adolescents aged 5–17 years should strive for at least 60 min of MVPA every day, limit recreational screen time to 120 min or less, and ensure adequate sleep duration (e.g., 9–11 h for children, 8–10 h for adolescents) within a 24-hour period [7]. These guidelines emphasize the importance of addressing the clustering and interactions among all aspects of 24-hour movement behaviors simultaneously to achieve optimal health outcomes [8].

Despite the numerous benefits associated with adhering to the 24-hour movement guidelines, a meta-analysis of 387,437 participants aged 3–18 years from 23 countries revealed a global adherence rate of only 7.1% [9]. This low compliance with the guidelines is concerning, especially considering that the overall adherence rate was 11.3% (95% confidence interval [CI]: 8.7–13.8%), with adherence rates of only 10.3% (95% CI 7.5–13.1%) and 2.7% (95% CI 1.8–3.6%) in children and adolescents, respectively. Furthermore, overall adherence varied significantly by region, with rates of 17.2% (95% CI 11.2–23.2%) in Africa, 3.8% (95% CI

J. F. López-Gil (✉)
One Health Research Group, Universidad de Las Américas, Quito, Ecuador
e-mail: josefranciscolopezgil@gmail.com

© The Author(s), under exclusive license to Springer Nature Switzerland AG 2024
A. García-Hermoso (ed.), *Promotion of Physical Activity and Health in the School Setting*, https://doi.org/10.1007/978-3-031-65595-1_2

2.8–4.8%) in Asia, 9.6% (95% CI 6.8–12.4%) in Europe, 7.9% (95% CI 6.7–9.1%) in North America, 10.9% (95% CI 8.4–13.4%) in Oceania, and 2.9% (95% CI 0.01–5.9%) in South America. Additionally, the meta-analysis revealed that overall adherence was significantly lower in girls (3.8%, 95% CI 3.2–4.3%) than in boys (6.9%, 95% CI 5.9–7.9%). These findings highlight the urgent need to increase PA levels, reduce screen time, and optimize sleep duration in preschoolers, children, and adolescents.

Early childhood education and care settings, such as child development centers, childcare facilities, crèches, nurseries, prekindergarten, kindergartens, long day care facilities, family day care facilities, and preschools, as well as educational settings, such as schools and school boards, with childcare and elementary, secondary, and postsecondary divisions, can be valuable allies in the health of the young population. These settings play a crucial role in promoting healthy behaviors among young people, as most of this population has spent time there for a certain period during their lifetime, and children spend half of their daily waking time at school [10]. Furthermore, schools present a conducive environment for reaching the majority of children, offering an evident setting for interventions that are independent of children's background characteristics, gender, socioeconomic status, or race/ethnicity [11]. Moreover, schools are an ideal setting for health promotion, as they can reach several other target groups, such as school staff, teachers, families, and even members of the local community [12]. The Commission on Ending Childhood Obesity has recognized the need to start preventing obesity early in life and acknowledges the important role that early childhood education and care settings play in shaping children's food and PA preferences and supporting caregivers and families [13]. However, there are currently no global standards for early childhood education and care settings or educational settings on PA, sedentary behavior (including screen time), or sleep duration [14].

2.2 Interactions and Interdependencies Among 24-Hour Movement Behaviors

2.2.1 Discussion on How Physical Activity, Screen Time, and Sleep Are Interconnected

The relationships between PA, screen time, and sleep are complex and interconnected rather than linear or independent [4]. These dimensions interact in unexpected ways, and a lack of PA, for instance, can negatively impact sleep quality, while excessive screen time can affect both the quantity and quality of nighttime rest [15]. During each period, individuals spend time sleeping, engaging in sedentary behavior, quietly standing, or engaging in PA [4]. Traditionally, epidemiologists have investigated these behaviors separately, considering them independent health risk factors [4].

Previous studies, however, emphasize the interdependence of these factors [4, 15]. For instance, a lack of PA may contribute to an increase in screen time, which, in turn, negatively affects sleep [16]. Conversely, insufficient sleep can decrease motivation for PA during the day [17]. In 2014, Pedišić [4] called attention to the statistical inadequacy of the isotemporal substitution model and other traditional multivariate methods when analyzing the associations of sleep, sedentary behavior, quiet standing, light-intensity PA, and MVPA with health outcomes. They proposed a shift in the research paradigm toward an integrated approach, suggesting that these factors should be analyzed as parts of a time-use composition using compositional data analysis. This framework, known as the activity balance model, highlights the importance of considering these dimensions holistically to better understand their impact on overall health [4].

2.2.2 Synergistic Effects of Positive Behaviors and the Compounding Impact of Negative Behaviors

Embracing healthy habits, such as integrating regular PA, mindfully controlling screen time, and prioritizing sufficient sleep, can produce beneficial synergies [8]. These behaviors complement each other, establishing a positive cycle that enhances overall health and well-being [1, 18]. Equally important is acknowledging the compounding effects of negative behaviors. For example, a lack of PA coupled with prolonged screen time and inadequate sleep can have a more pronounced and adverse influence on health than can each individual behavior alone [19].

Previous systematic reviews, both with and without meta-analyses, have attempted to determine the relationships between compliance with 24-hour movement guidelines and various health outcomes [1–3]. For example, a comprehensive review by Rollo et al. [3], which included a total of 51 studies from 20 different countries, concluded that meeting the 24-hour movement guidelines was associated with several positive health outcomes in children and youth. Specifically, meeting the guidelines was not linked to adiposity in toddlers; was favorably associated with health-related quality of life, social-cognitive development, or behavioral and emotional problems in preschoolers; and was associated with global cognition, health-related quality of life, and healthy dietary patterns in children. Additionally, meeting the guidelines was associated with favorable outcomes in terms of adiposity; fitness; and cardiometabolic, mental, social, and emotional health in children and youth. The review also revealed significant associations between the composition of 24-hour movement behaviors and indicators of adiposity and bone and skeletal health in preschoolers; health-related quality of life in children; adiposity, fitness, and cardiometabolic, social, and emotional health in children and youth; cardiometabolic health in adults; adiposity and fitness in adults and older adults; and mental health and risk of mortality in older adults.

On the other hand, a scoping review conducted by de Lannoy et al. [1] reported that a total of 55 articles focused on the relationships between combined movement behaviors and mental health, mental wellness, and mental illness. Within this scope, most of the studies reported a positive association, indicating a beneficial link between combined movement behaviors and mental wellness. Similarly, the majority of the studies reported a negative association between combined movement behaviors and indicators of mental illness.

Furthermore, a meta-analysis conducted by López-Gil et al. [2] revealed that adherence to the 24-hour movement guidelines was cross-sectionally associated with lower overall indicators of obesity. However, no longitudinal association was observed. When examining each obesity-related indicator independently, compliance with all three 24-hour movement guidelines was related to lower odds of overweight/obesity and obesity alone. Additionally, inverse relationships were identified between 24-hour movement guidelines and variables such as body mass index, body mass index z score, waist circumference, and body fat.

2.3 Global Guidelines and Variances

2.3.1 Overview of Guidelines Provided by Different Countries and the World Health Organization

Recommendations for the 24-hour movement behaviors of young children have been recently established [5, 7]. Canada took the lead in 2017 [7], followed by Australia [20]; subsequently, the World Health Organization (WHO) [6], New Zealand [21], South Africa [22], the United Kingdom [23], and Saudi Arabia [24] also embraced evidence-based guidelines for preschoolers (under 5 years), children and adolescents (aged 5–17 years), or both. Table 2.1 displays a summary of the different guidelines across various countries.

2.3.1.1 Canada

The initial evidence-based guidelines for children and adolescents (aged 5–17 years) regarding their 24-hour movement were introduced by Canada [7]. These guidelines, which address the entire day, were formulated by the Healthy Active Living and Obesity Group (HALO) of the Children's Hospital of Eastern Ontario (CHEO) Research Institute in collaboration with the Canadian Society for Exercise Physiology (CSEP), ParticipACTION, The Conference Board of Canada, the Public Health Agency of Canada, and a team of prominent researchers worldwide. The development process involved input from more than 700 national and international stakeholders. For children and adolescents (aged 0–17 years), these 24-hour movement guidelines include the following indications:

Table 2.1 Highlighting commonalities and variations in recommendations

Guideline aspect	Australia [25]	Canada [7]	New Zealand [21]	Saudi Arabia [24]	South Africa [22]	World Health Organization [6]
Age group	Early years (0–5 years) and children and adolescents (5–17 years)	Early years (0–4 years) and children and adolescents (5–17 years)	Early years (0–4 years)	Toddlers (1–2 years), preschoolers (3–5 years), children and adolescents (6–17 years)	Birth to 5 years (0–5 years)	Infants (less than 1 year) and children (1–2, 3–4 years)
Physical activity	Less than 1 year: be physically active several times a day in a variety of ways. For those not yet mobile, include at least 30 min in prone position (tummy time) spread throughout the day while awake. 1–2 years: 180 min/day in a variety of types of physical activities. 3–5 years: 180 min/day in a variety of types of physical activities, with a minimum of 60 min/day of vigorous play. 5–17: 60+ min/day (moderate to vigorous physical activity). Vigorous physical activities, and muscle and bone strengthening activities at least 3 days/week.	Less than 1 year: be physically active several times a day in a variety of ways. For those not yet mobile, include at least 30 min in prone position (tummy time) spread throughout the day while awake. 1–2 years: 180 min/day in a variety of types of physical activities. 3–4 years: 180 min/day in a variety of types of physical activities, with a minimum of 60 min/day of vigorous play. 5–17: 60+ min/day (moderate to vigorous physical activity). Vigorous physical activities, and muscle and bone strengthening activities at least 3 days/week.	0–4 years: Provide fun activities and include plenty of opportunities for active play.	1–2 years: 180 min/day. 3–5 years: 180 min/day in a variety of types of physical activities, with a minimum of 60 min/day of vigorous play. 6–17: 60+ min/day (moderate to vigorous physical activity). Vigorous physical activities, and muscle and bone strengthening activities at least 3 days/week.	0–1 year: be physically active several times a day in a variety of ways. For those not yet mobile, include at least 30 min in prone position (tummy time) spread throughout the day while awake. 1–2 years: 180 min/day in a variety of types of physical activities. 3–5 years: 180 min/day in a variety of types of physical activities, with a minimum of 60 min/day of vigorous play.	Less than 1 year: be physically active several times a day in a variety of ways. For those not yet mobile, include at least 30 min in prone position (tummy time) spread throughout the day while awake. 1–2 years: 180 min/day in a variety of types of physical activities. 3–4 years: 180 min/day in a variety of types of physical activities, with a minimum of 60 min/day of vigorous play.

(continued)

Table 2.1 (continued)

Guideline aspect	Australia [25]	Canada [7]	New Zealand [21]	Saudi Arabia [24]	South Africa [22]	World Health Organization [6]
Sedentary behavior/ screen time	Less than 1 year: not recommended. 1 year: ≤1 h/day. 2–4 years: ≤2 h/day.	Less than 1 year: not recommended. 1 year: ≤1 h/day. 2–4 years: ≤2 h/day.	0–1 year: not recommended. 2–5 years: ≤1 h/day.	1–2 years: not recommended. 3–5 years: ≤1 h/day. 6–17 years: ≤2 h/day.	0–2 years: not recommended. 3–5 years: ≤1 h/day.	Less than 1 year: not recommended. 1 year: ≤1 h/day. 2–4 years: ≤2 h/day.
Sleep duration	0–3 months: 14–17 h/day. 4–11 months: 12–16 h/day. 1–2 years: 11–14 h/day. 3–5 years: 10–13 h/day. 6–12 years: 9–12 h/day. 13–17 years: 8–10 h/day.	0–3 months: 14–17 h/day. 4–11 months: 12–16 h/day. 1–2 years: 11–14 h/day. 3–5 years: 10–13 h/day. 6–12 years: 9–12 h/day. 13–17 years: 8–10 h/day.	0–3 months: 14–17 h/day. 4–11 months: 12–16 h/day. 1–2 years: 11–14 h/day. 3–5 years: 10–13 h/day.	1–2 years: 11–14 h/day. 3–5 years: 10–13 h/day. 6–12 years: 9–12 h/day. 13–17 years: 8–10 h/day.	0–3 months: 14–17 h/day. 4–11 months: 12–16 h/day. 1–2 years: 11–14 h/day. 3–5 years: 10–13 h/day.	0–3 months: 14–17 h/day. 4–11 months: 12–16 h/day. 1–2 years: 11–14 h/day. 3–4 years: 10–13 h/day.

(a) Physical activity:

- For children younger than 5 years, it is recommended that they participate in a variety of physical activities throughout the day, totaling at least 180 min, with a minimum of 60 min involving vigorous play.
- Children aged 5 years and older should aim to accumulate a minimum of 60 min daily in moderate to vigorous physical activities, incorporating diverse aerobic exercises.

(b) Recreational screen time:

- The sedentary screen time of children under the age of 5 years should be limited to 1 hour or less per day.
- The recreational screen time should be restricted to a maximum of 2 h each day for children aged five and older.

(c) Sleep duration:

- Children under the age of 5 years require approximately 10–13 h of high-quality sleep, which may include the option of a nap. Maintaining consistent sleep and wake schedules is essential.
- Children aged 5 years and older were advised to maintain uninterrupted sleep for 9–11 h per night.

The guidelines also suggest that individuals who are not presently adhering to the 24-hour movement recommendations should gradually work toward incorporating them into their routine. Adherence to these guidelines has been linked to various positive outcomes, including improved body composition, cardiorespiratory and musculoskeletal fitness, academic performance, cognitive function, emotional regulation, prosocial behaviors, cardiovascular and metabolic health, and overall quality of life. The advantages of following these guidelines outweigh any potential risks. Additionally, these guidelines may be applicable to children and youth with disabilities or medical conditions; however, it is advisable to seek guidance from a healthcare professional for tailored advice in such cases.

2.3.1.2 Australia

The Australian *24-Hour Movement Guidelines for the early* years [25] and the *Australian 24-Hour Movement Guidelines for Children and Young People* [20] were developed using the Grading of Recommendations Assessment, Development and Evaluation-Adopt, adapt, adopt with minor changes, or exclude recommendations from a source guideline (GRADE-ADOLOPMENT) approach, a methodology inspired by the Grading of Recommendations Assessment, Development and Evaluation (GRADE) approach utilized by the Canadian Guideline Development Panel. Drawing from evidence presented in Canadian and updated Australian systematic reviews, the Guideline Development Group in Australia decided to embrace the Canadian recommendations. With only minor modifications to the phrasing of good practice statements, the Australian guidelines retained the wording of the Canadian guidelines, including the guidelines themselves, the preamble, and the title [20].

Babies (infants) under 1 year of age:

(a) Physical activity:

- Individuals were encouraged to be physically active several times a day through supervised interactive floor-based play, including crawling. For those not yet mobile, at least 30 min of tummy time, involving reaching, grasping, pushing, and pulling, should be incorporated and spread throughout the day while awake.

(b) Sedentary behavior:

- Restraining should be avoided for more than 1 h at a time (e.g., in a stroller, car seat, or highchair). Screen time is not recommended. When sedentary, they engage in activities such as reading, singing, puzzles, and storytelling with a caregiver.

(c) Sleep:

- The participants were asked to perform 14–17 h (for those aged 0–3 months) or 12–16 h (for those aged 4–11 months) of good-quality sleep, including naps.

Toddlers (1–2 years):

(a) Physical activity:

- At least 180 min of restraint are spent performing various physical activities, including energetic play, throughout the day.

(b) Sedentary behavior:

- Avoiding restraint for more than 1 h at a time or sitting for extended periods. For those younger than 2 years, no sedentary screen time is recommended. For those aged 2 years, limiting sedentary screen time to no more than 1 h is recommended; less time is needed. Engage in activities such as reading, singing, puzzles, and storytelling when sedentary.

(c) Sleep:

- The aim was for 11–14 h of good-quality sleep, including naps, consistent sleep, and wake-up.

Preschoolers (3–5 years):

(a) Physical activity:

- At least 180 min of PA, with a minimum of 60 min of energetic play, are spent throughout the day.

(b) Sedentary behavior:

- Avoiding restraint for more than 1 h at a time or sitting for extended periods. Limit sedentary screen time to no more than 1 h; less is better. Individuals should be encouraged to engage in activities such as reading, singing, puzzles, and storytelling when sedentary.

(c) Sleep:

- The aim of working for 10–13 h of good-quality sleep may include a nap, consistent sleep and wake-up.

These same guidelines indicate that, if unsure where to begin, parents are encouraged to make gradual changes, incorporate more movement, engage in quiet play, and establish healthy sleep habits over time. Positive changes can contribute to a healthier, happier, smarter, and stronger child.

On the other hand, to attain optimal health benefits, children and adolescents (aged 5–17 years) should strive for a recommended balance of high levels of PA, minimal sedentary behavior, and adequate daily sleep. The healthy 24-hour period included the following steps:

- Individuals perform more than 60 min of MVPA per day, primarily consisting of aerobic activities.
- Engaging in several hours of diverse light physical activities.
- The sedentary recreational screen time was restricted to no more than 2 h per day.
- Breaking up prolonged periods of sitting as frequently as possible.
- We aimed for uninterrupted sleep lasting 9–11 h per night for those aged 5–13 years and 8–10 h per night for those aged 14–17 years.
- Maintaining consistent bed and wake-up times.

Additionally, vigorous activities, as well as activities that strengthen muscles and bones, should be incorporated at least 3 days per week. For enhanced health benefits, sedentary time should be replaced with additional MVPA, while ensuring sufficient sleep.

2.3.1.3 The World Health Organization

The *WHO Guidelines on PA, sedentary behavior and sleep for children under 5 years of age* provide recommendations on the amount of time on a 24-hour day that young children under 5 years of age should spend being physically active or sleeping for their health and well-being, and the maximum recommended time these children should spend on screen-based sedentary activities or time restrained. They were developed using the best available evidence, expert consensus and consideration of values and preferences, acceptability, feasibility, equity, and resource implications.

Infants (younger than 1 year):

- Individuals should be physically active multiple times a day through interactive floor-based play, with at least 30 min of prone position (tummy time) for those not yet mobile.
- Restraint should be avoided for more than 1 h at a time, and sedentary screen time should be discouraged. Instead, they may engage in reading and storytelling with a caregiver.
- The aim was for 14–17 h of good quality sleep (0–3 months) or 12–16 h (4–11 months), including naps.

Children aged 1–2 years:

- At least 180 min of various physical activities, including moderate- to vigorous-intensity activities, accumulate throughout the day.
- Restraint should be limited to no more than 1 h, and sedentary screen time should be discouraged for 1-year-olds. For 2-year-olds, sedentary screen time should be restricted to no more than 1 h.
- Ensure 11–14 h of good quality sleep, including naps, with consistent sleep and wake-up times.

Children 3–4 years:

- Should be engaged in at least 180 min of various physical activities, with at least 60 min of moderate- to vigorous-intensity activities occurring throughout the day.
- Restraint should be avoided for more than 1 h, and sedentary screen time should be limited to no more than 1 h.
- The aim is for 10–13 h of good quality sleep, including a nap, with consistent sleep and wake-up times.

Conversely, for children and adolescents (aged 5–17 years), the WHO Guidelines on PA and sedentary behavior provide evidence-based public health recommendations for children, adolescents, adults, and older adults on the amount of PA (frequency, intensity, and duration) required to offer significant health benefits and mitigate health risks. For the first time, recommendations are provided on the associations between sedentary behavior and health outcomes, as well as for subpopulations, such as pregnant and postpartum women and people living with chronic conditions or disability. Although Canadian guidelines for children and adolescents aged 5–17 years have established specific cutoff points for PA, screen time, and sleep duration [7], the expert committee that developed the WHO guidelines considered that there was only sufficient evidence for the recommendation of PA and reducing sedentary time (without establishing a specific cutoff point) [26].

2.3.1.4 New Zealand

The Ministry of Health in New Zealand published *Sit Less, Move More, Sleep Well: Active Play Guidelines for Under Fives* [21] to assist health professionals, sports organizations, early childhood education centers, and others in providing advice on

PA for young children. This document offers population health recommendations for children under 5 years of age in New Zealand, emphasizing the significance of reducing sedentary behavior, increasing PA, and promoting healthy sleep habits. The guidelines are based on a review of international evidence tailored to the New Zealand context, as detailed in the *Review of Physical Activity Guidance and Resources for Under Fives* [27].

(a) Sit less:

- Regular breaks were encouraged for activities to limit a child's sitting time.
- The screen time for those under 2 years old was discounted, and the duration was restricted to less than 1 hour per day for children aged two and older, with an emphasis on minimizing screen use.
- The use of equipment that hinders free movement should be limited.

(b) Move more:

- Enjoyable activities that foster physical, social, emotional, and spiritual growth, aimed at least 3 hours daily for toddlers and preschoolers, were provided throughout the day.
- Incorporate opportunities for active play that:
  - Develop movement competence and confidence.
  - Offer sufficient challenges to enhance resilience and encourage creativity through exploration.
  - The interviews included questions about solo activities and interactions with parents, siblings, friends, and caregivers.
  - A variety of indoor and outdoor activities are featured, with a focus on those involving nature.

(c) Sleep well:

- It is important to ensure that babies (birth to 3 months) obtain 14–17 h of good-quality sleep daily, including daytime naps tailored to their physical and emotional needs.
- Infants (4–12 months old) were provided 12–15 h of good-quality sleep each day, and their daytime naps decreased as they approached 1 year of age.
- Ensured toddlers (1–2 years old) receive 11–14 h of good-quality sleep daily, including at least one daytime nap.
- Support preschoolers (3–4 years) in getting 10–13 h of good-quality sleep every day, maintaining consistent bedtimes and wake-up times.

2.3.1.5 South Africa

In 2018, the South African 24-Hour Movement Guidelines for Birth to Five Years were released [22]. To develop these guidelines, the GRADE-ADOLOPMENT approach was used, with certain practical adjustments, drawing inspiration from the Australian guidelines for the early years [28]. Similarly, a consensus panel comprising stakeholders in early childhood development and academics was established to contribute to the development process.

Infants (from birth to 1 year old)

(a) Moving:

- Individuals should engage in various physical activities multiple times a day, including interactive floor play such as crawling.
- For immobile babies, at least 30 min of tummy time spread throughout waking hours, along with activities such as reaching and grasping, are recommended. When sitting, babies should participate in stimulating activities with a caregiver, such as playing with safe toys, engaging in baby conversations, singing, and storytelling.

(b) Sitting:

- It is advised that babies not be confined or strapped in for more than 1 hour at a time, whether in a pram, highchair, or on a caregiver's back or chest. Screen time (including televisions, cell phones, tablets, video games, and computers) is not recommended.

(c) Sleeping:

- Adequate sleep is crucial, with babies aged 0–3 months requiring 14–17 h and those aged 4–11 months needing 12–16 h of good quality sleep, including naps during the day. Babies may sleep while strapped to a caregiver or while being held.

Toddlers (1–2 years old)

(a) Moving:

- Individuals should engage in at least 180 min of diverse physical activities, including energetic play throughout the day, with more being preferable.

(b) Sitting:

- When sitting, toddlers should participate in developmental activities such as reading, singing, playing games with blocks and puzzles, and storytelling with a caregiver. It is advised that toddlers not be confined or strapped in for more than 1 hour at a time, whether in a pram or highchair or on a caregiver's back or chest, and prolonged periods of sitting should be avoided. For toddlers younger than 2 years, screen time is not recommended. For those aged 2 years, screen time should be limited to no more than 1 h, with less being preferable.

(c) Sleeping:

- Adequate sleep is crucial, with toddlers requiring 11–14 h of good quality sleep, including naps during the day, and maintaining consistent sleep and wake-up times.

Preschoolers (3–5 years old)

(a) Moving:

- Preschoolers, typically aged 3–5 years, should engage in physical activities for a minimum of 180 min daily, with at least 60 min dedicated to energetic play that raises their heart rate, such as running, jumping, and dancing, spread throughout the day. Additional PA is encouraged for even greater benefits.

(b) Sitting:

- When sitting, preschoolers should participate in enriching activities such as reading, singing, puzzles, arts and crafts, and storytelling with caregivers and other children. It is recommended that preschoolers not be confined or strapped in for more than 1 hour at a time, and extended periods of sitting should be avoided. The screen time should be limited to no more than 1 h per day, with less being preferable.

(c) Sleeping:

- Adequate sleep is crucial, with preschoolers needing 10–13 h of good quality sleep, including a nap, if necessary, and maintaining consistent sleep and wake-up times.

2.3.1.6 Saudi Arabia

The Public Health Authority of Saudi Arabia unveiled the Twenty-Four-Hour Movement Practice Guidelines [24], a comprehensive set of recommendations designed to promote the well-being of Saudis across all age groups. The development panel utilized a customized Research and Development (RAND) appropriateness method and followed the GRADE-ADOLOPMENT approach to formulate the current recommendations for the guidelines [29]. These guidelines focus on three key aspects, PA, sedentary behavior, and sleep duration, aiming to provide a holistic approach to health over a 24-hour period. The guidelines are crafted to align with both international practices and local customs, ensuring cultural relevance and reflecting national evidence.

The release of the Saudi 24-hour movement guidelines signifies a significant contribution to Saudi Arabia's National Vision 2030. By providing a framework for healthy lifestyle practices, these guidelines offer valuable support for policymakers and decision-makers, facilitating the implementation of health-related objectives within the broader context of the national vision. The guidelines serve as a cornerstone for informed decision-making, rooted in evidence-based practices, as Saudi Arabia strives to achieve its health and well-being goals.

Toddlers (1–2 years old)

(a) Physical activity:

- Toddlers should engage in various physical activities totaling at least 3 h per day, including energetic and outdoor play, which can be spread throughout the day, with additional activities being beneficial (conditional).
- Examples of activities include walking, running, climbing, pulling, pushing, ball games, park activities (tricycle or bike riding), water activities, and tags.

(b) Sedentary behavior:

- Avoiding restraint of toddlers for more than 1 h at a time in a stroller, car seat, or highchair and discouraging prolonged sitting.
- Sedentary activities such as reading and storytelling should be encouraged when the child is not engaged in active play.
- Screen time for toddlers (1–2 years) is not recommended.
- For toddlers (2–3 years), sedentary screen time should be limited to no more than 1 h per day; less time is preferable.

(c) Sleep duration:

- The optimal duration of sleep for children aged 1–2 years is 11–14 h per day, including naps (strong recommendation).

Preschoolers (3–5 years old)

(a) Physical activity

- Preschoolers should participate in at least 3 h of various physical activities daily, including a minimum of 1 h of energetic and outdoor play throughout the day (conditional).
- The participants were advised to perform 1 h or more of MVPA appropriately for their age (conditional).
- Examples of activities include organized and free games; running, climbing, pulling, pushing, and ball games; park activities (tricycle or bike riding); water activities; and tags.

(b) Sedentary behavior

- Premature babies should be avoided for more than 1 h at a time in a stroller, car seat, or highchair.
- Having sedentary activities such as reading, storytelling, or coloring should be encouraged when the child is not actively playing.
- The sedentary screen time was limited to no more than 1 h per day for preschoolers; shorter durations were preferred.

(c) Sleep Duration

- The optimal duration of sleep for children aged 3–5 years is 10–13 h per day (including naps) (conditional).

Children and adolescents (6–17 years)

(a) Physical activity

- Children and adolescents (aged 6–17 years) should engage in a minimum of 1 h of MVPA per day, emphasizing aerobic activity (strong recommendation).
- The interventions included vigorous PA, muscle strengthening, and bone strengthening activities performed at least 3 days per week within the daily 1-hour minimum (strong recommendation).
- Participants participated in several hours of light PA per day (conditional).
- Examples of light activities include brisk walking, housework, recreational swimming, and free play.

(b) Sedentary behavior

- The recreational screen time should be limited to no more than 2 h per day, and prolonged sitting should be broken up whenever possible.

(c) Sleep duration and daytime naps

- Children (6–12 years) should aim for 9–12 h of good sleep per day, while adolescents (13–17 years) should target 8–10 h, both with consistent bedtimes and wake-up times.
- School-aged children (≥ 6 years) and adolescents should prioritize receiving recommended sleep at night (conditional).

Additionally, these guidelines provide several key considerations to supplement the recommendations for sleep duration in children:

- Meeting recommended sleep durations with consistent sleep patterns is associated with improved health outcomes, including higher attention, behavior, learning, memory, emotional regulation, quality of life, and overall mental and physical health.
- Regularly sleeping less than the recommended duration is linked to attention, behavior, and learning difficulties, as well as an increased risk of accidents, injuries, hypertension, obesity, diabetes, and depression.
- Adolescents with insufficient sleep are at a greater risk of self-harm, suicidal thoughts, and suicide attempts.
- Consistently sleeping more than the recommended duration may be associated with negative health outcomes such as hypertension, diabetes, obesity, and mental health issues.
- Parents who are concerned about their child's sleep quality, duration, or pattern are advised to consult with their family physician or pediatrician.

2.4 School Setting and 24-Hour Movement Behaviors

2.4.1 Role of School Setting in the Promotion of 24-Hour Movement Behaviors

Several scientific papers have investigated the influence of the school environment on 24-hour movement behaviors [30–33]. For example, Janda et al. [30] reported that children and adolescents exhibited more favorable 24-hour activity profiles on school days than on weekends. Additionally, a longitudinal study by García-Hermoso et al. [32] reported that participation in daily physical education (PE) lessons during adolescence was associated with increased odds of meeting weekly sessions of MVPA and all three guidelines compared to those reporting no days of PE lessons per week. The likelihood of meeting all three 24-hour movement guidelines also increased with each additional weekly hour of PE lessons, both during adolescence and adulthood, for both men and women. Considering the existing evidence regarding the health effects associated with 24-hour movement behaviors [1–3], it is reasonable to assume that shifts in behavior during the transition from primary to secondary school could influence the health and well-being of children [34]. Nonetheless, a scoping review, which included 37 studies, revealed that current interventions in schools do not encompass all aspects of 24-hour movement behaviors in children. This gap is particularly evident in the lack of intervention studies addressing sleep behavior [31].

Early childhood education and care facilities, along with educational settings, could have significant potential to shape the 24-hour movement behaviors of preschoolers, children, and adolescents [31, 35]. These settings are recognized as crucial environments for tackling various public health issues [36]. Schools could serve as a significant setting for providing comprehensive PA education to broad audiences, as children spend more time in school than in any other place except their homes [37]. Therefore, it may be essential to incorporate PA, including education, living spaces, and recreational activities, into every aspect of children's lives [37]. Despite this substantial presence, numerous studies have revealed concerning trends, with many children experiencing insufficient PA [33, 38] and excessive sedentary behavior [39] during their time in these settings. For instance, a systematic review reported that the duration of MVPA during school hours ranges from 3% to 22% (in children) and from 3% to 8% (in adolescents) [33] in this daily segment. Similarly, another systematic review reported that, on average, young people spent 63% of their time in school sedentary [39]. Given the compulsory schooling of preschoolers, children and adolescents in most countries and the large amount of time they spend in early childhood education and care facilities and educational settings, there is a significant opportunity for 24-hour movement behavior-related interventions [40, 41].

2.4.2 Factors Related to 24-Hour Movement Behaviors in the School Environment

Several factors influence 24-hour movement behaviors in the school environment, including the following:

- School policies. School policies that promote PA, such as those that establish minimum daily PA time or restrict the consumption of sugary drinks and unhealthy snacks, can have a positive impact on students' 24-hour movement behaviors [42].
- School curriculum. The integration of PA into the school curriculum through PE classes, extracurricular activities, or curricular integration programs can help students achieve the recommended levels of PA [32, 43].
- The physical environment. The physical environment of the school, such as the availability of spaces for PA, the safety of the environment, and accessibility, could also influence the 24-hour movement behaviors of students [44].
- The school climate. A positive school climate, which fosters participation and inclusion, may motivate students to be more active [45].

2.4.2.1 Strategies to Promote 24-Hour Movement Behaviors in the School Environment

Several strategies can be implemented in the school environment to promote 24-hour movement behaviors, including the following:

- Increasing the quality of time dedicated to PA in school. This can be achieved by increasing the duration of PE classes, offering more extracurricular activities, or integrating PA into other areas of the curriculum. Physical education endeavors to enhance not only physical health but also encompass aspects beyond it. Therefore, it is essential to strike a balance between maximizing active learning time and providing opportunities for instruction, feedback, and reflection [43].
- Creating a physical environment that promotes PA. This can be achieved by building or improving sports facilities, providing outdoor PA spaces, and promoting the safety of the school environment. In this sense, the WHO recommends including appropriate and supportive environments for PAs and increasing opportunities for PAs in schools [46].
- A positive school climate should be fostered. This can be achieved by creating a culture of respect and inclusion, promoting student participation in decision-making, and celebrating student achievement. Furthermore, actively involving students in the planning and implementation of PA initiatives, such as organizing events or sports competitions, can contribute to a positive and dynamic school environment [47]. Additionally, incorporating regular PA breaks within the classroom routine and encouraging collaborative PA can enhance social interactions among students, fostering a sense of community and well-being [48].

- Students and families should be educated about the importance of PA. This can be achieved through awareness campaigns, workshops, and educational programs. The literature presented significant evidence supporting the crucial role of family in shaping children's PA patterns, which underscores the significance of incorporating the entire family system as a key factor influencing and fostering healthy 24-hour movement behaviors in children and youth [49].

2.4.3 Successful Implementation Strategies for School-Based Interventions on 24-Hour Movement Behaviors in Young People

The development of effective strategies to inspire children to comply with 24-hour movement guidelines is a central concern in public health [20]. Consequently, upcoming interventions in school settings should embrace a holistic approach across diverse environments, aiming for sustained effects throughout the day, as proposed by Love et al. [50]. However, to date, few studies have addressed programs from schools to promote these behaviors.

Regarding preschoolers, Puder et al. [51] conducted interventions across 40 preschool classes in areas with a large migrant population in the German- and French-speaking regions of Switzerland (including 652 participants). The multidimensional, culturally tailored lifestyle intervention included a PA program, lessons on nutrition, media use (television and computers), and sleep, along with adaptation of the built environment. Significant enhancements were observed in reported PA, media use, and dietary habits within the intervention group. Furthermore, Ullevig et al. [52] conducted a clustered randomized controlled trial to assess the effects of an 8-month intervention involving multiple components on modifying behaviors related to energy balance in preschoolers. This intervention involved 12 Head Start centers and 325 parents. Parents in the intervention group, which included center-based and home-based components, reported higher levels of PA facilitated by adults and increased daily sleep duration for their children during weekdays (excluding weekends) and across the entire week, among other positive impacts on health-related behaviors, than parents from the only center-based intervention or the control group. Additionally, parents participating in the center-based intervention observed an increase in their children's total weekly sleep duration compared to those in the control group.

For school-aged children, studies have shown controversial results. For example, Pablos et al. [53] evaluated the effectiveness of the Healthy Habits Program for 158 children in the 5th and 6th grades. Over 8 months, the program aimed to foster a healthy lifestyle through school-based PA (including information about screen time and sleep duration). However, measurements conducted before and after the program revealed no significant improvements in PA, sedentary behavior, or sleep. Tapia-Serrano et al. [54] conducted a program consisting of ten one-hour weekly sessions focusing on health-related behaviors. Their study showed similar results, indicating a significant increase in adherence to the Mediterranean diet and weekday PA within the experimental group. Moreover, baseline differences in diet adherence and weekend PA between groups disappeared postintervention. These findings suggest that the school-based intervention effectively improved diet adherence and PA levels in children, which is consistent with previous research. The study by Donnelly et al. [55] evaluated the Happy Homework program, an 8-week home-focused intervention aimed at enhancing positive dietary behaviors, PA, and sleep habits in 158 children in four Scottish schools. These schools were randomly assigned to either the Happy Homework intervention group or the control group. Postintervention, the Happy Homework group showed significant increases in stepping time and sleep duration, along with elevated fruit and vegetable consumption.

Sevil et al. [56] investigated the impact of interventions implemented within schools on various health habits among 210 adolescents. These included behaviors related to PA, sedentary habits, sleep patterns, dietary choices, and substance use, such as alcohol and tobacco. The results indicated that students in the experimental group showed notable improvements in adhering to specific and overall combinations of 24-hour movement recommendations, reducing sedentary screen time, extending nap duration, and improving their overall dietary habits, including breakfast and soft drink consumption, compared to both of their counterparts in the control group. In addition, Champion et al. [57] introduced the eHealth intervention Health4Life, which aimed to address six key lifestyle risk behaviors across Australian secondary schools (including 6640 participants). However, their cluster randomized controlled trial revealed no significant differences between the intervention and control groups for any of the targeted lifestyle risk behaviors at the 24-month mark.

Therefore, there is a clear need for more robust interventions in school settings that adopt a holistic approach to promoting healthy behaviors across diverse environments and throughout the entire day [58]. This underscores the importance of future research and intervention development aimed at addressing the 24-hour movement guidelines to improve the overall health and well-being of children and adolescents.

2.5 Conclusion

2.5.1 Emphasis on the Collective Impact of 24-Hour Movement Behaviors on Health

To promote healthy lifestyles and prevent noncommunicable diseases, policymakers, educators, and parents must act during the critical early childhood period, when children are most receptive to external influences and lifestyle habits can have long-lasting effects. Early childhood, childhood, and adolescence are critical developmental periods in which children and their families and caregivers are most susceptible to external influences that can shape health and well-being throughout life [59]. Lifestyle habits (including 24-hour movement behaviors) could also contribute to preventing noncommunicable diseases later in life [14].

2.5.2 Calling to Action Policymakers, Educators, and Parents

Given the low prevalence of adherence to guidelines found worldwide [9], a strong call to action seems to be crucial. Policymakers are vital in creating and promoting environments that encourage healthy behaviors. Educational institutions play an important role in instilling healthy habits beginning at an early age and serve as a foundation for lifelong wellness [60]. The role of parents, who are the primary influencers, is essential in shaping favorable home environments that prioritize balanced 24-hour movement behaviors during the day [49]. The current time calls for action, and through collaborative efforts, the influence of an appropriate combination of 24-hour movement behaviors can be recognized and given prominence to prevent negative health outcomes.

References

1. de Lannoy L, Barbeau K, Vanderloo LM, Goldfield G, Lang JJ, MacLeod O, et al. Evidence supporting a combined movement behavior approach for children and youth's mental health – a scoping review and environmental scan. Ment Health Phys Act. 2023;24:100511.
2. López-Gil JF, Tapia-Serrano MA, Sevil-Serrano J, Sánchez-Miguel PA, García-Hermoso A. Are 24-hour movement recommendations associated with obesity-related indicators in the young population? A meta-analysis. Obesity. 2023;31(11):2727–39.
3. Rollo S, Antsygina O, Tremblay MS. The whole day matters: understanding 24-hour movement guideline adherence and relationships with health indicators across the lifespan. J Sport Health Sci. 2020:S2095254620300910.
4. Pedišić Z. Measurement issues and poor adjustments for physical activity and sleep undermine sedentary behaviour research—the focus should shift to the balance between sleep, sedentary behaviour, standing and activity. Kinesiology. 2014;46(1):135–46.
5. Tremblay MS, Chaput JP, Adamo KB, Aubert S, Barnes JD, Choquette L, et al. Canadian 24-hour movement guidelines for the early years (0–4 years): an integration of physical activity, sedentary behaviour, and sleep. BMC Public Health. 2017;17(S5):874.
6. World Health Organization. Guidelines on physical activity, sedentary behaviour and sleep for children under 5 years of age [Internet]. Geneva: World Health Organization; 2019 [cited 2022 Nov 1]. 33 p. Available from: https://apps.who.int/iris/handle/10665/311664.
7. Tremblay MS, Carson V, Chaput JP, Connor Gorber S, Dinh T, Duggan M, et al. Canadian 24-hour movement guidelines for children and youth: an integration of physical activity, sedentary behaviour, and sleep. Appl Physiol Nutr Metab. 2016;41(6 (Suppl. 3)):S311–27.
8. Carson V, Chaput JP, Janssen I, Tremblay MS. Health associations with meeting new 24-hour movement guidelines for Canadian children and youth. Prev Med. 2017;95:7–13.

9. Tapia-Serrano MA, Sevil-Serrano J, Sánchez-Miguel PA, López-Gil JF, Tremblay MS, García-Hermoso A. Prevalence of meeting 24-hour movement guidelines from pre-school to adolescence: a systematic review and meta-analysis including 387,437 participants and 23 countries. J Sport Health Sci. 2022;11(4):427–37.
10. Hegarty LM, Mair JL, Kirby K, Murtagh E, Murphy MH. School-based interventions to reduce sedentary behaviour in children: a systematic review. AIMS Public Health. 2016;3(3):520–41.
11. Åvitsland A, Ohna SE, Dyrstad SM, Tjomsland HE, Lerum Ø, Leibinger E. The process evaluation of a school-based physical activity intervention: influencing factors and potential consequences of implementation. HE. 2020;120(2):121–39.
12. Gugglberger L. A brief overview of a wide framework—health promoting schools: a curated collection. Health Promot Int. 2021;36(2):297–302.
13. World Health Organization. Report of the commission on ending childhood obesity [Internet]. Geneva: World Health Organization; 2016 [cited 2022 Jun 10]. 50 p. Available from: https://apps.who.int/iris/handle/10665/204176.
14. World Health Organization. Standards for healthy eating, physical activity, sedentary behaviour and sleep in early childhood education and care settings: a toolkit [Internet]. Geneva; 2021. Available from: https://iris.who.int/bitstream/handle/10665/345926/9789240032255-eng.pdf?sequence=1.
15. Pedišić Ž, Dumuid D, Olds TS. Integrating sleep, sedentary behaviour, and physical activity research in the emerging field of time-use epidemiology: definitions, concepts, statistical methods, theoretical framework, and future directions. Kinesiology. 2017;49(2):252–69.
16. Janssen X, Martin A, Hughes AR, Hill CM, Kotronoulas G, Hesketh KR. Associations of screen time, sedentary time and physical activity with sleep in under 5s: a systematic review and meta-analysis. Sleep Med Rev. 2020;49:101226.
17. Axelsson J, Ingre M, Kecklund G, Lekander M, Wright KP, Sundelin T. Sleepiness as motivation: a potential mechanism for how sleep deprivation affects behavior. Sleep. 2020;43(6):zsz291.
18. López-Gil JF, Tremblay MS, Tapia-Serrano MÁ, Tárraga-López PJ, Brazo-Sayavera J. Meeting 24 h movement guidelines and health-related quality of life in youths during the COVID-19 lockdown. Appl Sci. 2022;12(16):8056.
19. Chaput JP, Carson V, Gray C, Tremblay M. Importance of all movement behaviors in a 24 hour period for overall health. IJERPH. 2014;11(12):12575–81.
20. Okely AD, Ghersi D, Loughran SP, Cliff DP, Shilton T, Jones RA, et al. A collaborative approach to adopting/adapting guidelines. The Australian 24-hour movement guidelines for children (5-12 years) and young people (13-17 years): an integration of physical activity, sedentary behaviour, and sleep. Int J Behav Nutr Phys Act. 2022;19(1):2.
21. New Zealand Ministry of Health. Sit less, move more, sleep well: active play guidelines for under-fives Wellington. [Internet]. New Zealand: Ministry of Health; 2017. Available from: https://www.health.govt.nz/publication/sit-less-move-more-sleep-well-active-play-guidelines-under-fives#:~:text=Sit%20Less%2C%20Move%20More%2C%20Sleep%20Well%3A%20Active%20play%20guidelines%20for%20under%2Dfives%20(pdf%2C%20832%20KB).
22. Laureus Sport for Good Foundation. South African 24-hour movement guidelines for birth to five years: an integration of physical activity, sitting behaviour, screen time and Sleep Cape Town [Internet]. South Africa: Sports Science Institute of South Africa; 2018. Available from: https://www.laureus.co.za/wp-content/uploads/2018/11/EYMG-2-pager-ONLINE.pdf.
23. Chief Medical Officers UK. UK chief medical Officers' physical activity guidelines [Internet]. London, England: Department of Health and Social Care Llywodraeth Cymru Welsh Government, Department of Health Northern Ireland and the Scottish government, department of Health and social care; 2019. Available from: https://assets.publishing.service.gov.uk/government/uploads/system/uploads/attachment_data/file/832868/uk-chief-medical-officers-physical-activity-guidelines.pdf.

24. Public Health Authority. Twenty-four-hour movement practice guidelines for Saudi Arabia. An integration of physical activity, sedentary behavior, and sleep duration [Internet]. Saudi Arabia: Public Health Authority; 2017. Available from: https://faculty.ksu.edu.sa/sites/default/files/24hr_s_movement_practice_guidelines_for_saudi_arabia_1619026105.pdf.
25. Okely AD, Ghersi D, Hesketh KD, Santos R, Loughran SP, Cliff DP, et al. A collaborative approach to adopting/adapting guidelines - the Australian 24-Hour Movement Guidelines for the early years (birth to 5 years): an integration of physical activity, sedentary behavior, and sleep. BMC Public Health. 2017;17(S5):869.
26. Chaput JP, Willumsen J, Bull F, Chou R, Ekelund U, Firth J, et al. 2020 WHO guidelines on physical activity and sedentary behaviour for children and adolescents aged 5–17 years: summary of the evidence. Int J Behav Nutr Phys Act. 2020;17(1):141.
27. New Zealand Ministry of Health. Review of physical activity guidance and resources for under-fives: final report for the Ministry of Health [Internet]. New Zealand: Ministry of Health; 2015. Available from: https://www.health.govt.nz/system/files/documents/publications/review-physical-activity-guidance-resources-for-under-fives-apr16.pdf.
28. Draper CE, Tomaz SA, Biersteker L, Cook CJ, Couper J, De Milander M, et al. The South African 24-hour movement guidelines for birth to 5 years: an integration of physical activity, sitting behavior, screen time, and sleep. J Phys Act Health. 2020;17(1):109–19.
29. Alfawaz R, Aljuraiban G, AlMarzooqi M, Alghannam A, BaHammam A, Dobia A, et al. The recommended amount of physical activity, sedentary behavior, and sleep duration for healthy Saudis: a joint consensus statement of the Saudi Public Health Authority. Ann Thorac Med. 2021;16(3):239.
30. Janda D, Gába A, Vencálek O, Fairclough SJ, Dygrýn J, Jakubec L, et al. A 24-h activity profile and adiposity among children and adolescents: does the difference between school and weekend days matter? Muntaner Mas A, editor. PLoS One. 2023;18(5):e0285952.
31. Rodrigo-Sanjoaquín J, Bois JE, Aibar Solana A, Lhuisset L, Corral-Abós A, Zaragoza CJ. Are school-based interventions promoting 24-hour movement guidelines among children? A scoping review. Health Educ J. 2023;82(4):444–60.
32. García-Hermoso A, Ezzatvar Y, López-Gil JF. Association between daily physical education attendance and meeting 24-hour movement guidelines in adolescence and adulthood. J Adolesc Health. 2023:S1054139X23003245.
33. Grao-Cruces A, Velázquez-Romero MJ, Rodríguez-Rodríguez F. Levels of physical activity during school hours in children and adolescents: a systematic review. IJERPH. 2020;17(13):4773.
34. Chong KH, Dumuid D, Cliff DP, Parrish AM, Okely AD. Changes in 24-hour domain-specific movement behaviors and their associations with children's psychosocial health during the transition from primary to secondary school: a compositional data analysis. J Phys Act Health. 2022;19(5):358–66.
35. Hesketh KR, Lakshman R, Van Sluijs EMF. Barriers and facilitators to young children's physical activity and sedentary behaviour: a systematic review and synthesis of qualitative literature. Obes Rev. 2017;18(9):987–1017.
36. Inman DD, Van Bakergem KM, LaRosa AC, Garr DR. Evidence-based health promotion programs for schools and communities. Am J Prev Med. 2011;40(2):207–19.
37. World Health Organization. Promoting physical activity through schools: a toolkit. Geneva: World Health Organization; 2021.
38. Bourke M, Haddara A, Loh A, Carson V, Breau B, Tucker P. Adherence to the World Health Organization's physical activity recommendation in preschool-aged children: a systematic review and meta-analysis of accelerometer studies. Int J Behav Nutr Phys Act. 2023;20(1):52.
39. Egan CA, Webster CA, Beets MW, Weaver RG, Russ L, Michael D, et al. Sedentary time and behavior during school: a systematic review and meta-analysis. Am J Health Educ. 2019;50(5):283–90.
40. Wolfenden L, Barnes C, Jones J, Finch M, Wyse RJ, Kingsland M, et al. Strategies to improve the implementation of healthy eating, physical activity and obesity prevention policies,

practices or programmes within childcare services. Cochrane Public Health Group, editor. Cochrane Database Syst Rev [Internet]. 2020[cited 2024 Feb 10];2020(2). Available from: http://doi.wiley.com/10.1002/14651858.CD011779.pub3.
41. Story M, Kaphingst KM, French S. The role of child care settings in obesity prevention. Future Child. 2006;16(1):143–68.
42. Fournier E, Łuszczki E, Isacco L, Chanséaume-Bussiere E, Gryson C, Chambrier C, et al. Toward an integrated consideration of 24 h movement guidelines and nutritional recommendations. Nutrients. 2023;15(9):2109.
43. García-Hermoso A, Alonso-Martínez AM, Ramírez-Vélez R, Pérez-Sousa MÁ, Ramírez-Campillo R, Izquierdo M. Association of Physical Education with improvement of health-related physical fitness outcomes and fundamental motor skills among youths: a systematic review and meta-analysis. JAMA Pediatr. 2020;174(6):e200223.
44. Smith L, Foley L, Panter J. Activity spaces in studies of the environment and physical activity: a review and synthesis of implications for causality. Health Place. 2019;58:102113.
45. Rajbhandari-Thapa J, Metzger I, Ingels J, Thapa K, Chiang K. School climate-related determinants of physical activity among high school girls and boys. J Adolesc. 2022;94(4):642–55.
46. Bull FC, Al-Ansari SS, Biddle S, Borodulin K, Buman MP, Cardon G, et al. World Health Organization 2020 guidelines on physical activity and sedentary behaviour. Br J Sports Med. 2020;54(24):1451–62.
47. Berti S, Grazia V, Molinari L. Active student participation in whole-school interventions in secondary school. A systematic literature review. Educ Psychol Rev. 2023;35(2):52.
48. Peiris DLIHK, Duan Y, Vandelanotte C, Liang W, Yang M, Baker JS. Effects of in-classroom physical activity breaks on children's academic performance, cognition, health behaviours and health outcomes: a systematic review and meta-analysis of randomised controlled trials. IJERPH. 2022;19(15):9479.
49. Rhodes RE, Guerrero MD, Vanderloo LM, Barbeau K, Birken CS, Chaput JP, et al. Development of a consensus statement on the role of the family in the physical activity, sedentary, and sleep behaviours of children and youth. Int J Behav Nutr Phys Act. 2020;17(1):74.
50. Love R, Adams J, van Sluijs EMF. Are school-based physical activity interventions effective and equitable? A systematic review and meta-analysis of cluster randomised controlled trials. Lancet. 2018;392:S53.
51. Puder JJ, Marques-Vidal P, Schindler C, Zahner L, Niederer I, Bürgi F, et al. Effect of multidimensional lifestyle intervention on fitness and adiposity in predominantly migrant preschool children (Ballabeina): cluster randomised controlled trial. BMJ. 2011;343:d6195.
52. Ullevig SL, Parra-Medina D, Liang Y, Howard J, Sosa E, Estrada-Coats VM, et al. Impact of ¡Míranos! on parent-reported home-based healthy energy balance-related behaviors in low-income Latino preschool children: a clustered randomized controlled trial. Int J Behav Nutr Phys Act. 2023;20(1):33.
53. Pablos A, Nebot V, Vañó-Vicent V, Ceca D, Elvira L. Effectiveness of a school-based program focusing on diet and health habits taught through physical exercise. Appl Physiol Nutr Metab. 2018;43(4):331–7.
54. Tapia-Serrano MA, Sevil-Serrano J, Sánchez-Oliva D, Vaquero-Solís M, Sánchez-Miguel PA. Effects of a school-based intervention on physical activity, sleep duration, screen time, and diet in children. Revista de Psicodidáctica (English ed). 2022;27(1):56–65.
55. Donnelly S, Buchan DS, McLellan G, Roberts R, Arthur R. Exploring the feasibility of a cluster pilot randomised control trial to improve children's 24-hour movement behaviours and dietary intake: happy homework. J Sports Sci. 2023;41(19):1787–800.
56. Sevil J, García-González L, Abós Á, Generelo E, Aibar A. Can high schools be an effective setting to promote healthy lifestyles? Effects of a multiple behavior change intervention in adolescents. J Adolesc Health. 2019;64(4):478–86.
57. Champion KE, Newton NC, Gardner LA, Chapman C, Thornton L, Slade T, et al. Health4Life eHealth intervention to modify multiple lifestyle risk behaviours among adolescent students in Australia: a cluster-randomised controlled trial. Lancet Digit Health. 2023;5(5):e276–87.

58. López-Gil JF, García-Hermoso A, Smith L, Gallego A, Victoria-Montesinos D, Ezzatvar Y, et al. A cluster randomized controlled trial of the Archena Infancia Saludable project on 24-h movement behaviors and adherence to the Mediterranean Diet among schoolchildren: a pilot study protocol. Children. 2023;10(4):738.
59. Black MM, Walker SP, Fernald LCH, Andersen CT, DiGirolamo AM, Lu C, et al. Early childhood development coming of age: science through the life course. Lancet. 2017;389(10064):77–90.
60. Wenden EJ, Virgara R, Pearce N, Budgeon C, Christian HE. Movement behavior policies in the early childhood education and care setting: an international scoping review. Front Public Health. 2023;11:1077977.

Part II
Assessment and Evaluation of Physical Health and Skills in School Settings

Chapter 3
Physical Literacy Assessment: A Conceptualization and Tools

Andreas Fröberg and Suzanne Lundvall

3.1 Introduction

During the recent decade, the concept of physical literacy has gained increasing prominence worldwide. Physical literacy is nowadays included not only in research and practice but also in public health policies, and the popularity of the concept is anticipated to increase in the future. Despite this, however, there are several ongoing conceptual discussions that are permeated by competing approaches and country-specific traditions.

In essence, physical literacy initially emerged as a response to the limitations and inadequacies of traditional approaches to physical activity (PA), sports practices, and learning processes in physical education (PE). Physical literacy represents a fundamental shift in our understanding of human movement and its relationship with holistic development. More specifically, physical literacy challenges traditional views that emphasize physical fitness for sport, and health and well-being. Instead, a conceptualization of physical literacy recognizes a broader significance of our embodied dimension in everyday life and introduces a novel perspective on human movement. Physical literacy as a concept acknowledges previously overlooked aspects of our physical capabilities and their importance in human existence [1–3].

Alongside more established concepts, such as PE, and health and PE, physical literacy (as well as health literacy) have emerged, creating a somewhat confusing situation among researchers and practitioners [4]. In many ways, the concept of physical literacy and the idea of being physically literate bear similarities to, and may represent an alternative to, the idea of being physical educated. In this context,

A. Fröberg · S. Lundvall (✉)
Department of Food and Nutrition, and Sport Science, University of Gothenburg, Gothenburg, Sweden
e-mail: suzanne.lundvall@gu.se

some researchers have argued that the only difference—if any—between the two concepts is that physical literacy encourages more attention to cognitive outcomes rather than movement and psychomotor outcomes [5]. Despite the similarities, the potential of physical literacy, however, may include re-definitions of how individuals engage with PA as a lifelong journey, transcending the acquisition of motor skills to encompass a broader and more profound sense of motivation, confidence and physical competence, and knowledge and understanding.

In this context, the purpose of this chapter is to explore what is currently known regarding physical literacy assessment tools, the validity of the tools, and the association between physical literacy and PA participation and health and well-being among school-aged children and adolescents. The chapter begins with an introduction to the concept of physical literacy, its origins, attributes, as well as the challenges that surround its conceptualization and implementation. Thereafter, we provide an overview and a (critical) discussion based on two reviews of assessment tools developed for children and adolescents that make explicit references to physical literacy.

3.2 The Concept of Physical Literacy

The earliest published references to the term "physical literacy" appeared in the American literature during the 1880s [6]. Ever since, multiple perspectives on the concept of physical literacy have existed. In an analysis of more than 150 peer-reviewed papers published throughout approximately 100 years, three different, albeit overlapping, physical literacy ideologies were identified [7]. The first two ideologies emerged in the 1920s and 1950s and were physical literacy as health-promoting PA, and physical literacy as motor competence, respectively. The third ideology—physical literacy as phenomenological embodiment—emerged during 1990s when Margaret Whitehead re-introduced physical literacy in the field of PE.

The concept of physical literacy as discussed nowadays is often credited to the seminal work of Margaret Whitehead. In the early 1990s, Whitehead articulated a vision of PE that extended beyond the confines of various sports and structured games [8], and one of the first papers to outline a provisional context for a definition of PL was published in 2001 [9]. In the first book to explore the meaning of concept of physical literacy in depth, Whitehead [2] rationalized the philosophical underpinning as an interweaving of monism, existentialism, and phenomenology that together create a holistic understanding of physical literacy and its significance in human life. From the perspective of monism, physical literacy recognizes the lived embodiment as essential to aspects of human existence, and that body and mind are interdependent and indivisible. The monism perspective of physical literacy is further supported by existentialism which contends that all individuals is a creation of their interactions and life experiences. In this sense, existentialism emphasizes the unique nature of the human experience where individuals not only define their own meaning and purpose in their physical activities but also take the ability and ownership of their bodies to, in a productive way, interact and communicate with/in/through the world and make choices that align with their values. Here, phenomenology, a philosophical perspective that focuses on the study of human consciousness and subjective experience, may support us to understand how individuals perceive and experience their own bodies and physical activities. Phenomenology suggests that our personal experiences shape us, and that our perception, through our embodied nature, gives rise to distinct perspectives and worldviews.

In line with above, Whitehead's [1, 2] pioneering contributions conceptualized physical literacy as a developmental process—a journey—encompassing a multifaceted range of attributes, including not only competence in the physical dimensions but also in the affective and cognitive dimensions. Whitehead also refers to physical literacy as a capability to recognize the potential that is inherently present among all human beings. This conceptualization marked a paradigmatic shift from the traditional approach to PE, which often (and perhaps still do) placed excessive emphasis on sport-related techniques and skill, performance, and competition. According to Whitehead [1], the traditional approach to PE deserted those who did not possess exceptional skills or talents, and left children and adolescents unprepared to engage in lifelong physical activities beyond the logics of sports and structured games.

Until today, the possible implications of physical literacy have not only been discussed explicitly in the relation to PE [10] but also to the wider fields of PA, sports, and, lately, also public health [11]. The growing number of peer-reviewed papers in recent years suggest an increased interest in the concept of physical literacy among researchers [12, 13]. The growing interest is also notable in the context of policy. For example, in the 2013 revision of United States national PE content standard, physical literate replaced physical educated, apparently without any consultative processes with stakeholders or critique or criticism of the original label [5].

Despite its considerable potential, the concept of physical literacy is not without its share of challenges, and several issues have been, and are still, debated in the field of physical literacy. One critical issue that has gained considerable attention among researchers and practitioners is that of what physical literacy is, or should be, its educative role and how to define the concept [14].

In conceptualizing physical literacy, Whitehead used the term "physical" to describe the physical or embodied dimension of individuals. The term "literacy," typically used to describe communication, was chosen to depict human characteristics of doing, responding, and understanding, while taking into consideration the interaction with the environment [15]. In non-English speaking countries, there are linguistic issues where adequate translation for physical literacy is a challenge [16]. The challenge extends beyond adequately translating and making sense of the term "literacy" as it becomes even more problematic when combined with "physical" [17].

The precise definition of physical literacy is not static but remains a subject of ongoing discussion. Researchers and practitioners seem to refine their understanding of physical literacy, leading to both development and introduction of alternative definitions and revisions of already existing ones. Consistent with this, the peer-reviewed literature shows that several definitions coexist both in research and across leading international organizations and stakeholders within the physical literacy community [18–22]. For example, in the process of formulating the physical literacy consensus statement for England, 23 different definitions of physical literacy were found in the academic and grey literature sources. These definitions varied in terms of breadth and complexity [23]. Nonetheless, many used definitions have what has typically been referred to as a "Whiteheadian" perspective, thus resembling the definition originally proposed by Whitehead. In the first book to explore the meaning of the concept, Whitehead [1] defined physical literacy as:

> As appropriate to each individual's endowment, physical literacy can be described as the motivation, confidence, physical competence, knowledge and understanding to maintain PA throughout the life course.

Later, Whitehead refined the definition and highlighted the long-term engagement in PA. In the book *Physical literacy across the world* [3], she defined physical literacy (p. 8):

> As appropriate to each individual, physical literacy can be described as the motivation, confidence, physical competence, knowledge and understanding to value and take responsibility *for engaging in PA for life.*

Since 2017, a similar definition has been used by the International Physical Literacy Association (IPLA) [24], as endorsed by the committee president Whitehead:

> The motivation, confidence, physical competence, knowledge and understanding to value and take responsibility for engagement in physical activities for life.

The coexistence of multiple definitions of physical literacy may be attributed to several factors. The interdisciplinary nature of physical literacy, considering not only physical but also affective and cognitive dimensions related to PA, draws from various disciplines and interdisciplinary collaboration. Researchers and practitioners, as well as other stakeholders, may approach physical literacy from different perspectives, and emphasize the importance of individual domains differently [25]. Each field, whether it is, for example, PE or public health, also bring its unique perspectives and priorities to the concept, leading to divergent context-specific definitions that may be tailored to align with the specific needs and objectives. Therefore, one or two physical literacy dimensions may be prioritized over others, or even emphasized differently, leaving a variety of definitions that coexist but reflect the specific perspectives and intents of the stakeholders.

It should be noted that there are some attempts in establishing a universal definition of the concept of physical literacy, reflecting consensus statement from stakeholders in countries, such as England, Australia, and Canada; however, some differences remain [23, 26, 27]. While the existence of multiple definitions allows for a richer and more adaptable concept that can be tailored to meet the needs of various stakeholders across various contexts, it remains a challenge in achieving consensus and building solid theoretical foundations.

3.2.1 The Physical Literacy Attributes

As suggested by Whitehead [2], physical literacy comprises six interconnected attributes. Following the philosophical underpinning, physical literacy should be understood as a holistic concept where these attributes are interconnected and inseparable [1]. The key attributes are (a) Motivation, (b) Confidence and physical competence, and (c) Effective interaction with a wide range of environments. These key attributes are mutually reinforcing and relate to each other in a sense that motivation may encourage participation in PA, which can promote confidence and physical competence. In turn, development of confidence and physical competence may sustain or increase motivation. In addition, development of confidence and physical competence may facilitate effective interaction with a wide range of environments that, in turn, promote motivation that may further encourage exploration and effective interaction with diverse environments.

Furthermore, as the interconnected key attributes are nurtured, the following additional attributes are assumed to develop: (d) Sense of self and self-confidence, (e) Self-expression and communication with others, and (f) Knowledge and understanding. For example, those individuals who engage in rewarding physical activities may develop a positive sense of self and enhanced self-confidence. A deep awareness of the embodied dimension may also facilitate fluent self-expression and empathetic communication (or interaction) with others, whereas participation in physical activities across a wide range of environments may enrich knowledge and understanding [1]. The relation between all attributes of physical literacy is shown in Fig. 3.1.

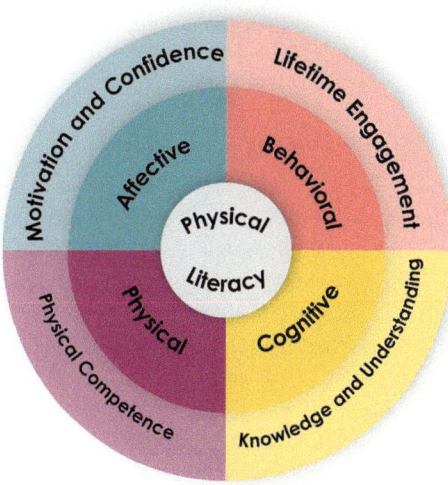

Fig. 3.1 The relation between all six attributes of physical literacy

Based on these attributes, [1] also describes the characteristics of physically literate individuals. These individuals are described to "move with poise, economy and confidence in a wide variety of physically challenging situations," and they are "perceptive in 'reading' all aspects of the physical environment, anticipating movement needs or possibilities and responding appropriately to these with intelligence and imagination." They also have "a well-established sense of self as embodied in the world," and they will "engender positive self-esteem and self-confidence" and have the "ability to identify and articulate the essential qualities that influence the effectiveness of their own movement performance and will have an understanding of the principles of embodied health with respect to basic aspects such as exercise, sleep and nutrition."

Drawing from Whitehead's description, some recent conceptualization of physical literacy comprises four interrelated key elements (rather than attributes) that consider the physical, affective, cognitive, and behavioral dimensions. In Canada's Physical Literacy Consensus Statement [28], describe physical competence (physical domain) as "an individual's ability to develop movement skills and patterns, and the capacity to experience a variety of movement intensities and durations. Enhanced physical competence enables an individual to participate in a wide range of physical activities and settings." Motivation and confidence, that represent the affective domain, was described as "an individual's enthusiasm for, enjoyment of, and self-assurance in adopting PA as an integral part of life." Furthermore, knowledge and understanding (cognitive domain) "includes the ability to identify and express the essential qualities that influence movement, understand the health benefits of an active lifestyle, and appreciate appropriate safety features associated with PA in a variety of settings and physical environments." Finally, engagement in physical activities for life (behavioral domain) was described as "an individual taking personal responsibility for physical literacy by freely choosing to be active on a regular basis. This involves prioritizing and sustaining involvement in a range of meaningful and personally challenging activities, as an integral part of one's lifestyle."

3.2.2 Physical Literacy During Childhood

Each of the physical literacy attributes, including motivation, confidence, and physical competence, knowledge and understanding, can be nurtured during all stages of life. During childhood, these attributes or key elements provide the foundation for enhancing the development of physical literacy. During childhood, physical development is an ongoing process that involves growth and development of not only the physical body (e.g., skeleton, muscles, and nervous systems) but also other aspects critical for development of physical literacy. In the context of physical literacy, these have been described as movement vocabulary (i.e., the spectrum of movements, e.g., balancing and locomotion, such as crawling, climbing, skipping, running, etc.), movement memory (i.e., the internalizing of movement experience), and movement quality (i.e., movement with poise and sound coordination and accuracy) [29].

As a natural and integrated aspect of childhood development, play serves several important functions for the growing child, including development of physical, cognitive, and social skills, as well as creativity and imagination. Play is therefore deemed critical for the development of movement vocabulary, movement memory, and movement quality [29]. A mixture of free play, where children engage at will and follow their own initiative, and guided and formal play, as encouraged, challenged, and supported by knowledgeable adults, conducted across a wide range of environments and with different resources (natural or manufactured), is expected to enrich and nurture physical literacy attributes [29].

Moreover, significant others play an important role in developing and maintaining physical literacy throughout the course of life. During childhood, these significant others include adults, especially parents/legal guardians, and teachers due to their consistent engagement and interaction with children [30]. Fostering a sense of enjoyment within the context of PA is vital for the development of physical literacy. In this sense, it is imperative that significant others engage with children on an individual basis and prioritize the involvement of them in planning and guidance. In addition, significant others should make every effort to foster a positive attitude toward PA and use movement skills in a context rather in isolation and mitigate any sense of inadequacy among children. While ample opportunities for engagement in a wide range of physical activities across a wide range of environments are essential, the importance of a motivating and supportive approach toward participants cannot be exaggerated. Although the nature of these opportunities may change as individuals progress from childhood to early adulthood and, further, into adulthood, the necessity for empathetic encouragement remains a crucial factor at every stage of life [30].

Among those who engage and interact with children, teachers and coaches play a crucial role in the development of physical literacy among children. As a collective, teachers and the whole school can provide structured instruction and guidance (e.g., constructive feedback), supporting the development of physical competence in a safe and effective manner. Many teachers, especially PE teachers, possess the knowledge on how to unpack complex movements, making it easier for children to learn and refine their physical skills. Teachers can also work toward ensuring inclusivity and may serve as positive role models that inspire and motivate participation in physical activities, ultimately making children more engaged and enthusiastic about being physically active [30]. The question remains how school environment and leisure time activities can or cannot develop and implement a culture of physical literacy where it may also be possible to evaluate the contribution of physical literacy. In the following section, we explore what is currently known regarding physical literacy assessment tools, and the validity of these tools. In doing so, we first provide an overall introduction to physical literacy assessment.

3.3 Physical Literacy Assessment

Due to the potential of the concept, there has been an increased interest in assessing (i.e., monitoring, evaluating, and/or observing) physical literacy, especially among children and adolescents. To assess physical literacy among children and adolescents may be critical because it provides essential information and insights for understanding their physical competence and readiness to engage in PAs. Furthermore, physical literacy assessment is crucial for monitoring the progress and development of physical literacy attributes during childhood. Such information provides guidance when designing, adapting, and implementing educational strategies to develop and maintain physical literacy over time.

The assessment of physical literacy has been debated, especially in the context of PE [27, 31, 32]. Some have raised certain concerns about the lack of critique against physical literacy assessment, as well as the feasibility and trustworthiness of available assessment tool [32]. Nonetheless, researchers and practitioners have put effort toward developing valid, reliable, and feasible physical literacy assessment tools among different populations. To be aware of is that physical literacy can be understood from either an idealist or pragmatic philosophical perspective. These contrasting philosophical perspectives have different points of departure in terms of what and how to assess physical literacy [7, 33].

From an idealist philosophical perspective, physical literacy is perceived as a valuable end in itself. The holistic nature of the concept of physical literacy is emphasized, with its interconnected attributes that encompass not only physical but also affective and cognitive dimensions. According to idealists, single attributes, or dimensions of physical literacy, such as physical competence, should not be assessed in isolation. Therefore, in-depth interviews, reflections, and observations may be deemed appropriate qualitative research methods for physical literacy assessment. Pragmatists, however, may perceive physical literacy as means to other ends, such as making healthier individuals through increased PA, and therefore stress that research should be evaluated based on its practical implication. As such, any assessments tool should align with evidence-based practice [33]. From a pragmatic philosophical perspective, physical literacy may be assessed with both qualitative and quantitative research methods. In this context, some researchers also argue that physical literacy assessment may include measure of performance within each domain since it is challenging to assess the philosophical nature of physical literacy, in this case, a dynamic, ongoing process, similar to an individualized holistic journey [34].

3.3.1 Deconstruction of Physical Literacy into Components

Today, available assessment tools are designed to encompass varying numbers of dimensions of physical literacy, ranging from one single dimension to all three dimensions. Whether assessment tools encompass one or multiple dimensions depends, for example, on the operationalized definition of physical literacy and thus depicting the underlying philosophical underpinnings, as well as the context in which the procedure is undertaken.

When assessing physical literacy, researchers often deconstruct or analyze attributes and domain of physical literacy into various components (i.e., the specific variable under assessment). This process of operationalizing the domains of physical literacy into components allows for a detailed and comprehensive examination of specific skills, behaviors, knowledge and understandings, and attitudes related to and relevant for physical literacy [19, 20, 33]. In the peer-reviewed literature, the physical domain of physical literacy has been operationalized as fundamental motor competence, fundamental and complex movement skills, coordination, PA, physical fitness, such as aerobic endurance, muscular endurance and strength, and flexibility. These components have typically been assessed with objective criterion-based tests, comprehensive test batteries, and objective devices, such as pedometers and accelerometers [20]. Assessment tools for the affective domain encompass, for example, motivation and confidence, sense of self and self-confidence, and perceived physical competence. These components have typically been assessed through self-report questionnaires. Self-report questionnaires have also frequently been used to assess components for the cognitive domain of physical literacy, such as knowledge and understanding [20].

At present, several reviews of the peer-reviewed literature (e.g., systematic reviews and scoping reviews), published from 2021 and onwards have synthesized physical literacy assessment tools. These reviews have identified between 22 and 88 papers that described six to 52 assessment tools [20, 21, 35–37]. The contrasting findings in terms of numbers of identified papers and described assessment tools may be explained by the fact that some reviews have included tools that assess individual attributes and dimensions of physical literacy. Two examples of such tools are EUROFIT and FITNESSGRAM that are used to assess physical fitness in terms of aerobic and muscular endurance, thus only focusing on the physical domain of physical literacy [36]. Even though these tools serve a significant purpose when assessing physical fitness, they were not developed in the context of physical literacy, neither do they make explicit references to physical literacy. Below we provide an overview of commonly used assessment tools that make explicit references to physical literacy among school-aged children and adolescents in Table 3.1.

The overviewed assessment tools differ in terms of specific age-group targeted, definition of physical literacy, and assessed categories and domains. Most assessment tools were, however, developed using the definition proposed by IPLA, and the tools include assessment of categories and domains that typically is discussed in the field of physical literacy. Most of the tools are completed by the participants through self-report measurements. Although the number of items varies considerably, self-report measurements are the most feasible to administer in, as they can be used to collect data in large sample of children and adolescents.

Furthermore, the three comprehensive assessment tools Canadian Assessment of Physical Literacy (version 2) (CAPL-2), Passport for Life (PFL), and Physical Literacy Assessment for Youth (PLAY) include, among others, measurements of

Table 3.1 Assessment tools (in alphabetical order) that make explicit references to physical literacy among school-aged children and adolescents

Tool (abbreviation), country, and age-group	Definition or explanation of physical literacy	Assessed categories and/or domainsa	Description of measures	Description of data and/or scale	Equipment and/or requirements
Adolescent Physical Literacy Questionnaire (APLQ) [38] Iran 12–18 years	The motivation, confidence, physical competence, knowledge and understanding to value and take responsibility for engagement in physical activities for life	Psychological and behavioral, knowledge and awareness, and physical competence and activity	In total, 25 items, self-report, completed by the participant. Psychological and behavioral: $n = 11$ items Knowledge and awareness: $n = 7$ items Physical competence and activity: $n = 7$ items	5-point scale (from "strongly agree" to "strongly disagree")	Paper and pencil
Canadian Assessment of Physical Literacy, version 2 (CAPL-2) [39–42] Canada 8–12 years	The motivation, confidence, physical competence, knowledge and understanding to value and take responsibility for engagement in physical activities for life	Physical competence, motivation and confidence, knowledge and understanding, and daily behavior	Physical competence: movement skill, objective, completed by qualified assessors; $n = 1$ skill; fitness skills, objective, completed by qualified assessors: $n = 2$ skills Motivation and confidence: self-report, completed by the participant: $n = 12$ items Knowledge and understanding: self-report, completed by the participant: $n = 5$ items Daily behavior: self-report, completed by the participant: $n = 1$ item; steps-per-day, objective, completed through pedometer	Physical competence: movement skills: 2-point scale (from "performed" to "not correctly performed") and 14-point scale (from "<14 s" to ">30 s"); fitness skills: 10-point scale ($n = 2$ versions) (1: from "<5 laps" to ">49 laps"; 2: from "<20 s" to ">110 s") Motivation and confidence: two-stage dichotomous choice process (stage 1: participant selects a sentence that is more like them; stage 2: participant selects a box if it is "really true" or "sort of true"), and 5-point scales ($n = 2$ versions) (1: from "not true for me" to "very true to me"; 2: from "not like me at all" to "really like me") Knowledge and understanding: 4 options each, and fill in the missing words (story) Daily behavior: self-report. 5-point scale (from "0 or 1 days" to "6 or 7 days"; steps-per-day: 25-point scale (from "1000–1999 steps/day" to "18,000–30,000 steps/day") *Note*: overall scored and labeled as: "beginning," "processing", "achieving", or "excelling"	Physical competence: Qualified (trained) assessors, floor space, tape, hula hoops, cones, soccer ball, squelet ball or soft ball, cardboard wall, gym hall, CD player, Fitnessgram PACER (beep) CD, mats, stopwatch Knowledge and understanding: paper and pencil Daily behavior: paper and pencil, and pedometers

Passport for Life (PFL) [43] Canada Children and adolescents	The motivation, confidence, physical competence, knowledge and understanding to value and take responsibility for engagement in physical activities for life	Fitness skills, movement skills, living skills, and active participation	Fitness skills, objective, completed by qualified assessors: $n = 3$ skills Movement skills, objective, completed by qualified assessors: $n = 3$ skills Living skills, self-report, completed by the participant. $n = 49$ items (domains: feelings, thinking, and relating) Active participation, self-report, completed by the participant: $n = 46$ items (domains: moderate-to-vigorous physical activity, perceived fitness level, hours of daily sleep time, hours of daily sedentary screen time, barriers to physical activity, participation in diverse physical activities and environments, and interest in participating in more diverse physical activities)	Fitness skills: 4-point scale (scored and labeled as: "emerging," "developing," "acquired," or "accomplished") Movement skills: 4-point scale (scored and labeled as: "emerging," "developing," "acquired," or "accomplished") Living skills, 4-point scale (from "never" to "all of the time") Active participation: 5-point scale (from "strongly disagree" to "strongly agree"); 8-point scale (from "0" to "every day"), 12-point scale (from "0 h" to ">10 h"), and 14-point scale (from "0 h" to ">12 h")	Fitness and movement skills: qualified (trained) assessors, a large wall, floor space, tape, agility ladder, pylons, balls, and boxes Living skills and active participation: paper and pencil
Perceived Physical Literacy Inventory (PPLI) [44] China 11–19 years	Physical literacy is a specific intelligence that includes the motivation, confidence, physical competence, and knowledge and understanding to value and take responsibility for maintaining purposeful physical pursuits and activities throughout the course of one's life	Self-expression and communication with others, sense of self and self-confidence, knowledge and understanding	In total, 9 items, self-report, completed by the participant. Self-expression and communication with others: $n = 3$ items Sense of self and self-confidence: $n = 3$ items Knowledge and understanding: $n = 3$ items	5-point scale (from "strongly disagree" to "strongly agree")	Paper and pencil

(continued)

Table 3.1 (continued)

Tool (abbreviation), country, and age-group	Definition or explanation of physical literacy	Assessed categories and/or domainsa	Description of measures	Description of data and/or scale	Equipment and/or requirements
Perceptions of Physical Literacy for Middle-School Students (PPLMS) [45] USA 11–13 years	As appropriate to each individual's endowment, physical literacy can be described as the motivation, confidence, physical competence, knowledge and understanding to maintain physical activity throughout the lifecourse	Intrinsic motivation, confidence (affectivity of physical activity), perceived physical competence, knowledge and understanding, and engagement in physical activity	In total, 22 items, self-report, completed by the participant. Intrinsic motivation, confidence (affectivity of physical activity): $n = 8$ items Perceived physical competence: $n = 5$ items Knowledge and understanding: $n = 5$ items Engagement in physical activity: $n = 4$ items	6-point scale (from "definitely not likely" to "definitely likely")	Paper and pencil
Physical Literacy Assessment for Youth—4 versions (PLAY) [46, 47] Play*basic* Play*fun* Play*self* Play*coach* Canada 5 years or older	The motivation, confidence, physical competence, and understanding to value and take responsibility for engagement in physical activity for life	Movement competence, confidence, motivation, and behavior	Play*basic*. Movement competence: $n = 5$ movement skills, objective, completed by qualified assessors Play*fun*. Movement competence: $n = 18$ movement skills, objective, completed by qualified assessors Play*self*: 22 items, self-report, completed by the participant. Environments (land, water, ice, and snow): $n = 6$ items; physical literacy self-description: $n = 12$ items; relative ranking of literacies: $n = 3$ items; fitness: $n = 1$ item Play*coach*: 17 items, proxy report, completed by coaches. Physical literacy visual analogue scale; $n = 1$ item: environment: $n = 6$ items; confidence, motivation and comprehension: $n = 3$ items; motor competence: $n = 11$ items; fitness: $n = 1$ item	Play*basic*: Visual analogue scale (from "0" to "100", scored and labeled as: "initial," "emerging," "competent," or "proficient") Play*fun*: Visual analogue scale (from "0" to "100", scored and labeled as: "initial," "emerging," "competent," or "proficient") Play*self*: 4-point scales ($n = 4$ versions) (1: from "never tried" to "excellent"; 2: from "not true at all" to "very true"; 3: from "strongly disagree" to "strongly agree," and 4: from "agree" to "disagree") Play*coach*: Visual analogue scale (from "0" to "100" to score overall level of physical literacy); and 4-point scale (from "poor" to "excellent")	Play*basic*: Qualified assessors, markers, pylons, a large wall, and balls (a tennis ball and a soccer ball, or similar). Play*fun*: Qualified assessors, markers, pylons, a large wall, balls (a tennis ball, a soccer ball, a basketball, or similar), a baseball tee, a baseball bat, a basketball, and floor space Play*self*: Paper and pencil Play*coach*: Paper and pencil (note: Play*coach* should be used along with the other PLAY tools)

Instrument	Definition	Categories/dimensions[a]	Items	Scale/scoring	Administration
International Physical Literacy Association—Physical Literacy Charting Tool (IPLA) [48] UK Children and adolescents	The motivation, confidence, physical competence, knowledge and understanding to value and take responsibility for engagement in physical activities for life	Motivation, confidence, physical competence, and knowledge and understanding	In total, 12 items, self-report, completed by the participant. Motivation: $n = 3$ items Confidence: $n = 3$ items Physical competence: $n = 3$ items Knowledge and understanding: $n = 3$ items	5-point scale (from "unaware of or dismissing potential" to "maximizing potential")	Paper and pencil
Physical Literacy in Children Questionnaire (PL-C Quest) [49, 50] Australia 5–12 years	The motivation, confidence, physical competence, knowledge and understanding to value and take responsibility for engagement in physical activities for life	Physical dimension, psychological dimension, social dimension, and cognitive dimension	In total, 30 items, self-report, completed by the participant. Physical dimension: $n = 12$ items Psychological dimension: $n = 7$ items Social dimension: $n = 4$ items Cognitive dimension: $n = 7$ items	Two-stage dichotomous choice process: Stage 1: participant selects an image appropriate for them; Stage 2: participant selects a descriptive text correct for them	Computer or tablet
Physical Literacy self-Assessment Questionnaire (PLAQ) [51] China 8–12 years	The motivation, confidence, physical competence, knowledge, and understanding to maintain physical activity throughout the lifecourse	Physical competence, affective domain, knowledge and understanding, and behavior of physical activity	In total, 44 items, self-report, completed by the participant. Physical competence: $n = 9$ items Affective domain: $n = 13$ items Knowledge and understanding: $n = 11$ items Behavior of physical activity: $n = 11$ items	5-point scale (from "strongly disagree" to "strongly agree")	Paper and pencil
Portuguese Physical Literacy Assessment Questionnaire (PPLA-Q) [52, 53] Portugal 15–18 years	Contemplating integrated learning in the motor, cognitive, affective, and social domains, to empower students to engage in significant physical activity, and actively participate in the movement culture throughout their lives	Psychological, social, and cognitive	In total, 99 items, self-report, completed by the participant. Psychological: $n = 46$ items Social: $n = 43$ items Cognitive: $n = 10$ items	Psychological and social: 5-point scale (from "not at all" to "totally") Cognitive: Selecting the correct statement/option	Paper and pencil

[a] Interpreted from the categories/dimensions stated by the authors

movement and fitness skills with test procedures that require qualified assessors (training videos and manual are usually available through websites). The assessment procedure as part of these tools could be completed using the space and resources (equipment) available in typical school environments [36]. In these tools, the assessed skills (movement and other skills or behaviors) among children and adolescents are scored and compared against pre-specified criterion and labeled as "beginning," "processing," "achieving," or "excelling" (CAPL-2), "emerging," "developing," "acquired," or "accomplished" (PFL), or "initial," "emerging," "competent," or "proficient" (PLAY*fun*).

In CAPL-2, the Canadian Agility and Movement Skill Assessment (CAMSA) is used to measure fundamental, combined, and complex movement skills. The CAMSA involves completing seven movement skill tasks (two-foot jumping, sliding, catching, throwing, skipping, one foot hopping, and kicking). CAPL-2 also measures fitness as aerobic endurance (through PACER test), and muscular endurance (through plank). Furthermore, CAPL-2 is currently the only assessment tool to include objective measurement of PA (i.e., pedometer-determined steps-per-day). Furthermore, the PFL tool involves assessment of movement skills, such as locomotion (run, cross over, shuffle, backpedal), object control (run, throw, and catch) and object manipulation (run, punt, and catch), and fitness skills (hexagon hop, plank, four-station circuit). Another comprehensive assessment tool is PLAY*fun* that involves assessment of 18 movement skills. These movement skills include running (running a square, run there and back, run, jump, then land on two feet), locomotor (crossovers, skip, gallop, hop, and jump), object control of both upper body (overhand throw, strike with stick, one-handed catch, and hand dribble stationary and moving forward) and lower body (kick ball and foot dribble moving forward), as well as balance, stability and body control (balance walk forward and backward, drop to the ground and back up, and lift and lower).

Although there are currently no universally accepted standards, a recent analysis indicated that the PFL and four assessment tools based on self-report assessment—Adolescent Physical Literacy Questionnaire (APLQ), Physical Literacy in Children Questionnaire (PL-C Quest), Portuguese Physical Literacy Assessment Questionnaire (PPLA-Q), and Perceptions of Physical Literacy for Middle-School Students (PPLMS)—have evidence for at least three of the five validity aspects (content validity, face validity, internal structure, relations with other variables, and screening potential) [35].

3.4 Physical Literacy and Outcomes

In this last section of this chapter, we explore the association between physical literacy and PA participation and health and well-being among school-aged children and adolescents.

Physical literacy has been proposed to associate with several outcomes, such as PA, sport participation, and an overall active lifestyle, as well as other health behaviors and outcomes [19]. So far, these associations have mainly been theoretical assumptions and not empirically supported. Although research about the association between physical literacy and associated health outcomes is still in its infancy, however, some empirical studies among children and adolescents exist. For example, a scoping review by [54] identified 12 empirical studies that have explored physical literacy in the context of health. Eight of these explored the association between physical literacy and health behaviors and outcomes among children and adolescents, with a predominant focus on the physical domain. Physical literacy was assessed with some of the tools overviewed earlier in this chapter, namely, the Perceived Physical Literacy Inventory (PPLI), CAPL and CAMSA, PFL, and PLAY*basic* and PLAY*fun* (see Sect. 3.3.1). The overall findings in the reviewed studies were that physical literacy was associated with more PA, less sedentary behavior, and more favorably anthropometric measurements (e.g., body weight, waist circumference, and body mass index) and measures of cardiorespiratory fitness. Due to the cross-sectional design of the studies, however, there was no evidence of casual associations between physical literacy and health behavior and outcomes [54]. The findings for a positive cross-sectional association between physical literacy and PA is further supported by a systematic review that predominantly included studies with children and adolescents [55]. Furthermore, some recent studies overall confirm these positive associations between physical literacy and health behavior and outcomes [56–63].

Similar to the above, overviews of interventions with physical literacy as the major theoretical underpinning or physical literacy as the outcome of interest show that the most frequently assessed domain is physical competence, with less attention to motivation and confidence, and knowledge and understanding [64, 65]. Despite that most interventions adopted a holistic approach to the concept, about one-third involved content relevant for all physical literacy domains [64]. In one overview, 48 interventions were identified, yet only three included outcomes for all physical literacy domains [65].

Even though few empirical studies have explored physical literacy in the context of health to date, Cairney et al. [66] made one of the first attempts to present an evidence-based model to illustrate the potential relation between physical literacy, PA, and health outcomes across the life course, while emphasizing the idea of physical literacy as a lifelong journey. In doing so, they undertook a pragmatic approach, arguing that physical literacy assessment may include measure of performance within each domain, hence separating elements for empirical consideration. In summary, the model emphasizes the importance of considering the dynamic interrelationships between the components of physical literacy and their impact on health outcomes, highlighting a more holistic approach rather than a simple and additive consideration of individual components.

The authors argue that the model approaches physical literacy as a holistic concept. In this sense, physical literacy is conceptualized as a cycle involving four dynamic, interrelated elements: (a) movement competence, (b) confidence and motivation, (c) social participation, and (d) affective outcomes (e.g., happiness and enjoyment). Furthermore, the model positions knowledge outside the cycle as it is deemed both an outcome of engagement and a contributing factor for further engagement [66]. To illustrate the potential relation, physical literacy and its dynamic, interrelated elements are viewed as a determinant of not only health but also PA behavior. In this sense, health is achieved through a fully mediated model that incorporates the favorable physiological changes stemming from both short- and long-term engagements in PA [66]. The model also acknowledges that PA improves physiological attributes, such as aerobic fitness and muscular strength, and that improvements in these physiological dimensions can positively influence future PA participation. Furthermore, the model acknowledges the possible moderating effects influenced by individual and socioenvironmental factors to the association between physical literacy and PA. Accordingly, individual factors, such as sex, age, and socioeconomic status, may influence the transition between physical literacy and participation in PA. In a similar vein, socioenvironmental factors, such as neighborhood environment and climate, may influence opportunities to engage in PA [66].

3.5 Discussion

During the recent decade, the concept of physical literacy has gained increasing prominence worldwide. Introduced by Whitehead in the early 1990s, physical literacy was conceptualized as a developmental process encompassing competence in the physical, affective, and cognitive dimensions that should be understood in a holistic manner where the attributes are interconnected and inseparable. Even though physical literacy originally was considered as having value in its own right, there has been an increased interest in assessing physical literacy during the last years. The assessment tools overviewed in this chapter (see Sect. 3.3.1) have different points of departure as different categories and domains of physical literacy are assessed, both with self-report and objective measures. Upon deciding which assessment tool to use, some considerations should be made in relation to not only validity and reliability but also overall feasibility. Although self-report measurements arguably are the most feasible to administer, three comprehensive assessment tools also include measurements of movement and fitness skills with test procedures. These test procedures require qualified assessors, space, and resources (equipment).

Indeed, to assess physical literacy is not without intricate challenges. The multidimensional nature of the concept of physical literacy has contributed to the proliferation of diverse meanings and interpretations, and the lack of universally established standards makes it challenging to develop assessment tools and interpret the assessed outcomes. The multidimensionality of the concept makes it challenging to create a single, comprehensive assessment tool that adequately captures all aspects of physical literacy. Researchers and practitioners have tried to operationalize the domains of physical literacy into components that allow to create a structured framework for assessment, assessing single components, such as fundamental motor skills. This may not only generate a fragmented view of the overall physical literacy but also risk disregarding the holistic nature of the concept. An added risk is also if the assessments scores are utilized for the purpose of comparing physical literacy across individuals; this could potentially threaten, for example, motivation and self-confidence among children and adolescents. This could also contradict the perspective of viewing physical literacy as a continuous process and not as a goal, fostering of a disposition providing a wide range of experiences [1, 3].

It may also be argued that some tools assess movement skills, typically fundamental, combined, and complex movement skills, that relate closely to the logics of sports. For example, movement skills, such as catching, throwing, kicking, and dribbling, skills that can be ascribed to various sports. On the other hand, it may be argued that these movement skills are fundamental to the engagement in play, a natural and integrated aspect of childhood development that serve several important functions for the growing child, not least the development of physical competence. Several of the assessment tools also include measures of skills that, as far as we are concerned, are critical for participation in physical activities beyond sports. Some examples of these skills include jumping, running, and balancing. To be aware of, however, is that the assessment tools focus on these skills in isolation and also lack skills that interplay with a broader range of movement skills, such as rotating, hanging and climbing. Still, these assessment tools, if handled with caution, can be used to provide an overview of what opportunities for practicing fundamental skills that children and adolescents would benefit from to make possible a development of movement capacities. In turn, this may provide children and adolescents with a broad repertoire of movement patterns that they can utilize in a social cultural context. Again, we stress the fact that creating a single, comprehensive assessment tool that adequately captures all aspects of physical literacy is challenging. In this sense, a critical question is—*if* physical literacy should be assessed at all—and what alternative movement skills or interaction with the environment that should be included as part of a tool to align more closely with the concept of physical literacy.

The growing interest in the concept of physical literacy is partially to be understood against the backdrop of global challenges related to physical inactivity and increased health issues among children and adolescents [67–69]. Through this lens, the potential of physical literacy is perceived as a holistic approach to motivation, confidence, physical competence, knowledge and understanding to value and take responsibility for engaging in PA for life. Although physical literacy has been proposed to associate with PA and other health behaviors and outcomes, these associations have so far mainly been theoretical assumptions. While there is some evidence to suggest associations between physical literacy and PA, as well as other health behaviors and outcomes (see Sect. 3.4), additional research, especially of longitudinal research design, is needed to enhance our understanding of how these associations manifest (e.g., causal or bidirectional) among children and adolescents across ages-groups and contexts.

References

1. Whitehead M. The concept of physical literacy. In: Whitehead M, editor. Physical literacy: throughout the lifecourse. Oxford: Routledge; 2017. p. 10–20.
2. Whitehead M. Philosophical underpinning of physical literacy. In: Whitehead M, editor. Physical literacy: throughout the lifecourse. 1st ed. Florence: Routledge; 2017.
3. Whitehead M, editor. Physical literacy across the world. London: Routledge; 2019.
4. Lynch T, Soukup GJ. "Physical education", "health and physical education", "physical literacy" and "health literacy": global nomenclature confusion. Cogent Educ. 2016;3(1):1217820.
5. Lounsbery MAF, McKenzie TL. Physically literate and physically educated: a rose by any other name? J Sport Health Sci. 2015;4(2):139–44.
6. Cairney J, Kiez T, Roetert EP, Kriellaars D. A 20th-century narrative on the origins of the physical literacy construct. J Teach Phys Educ. 2019;38(2):79–83.
7. Young L, Alfrey L, O'Connor J. Moving from physical literacy to co-existing physical literacies: what is the problem? Eur Phys Educ Rev. 2023;29(1):55–73.
8. Whitehead M. Physical literacy. Unpublished paper given at IAPESWG Congress, Melbourne. 1993.
9. Whitehead M. The concept of physical literacy. Eur J Phys Educ. 2001;6(2):127–38.
10. Claudia WMY. The physical education pedagogical approaches in nurturing physical literacy among primary and secondary school students: a scoping review. Int J Educ Res. 2022;116:102080.
11. Carl J, Jaunig J, Kurtzhals M, Müllertz ALO, Stage A, Bentsen P, et al. Synthesising physical literacy research for 'blank spots': a systematic review of reviews. J Sports Sci. 2023;41(11):1056–72.
12. Mendoza-Muñoz M, Vega-Muñoz A, Carlos-Vivas J, Denche-Zamorano Á, Adsuar JC, Raimundo A, Salazar-Sepúlveda G, Contreras-Barraza N, Muñoz-Urtubia N. The bibliometric analysis of studies on physical literacy for a healthy life. Int J Environ Res Public Health. 2022;19(22):15211. https://doi.org/10.3390/ijerph192215211.
13. Urbano-Mairena J, Castillo-Paredes A, Muñoz-Bermejo L, Denche-Zamorano Á, Rojo-Ramos J, Pastor-Cisneros R, et al. A bibliometric analysis of physical literacy studies in relation to health of children and adolescents. Children. 2023;10(4):660.
14. Young L, O'Connor J, Alfrey L. Mapping the physical literacy controversy: an analysis of key actors within scholarly literature. Phys Educ Sport Pedagogy. 2023;28(6):658–74.
15. Whitehead M. Introduction. In: Whitehead M, editor. Physical literacy: throughout the lifecourse. Oxford: Routledge; 2017. p. 10–20.
16. Carl J, Bryant AS, Edwards LC, Bartle G, Birch JE, Christodoulides E, Emeljanovas A, Fröberg A, Gandrieau J, Gilic B, van Hilvoorde I, Holler P, Iconomescu TM, Jaunig J, Laudanska-Krzeminska I, Lundvall S, De Martelaer K, Martins J, Mieziene B, et al. Physical literacy in Europe: the current state of implementation in research, practice, and policy. J Exerc Sci Fit. 2023;21(1):165–76. https://doi.org/10.1016/j.jesf.2022.12.003.
17. Durden-Myers EJ, Bartle G, Whitehead ME, Dhillon KK. Exploring the notion of literacy within physical literacy: a discussion paper. Front Sports Act Living. 2022;3(4):853247.
18. Bailey R, Glibo I, Koenen K, Samsudin N. What is physical literacy? An international review and analysis of definitions. Kinesiol Rev. 2023;12(3):247–60.
19. Edwards LC, Bryant AS, Keegan RJ, Morgan K, Jones AM. Definitions, foundations and associations of physical literacy: a systematic review. Sports Med. 2017;47(1):113–26.
20. Grauduszus M, Wessely S, Klaudius M, Joisten C. Definitions and assessments of physical literacy among children and youth: a scoping review. BMC Public Health. 2023;23(1):1746.
21. Jean De Dieu H, Zhou K. Physical literacy assessment tools: a systematic literature review for why, what, who, and how. Int J Environ Res Public Health. 2021;18(15):7954.
22. Shearer C, Goss HR, Edwards LC, Keegan RJ, Knowles ZR, Boddy LM, et al. How is physical literacy defined? A contemporary update. J Teach Phys Educ. 2018;37(3):237–45.

23. Hurter L, Essiet I, Dunca M, Roberts W, Lewis K, Goss H, et al. Physical literacy consensus for England: evidence review [Internet]. Liverpool John Moores University; 2022. Available from: https://researchonline.ljmu.ac.uk/id/eprint/17272/.
24. International Physical Literacy Association (IPLA). 2017. https://www.physical-literacy.org.uk/. Accessed 10 Oct 2023.
25. Belton S, Connolly S, Peers C, Goss H, Murphy M, Murtagh E, et al. Are all domains created equal? An exploration of stakeholder views on the concept of physical literacy. BMC Public Health. 2022;22(1):501.
26. Keegan R, Barnett L, Dudley D. Physical literacy: informing a definition and standard for Australia, vol. 1. 1st ed. Australian Sports Commission; 2017. 38 p.
27. Tremblay MS, Longmuir PE. Conceptual critique of Canada's physical literacy assessment instruments also misses the mark. Meas Phys Educ Exerc Sci. 2017;21(3):174–6.
28. Tremblay MS, Costas-Bradstreet C, Barnes JD, et al. Canada's Physical Literacy Consensus Statement: process and outcome. BMC Public Health. 2018;18(Suppl 2):1034. https://doi.org/10.1186/s12889-018-5903-x.
29. Maude P. Physical literacy and the young child. In: Whitehead M, editor. Physical literacy: throughout the lifecourse. Florence: Routledge; 2010.
30. Whitehead M. Promoting physical literacy within and beyond the school curriculum. In: Whitehead M, editor. Physical literacy: throughout the lifecourse. Florence: Routledge; 2010.
31. Lundvall S. Physical literacy in the field of physical education – a challenge and a possibility. J Sport Health Sci. 2015;4(2):113–8.
32. Robinson DB, Randall L. Marking physical literacy or missing the mark on physical literacy? A conceptual critique of Canada's physical literacy assessment instruments. Meas Phys Educ Exerc Sci. 2017;21(1):40–55.
33. Edwards LC, Bryant AS, Keegan RJ, Morgan K, Cooper SM, Jones AM. 'Measuring' physical literacy and related constructs: a systematic review of empirical findings. Sports Med. 2018;48(3):659–82.
34. Allan V, Turnnidge J, Côté J. Evaluating approaches to physical literacy through the lens of positive youth development. Quest. 2017;69(4):515–30.
35. Barnett LM, Jerebine A, Keegan R, Watson-Mackie K, Arundell L, Ridgers ND, et al. Validity, reliability, and feasibility of physical literacy assessments designed for school children: a systematic review. Sports Med. 2023;53(10):1905–29.
36. Shearer C, Goss HR, Boddy LM, Knowles ZR, Durden-Myers EJ, Foweather L. Assessments related to the physical, affective and cognitive domains of physical literacy amongst children aged 7–11.9 years: a systematic review. Sports Med Open. 2021;7(1):37.
37. Young L, O'Connor J, Alfrey L, Penney D. Assessing physical literacy in health and physical education. Curric Stud Health Phys Educ. 2021;12(2):156–79.
38. Mohammadzadeh M, Sheikh M, Houminiyan Sharif Abadi D, Bagherzadeh F, Kazemnejad A. Design and psychometrics evaluation of Adolescent Physical Literacy Questionnaire (APLQ). Sport Sci Health. 2022;18(2):397–405.
39. Gunnell KE, Longmuir PE, Barnes JD, Belanger K, Tremblay MS. Refining the Canadian assessment of physical literacy based on theory and factor analyses. BMC Public Health. 2018;18(2):1044.
40. Gunnell KE, Longmuir PE, Woodruff SJ, Barnes JD, Belanger K, Tremblay MS. Revising the motivation and confidence domain of the Canadian assessment of physical literacy. BMC Public Health. 2018;18(2):1045.
41. Longmuir PE, Gunnell KE, Barnes JD, Belanger K, Leduc G, Woodruff SJ, et al. Canadian assessment of physical literacy second edition: a streamlined assessment of the capacity for physical activity among children 8 to 12 years of age. BMC Public Health. 2018;18(2):1047.
42. Longmuir PE, Woodruff SJ, Boyer C, Lloyd M, Tremblay MS. Physical literacy knowledge questionnaire: feasibility, validity, and reliability for Canadian children aged 8 to 12 years. BMC Public Health. 2018;18(2):1035.

43. Lodewyk KR. Early validation evidence of the canadian practitioner-based assessment of physical literacy in secondary physical education. Phys Educat. 2019;76(3):634–60.
44. Sum RKW, Cheng C-F, Wallhead T, Kuo C-C, Wang F-J, Choi S-M. Perceived physical literacy instrument for adolescents: a further validation of PPLI. J Exerc Sci Fit. 2018;16(1):26–31.
45. Dong X. Measuring middle-school students' physical literacy: instrument development [Ed.D.]. Miami Shores: Barry University; 2021.
46. Caldwell HA, Di Cristofaro NA, Cairney J, Bray SR, Timmons BW. Measurement properties of the Physical Literacy Assessment for Youth (PLAY) tools. Appl Physiol Nutr Metab. 2020;46(6):571–8.
47. Sport for Life. Physical literacy assessment for youth. https://sportforlife.ca/.
48. International Physical Literacy Association (IPLA). Physical literacy charting tool. 2018. https://www.physical-literacy.org.uk/library/charting-physical-literacy-journey-tool/.
49. Barnett LM, Mazzoli E, Bowe SJ, Lander N, Salmon J. Reliability and validity of the PL-C Quest, a scale designed to assess children's self-reported physical literacy. Psychol Sport Exerc. 2022;60:102164.
50. Barnett LM, Mazzoli E, Hawkins M, Lander N, Lubans DR, Caldwell S, et al. Development of a self-report scale to assess children's perceived physical literacy. Phys Educ Sport Pedagog. 2022;27(1):91–116.
51. YongKang W, QianQian F. The Chinese assessment of physical literacy: based on grounded theory paradigm for children in grades 3–6. PLoS One. 2022;17(9):e0262976.
52. Mota J, Martins J, Onofre M. Portuguese Physical Literacy Assessment Questionnaire (PPLA-Q) for adolescents: validity and reliability of the psychological and social modules using Mokken scale analysis. Percept Mot Skills. 2023;130(3):958–83.
53. Mota J, Martins J, Onofre M. Portuguese Physical Literacy Assessment Questionnaire (PPLA-Q) for adolescents (15–18 years) from grades 10–12: development, content validation and pilot testing. BMC Public Health. 2021;21(1):2183.
54. Cornish K, Fox G, Fyfe T, Koopmans E, Pousette A, Pelletier CA. Understanding physical literacy in the context of health: a rapid scoping review. BMC Public Health. 2020;20(1):1569.
55. Dlugonski D, Gadd N, McKay C, Kleis RR, Hoch JM. Physical literacy and physical activity across the life span: a systematic review. Transl J Am Coll Sports Med. 2022;7(3):e000201. Available from: https://journals.lww.com/10.1249/TJX.0000000000000201.
56. Brown DMY, Dudley DA, Cairney J. Physical literacy profiles are associated with differences in children's physical activity participation: a latent profile analysis approach. J Sci Med Sport. 2020;23(11):1062–7.
57. Domínguez-Martín G, Tárraga-López PJ, López-Gil JF. Cross-sectional association between perceived physical literacy and mediterranean dietary patterns in adolescents: the EHDLA study. Nutrients. 2023;15(20):4400.
58. Liu Y, Hadier SG, Liu L, Hamdani SMZH, Hamdani SD, Danish SS, et al. Assessment of the Relationship between body weight status and physical literacy in 8 to 12 year old Pakistani school children: the PAK-IPPL cross-sectional study. Children. 2023;10(2):363.
59. Melby PS, Elsborg P, Bentsen P, Nielsen G. Cross-sectional associations between adolescents' physical literacy, sport and exercise participation, and wellbeing. Front Public Health. 2023;28(10):1054482.
60. Nezondet C, Gandrieau J, Nguyen P, Zunquin G. Perceived physical literacy is associated with cardiorespiratory fitness, body composition and physical activity levels in secondary school students. Children. 2023;10(4):712.
61. Pastor-Cisneros R, Carlos-Vivas J, Muñoz-Bermejo L, Adsuar-Sala JC, Merellano-Navarro E, Mendoza-Muñoz M. Association between physical literacy and self-perceived fitness level in children and adolescents. Biology. 2021;10(12):1358.
62. Tang Y, Algurén B, Pelletier C, Naylor PJ, Faulkner G. Physical Literacy for Communities (PL4C): physical literacy, physical activity and associations with wellbeing. BMC Public Health. 2023;23(1):1266.

63. Mendoza-Muñoz M, Barrios-Fernández S, Adsuar JC, Pastor-Cisneros R, Risco-Gil M, García-Gordillo MÁ, et al. Influence of body composition on physical literacy in Spanish children. Biology. 2021;10(6):482.
64. Carl J, Barratt J, Töpfer C, Cairney J, Pfeifer K. How are physical literacy interventions conceptualized? – a systematic review on intervention design and content. Psychol Sport Exerc. 2022;58:102091.
65. Carl J, Barratt J, Wanner P, Töpfer C, Cairney J, Pfeifer K. The effectiveness of physical literacy interventions: a systematic review with meta-analysis. Sports Med. 2022;52(12):2965–99.
66. Cairney J, Dudley D, Kwan M, Bulten R, Kriellaars D. Physical literacy, physical activity and health: toward an evidence-informed conceptual model. Sports Med. 2019;49(3):371–83.
67. Aubert S, Barnes JD, Demchenko I, Hawthorne M, Abdeta C, Abi Nader P, et al. Global matrix 4.0 physical activity report card grades for children and adolescents: results and analyses from 57 countries. J Phys Act Health. 2022;19(11):700–28.
68. Guthold R, Stevens GA, Riley LM, Bull FC. Global trends in insufficient physical activity among adolescents: a pooled analysis of 298 population-based surveys with 1·6 million participants. Lancet Child Adolesc Health. 2020;4(1):23–35.
69. Van Sluijs EMF, Ekelund U, Crochemore-Silva I, Guthold R, Ha A, Lubans D, et al. Physical activity behaviours in adolescence: current evidence and opportunities for intervention. Lancet. 2021;398(10298):429–42.

Chapter 4
Assessment of Physical Activity in Children and Adolescents

Jairo H. Migueles and Patricio Solis-Urra

4.1 Introduction

4.1.1 Defining Physical Activity

Physical activity, a term commonly referenced since 1985 in a seminal work by Caspersen et al. [1], is broadly described as "any bodily movement produced by skeletal muscles that results in energy expenditure." In practical terms, we often categorize the activities of our daily lives as either sedentary behavior or PA based on posture and energy expenditure. Sitting or lying down with an energy expenditure less than 1.5 times our resting metabolic rate is considered sedentary behavior, while any activity surpassing this threshold and involving bodily movement is classified as PA. The categorization further defines the intensity of PA, with the most established categories of light, moderate, and vigorous intensity based on the energy expenditure produced by the activity. Physical activity is sometimes used interchangeably with exercise, even though not all PA is exercise. Physical exercise refers to structured, planned, and purposeful PA, while incidental PA is usually the result of daily activities at home, at work, or during transportation.

One may already note that defining PA is a nuanced task that goes beyond movement and energy expenditure. Like any other behavior, comprehending PA requires understanding how, when, how often, and where. In other words, PA is bodily movement, yet the context in which such movement occurs is highly relevant. This led the field to establish what we refer to as the dimensions and the domains of PA. The four dimensions of PA include intensity, type (or mode),

---

J. H. Migueles (✉) · P. Solis-Urra
Department of Physical Education and Sports, Faculty of Sport Sciences, Sport and Health University Research Institute (iMUDS), University of Granada, Granada, Spain
e-mail: jairo@jhmigueles.com

volume, and frequency. The domains include occupational, domestic, transportation, and leisure time. Measuring the dimensions of PA is relevant for defining behavior, and assessing these domains is especially relevant for promoting behavioral change based on the context in which it occurs. Thus, talking about measuring PA is more than just quantifying the energy expenditure of bodily movement; a holistic measure of PA should provide information on the dimensions and domains of this behavior.

4.1.2 Significance of Measuring Physical Activity

After having established the notions of PA, our focus now turns to why measuring this behavior is of relevance, and we will address this question with a special focus on children and adolescents.

As summarized in the latest report of the World Health Organization (WHO) on PA, there are myriad benefits that this behavior confers on the health and well-being of children and adolescents [2]. This report led to the establishment of guidelines for PA that recommend at least 60 min per day of moderate-to-vigorous PA (MVPA) for children and adolescents older than 5 years. For children under 5 years of age, the recommendation is twofold: a total of 180 min per day of PA of any intensity, of which at least 60 min should reach a MVPA intensity.

The underpinnings of these guidelines draw from a robust body of scientific literature revealing a cascade of positive effects on both the physical and mental health of children and adolescents. These positive effects might be observed immediately after a single bout of PA, or in the long term, even some of the adverse effects could even become chronic and potentially influence the later life of the youths.

The measurement of PA in children and adolescents is key to identifying compliance with public health recommendations, identifying, and promoting interventions among groups at risk, or serving as a roadmap for designing interventions that effectively enhance PA levels among this population. Therefore, the measurement of PA is crucial for evaluating the degree of success of such interventions. Moreover, increasing the precision of the measurement of PA would assist future versions of the PA guidelines in providing more detailed recommendations for children and adolescents and for different subgroups of this demographic.

4.2 Methods for Measuring Physical Activity

This chapter is dedicated to exploring the behavioral aspect of PA (i.e., movement), intentionally excluding the methods used to assess its physiological consequences. Specifically, the measurement of energy expenditure, or heart rate as a response to the realization of PA, is not discussed. The physiological reactions of an organism are influenced by various factors beyond mere movement, including age, sex, body weight, and body composition. Moreover, these methods are often impractical for extended application over multiple days, a necessity when quantifying a behavior prone to variation across days and weeks. Direct observation is another method that can also fall into the category of methods unsuitable for relatively long-term use.

It is important to clarify that this chapter does not aim to comprehensively detail every method for measuring PA and its associated characteristics. Instead, its purpose is to provide a summary of useful methods that are feasible, valid, and reliable in yielding meaningful insights into the PA patterns of children and adolescents.

The instruments designed to measure free-living PA over extended periods are broadly classified into two categories: report-based and device-based methods (Fig. 4.1).

4.2.1 Reporting-Based Methods

This category encompasses self-report questionnaires, parental reports, and interviews. These instruments primarily seek to assess aspects such as volume, intensity, type, and domain of PA, relying on participants' memories or self-perceptions or insights from individuals familiar with the contexts in which children are engaged.

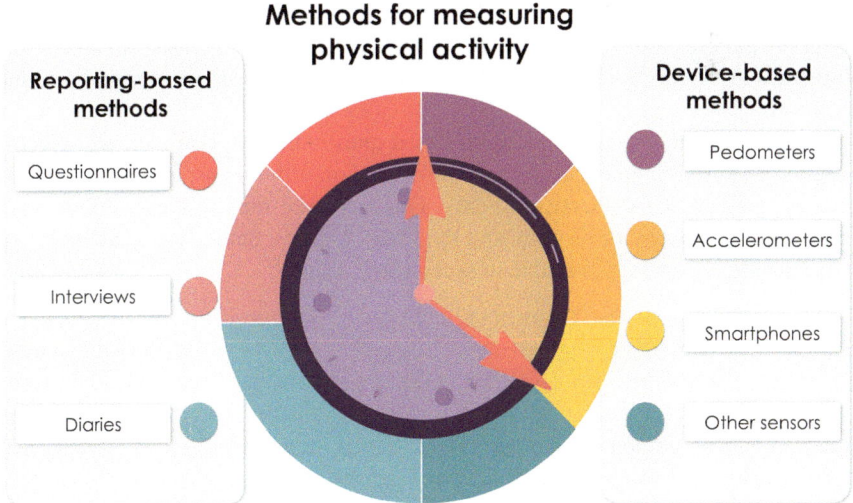

Fig. 4.1 Types of methods for measuring physical activity

4.2.2 Recall-Based Questionnaires

Recall-based questionnaires usually propose a set of questions related to PA that participants should answer based on their PA patterns in the previous days, weeks, or even years. Therefore, this method relies on participants' memory capacity and their perceptions of the PA performed to provide an estimate of this behavior.

Questionnaires are popular in settings that require assessing PA in large populations. The main advantage of this method is the time effectiveness of its application, as it is able to provide a quick estimate of different aspects of PA in a few minutes. Another advantage is their flexibility to be applied in paper-and-pencil or digital ways, adapting to different needs and participants' characteristics. It is also worth noting that this is the method of choice for surveilling the prevalence of the population meeting the PA recommendations worldwide. Even though the accuracy of these methods may be limited, they can still provide important information. Finally, questionnaires might be used to assess certain aspects of PA that device-based measures struggle to capture, for example, the dimension of PA (e.g., household, leisure, occupational, transportation) or the specific type (i.e., walking, cycling, running, among others) of PA that has been conducted.

The main limitation of these questionnaires is that their validity has been questioned, and there is no consensus on which one is best to use. The main biases that affect the recall-based questionnaires are recall and subjective biases. These two factors are of special relevance in children under 10 years of age since their memory capacity might be limited to reporting what they did in the days before the questionnaire was administered and their capacity to self-rate their PA level. To address these limitations, it is common for parents, legal guardians, or teachers of children to be responsible for completing the questionnaire. Nevertheless, the children's usual PA patterns are intermittent, with short bouts of high-intensity activities that might last less than 10 s. This type of activity is extremely difficult to remember and to report.

There are many examples of recall-based questionnaires; however, we selected several broadly used questionnaires that focused on different aspects of PA for this chapter: the PAQ-C/A (Physical Activity Questionnaire for Children/Adolescents), the YAP (Youth Activity Profile), and the ACS (Active Commuting to School). All these questionnaires are available in several languages.

PAQ-C and PAQ-A *The Physical Activity Questionnaire-Children* (PAQ-C) and the Physical Activity Questionnaire-Adolescent (PAQ-A) are instrumental tools designed to assess the PA levels of children (8–14 years old) and adolescents (15–18 years old), respectively, over the past 7 days within the school term. These questionnaires are integral members of the "PAQ" family, a comprehensive set utilized across age groups, from children to adults, and widely employed in both national and international surveillance systems. While the PAQ-C and PAQ-A share a fundamental similarity, the key distinction lies in their treatment of school recesses. Each questionnaire comprises ten items, with nine devoted to evaluating the extent of PA and the tenth gauging whether any unforeseen events hindered the child's regular activities during the preceding week. The resulting score on the questionnaire ranged from 1 to 5, with higher scores indicating elevated activity levels. The inquiries cover various dimensions, including the type of activity, participation in physical education (PE) lessons, engagement in leisure time activities, and the specific times of the day when participants are most active. These questionnaires play a crucial role in surveillance, allowing for facile comparisons with other populations [3] and survey data. This standardization ensures consistency in evaluating PA levels, making these tools invaluable for researchers, policymakers, and health professionals engaged in the promotion of active lifestyles among children and adolescents.

Youth Activity Profile (YAP) The YAP is a valuable tool designed to capture a detailed snapshot of sedentary behavior and PA in children and adolescents over the preceding 7 days. Its scope extends across various time frames, meticulously examining different aspects of daily life: before going to school, on the way to and from school, at school (with sub windows for breaks and PE lessons), after school, during the evening, and on weekends. The questionnaire is available in paper and pencil formats and online at https://www.youthactivityprofile.org/. There are a total of 15 items, including questions about PA and sedentary time, with a focus on frequency rather than intensity or type. The weekend dimension was added to the output data, which were not available in the PAQ-C or PAC-A questionnaire. The validity of the YAP has been rigorously tested across diverse populations using device-based methods as a reference, revealing strong agreement between methods at the populational level (not at the individual level). Moreover, the questionnaire has demonstrated good reliability for application in both children and adolescents.

Active Commuting to School (ACS) The ACS questionnaire is a child-friendly tool designed to swiftly measure PA during school commutes for children and adolescents. It begins by gathering essential information and estimating the distance between home and school. Two straightforward questions were asked about the typical mode of travel to and from school, with options such as "walking," "bicycle," and "car." Extending this questioning to cover the past 5 days, the ACS provides a nuanced understanding of specific travel modes. In addition to self-reports, the ACS has proven validity in determining commuting habits. Notably, it can calculate travel distance, offering valuable insights into the level of PA during the journey. In essence, the ACS is a holistic tool that seamlessly blends simplicity with depth, making it invaluable for assessing and promoting PA in the lives of children and adolescents.

4.2.3 Interviews

A more flexible approach to gauging diverse aspects of PA involves conducting interviews. These individual interviews can be customized to extract additional insights, such as details about the nature of PA or the motivations driving engagement.

However, interviews share some drawbacks with recall-based questionnaires, predominantly relying on participants' memories of past PA habits. This introduces self-perception and recall bias. Moreover, the interviews faced distinct limitations. The questionnaires lacked replicability and transparency, as not only the questions but also how they were presented may influence participant responses, impacting the accuracy of PA measurements. An additional constraint is the increased workload for researchers. When one-on-one interviews are conducted, they can be time-consuming, making this method less common than questionnaires. Typically, interviews find utility in qualitative research with a restricted participant pool.

4.2.4 Diaries

The last reported method that is described in this chapter is the use of diaries of activity. In this case, the burden is extremely increased for both the participants and the researchers. This method usually requires that the participants fill in an epoch-based diary indicating the type of activity that they have done; usually, the epoch window is 15 min or longer.

These questionnaires are argued to be more accurate than questionnaires because they are less prone to recall bias. However, the burdens that they impose both for participants and for researchers make them less feasible than questionnaires and, in the last instance, less used in research or school settings.

4.2.5 Device-Based Methods

Device-based methods include wearable devices, a product of recent technological advancements. Examples include pedometers, accelerometers, geolocation systems (GPSs), and inertial units. These devices offer a technological edge in capturing and quantifying PA in a manner that aligns with the demands of contemporary research and monitoring methodologies.

4.2.6 Pedometers

The pedometers marked the initial foray into objectively measuring PA levels [4]. Worn by participants, these devices track the number of steps taken at specific intervals. Pedometers assume that the primary source of daily PA is ambulatory, encompassing walking or running. This assumption has been validated by numerous investigations across diverse populations, rendering pedometers a reliable means of objectively measuring the majority of PA. However, limitations arise when considering activities such as swimming or cycling, as well as gauging the intensity of climbing stairs or slopes. Pedometers only register step counts and do not account for the energy cost associated with each step, leading to potential underestimation in these scenarios.

Despite their limitations, pedometers remain in use today both for assessing and promoting PA. The information they provide, such as steps taken throughout the day, is easily interpretable, making it conducive to goal setting—such as achieving a specific number of steps per day. Traditionally, pedometers feature a spring-suspended arm that moves in response to the vertical impacts generated during walking, registering a step when the impact exceeds a certain threshold. Building on this concept, modern pedometers incorporate piezoelectric materials, enabling signal digitization, increased memory capacity, and extended battery life—all while maintaining the cost-effectiveness of these instruments.

A significant limitation of pedometers in current use is the absence of a timestamp accompanying recorded steps. Most pedometers provide only the total number of steps without indicating when these steps were taken. Consequently, it becomes challenging to discern the timing of PA during specific periods of the day. For instance, it is not feasible to determine how many steps were accumulated during the commute to and from school. Moreover, the absence of a timestamp means that we cannot calculate the step cadence—the number of steps taken per minute. This information is crucial for assessing whether children are performing the recommended 60 min of PA at a rate indicative of moderate or vigorous PA. However, certain pedometer models have started incorporating estimations of the step rate within their measurements, addressing this limitation to some extent.

In summary, pedometers offer several advantages, including their ability to provide straightforward records of the most common form of PA across diverse populations. The steps per day derived by pedometers are easily interpretable, facilitating the setting of goals to enhance PA levels. Additionally, pedometers are highly cost-effective and accessible devices for the majority of individuals [5]. However, the main limitations of pedometers lie in their inability to distinguish between different types of activities and the absence of a time record, hindering the classification of step cadence or identification of activity periods throughout the day.

4.2.7 Accelerometers

The advent of accelerometers represents a significant advancement in measuring PA. These motion sensors record signals of magnitude and frequency of body acceleration, enabling the identification of movement frequency, intensity, and duration [6]. Accelerometers are being increasingly used over self-reports due to their ability to minimize biases, particularly in children and adolescents, even though they are accused of lacking contextual information. Accelerometers offer a highly sensitive measurement of body accelerations throughout the day, providing valuable insights into the intensity and duration of PA. Ongoing advancements in this technology allow for precise tracking of time spent in activities at different intensities—whether light, moderate, or vigorous. This capability makes it straightforward to assess whether a child or adolescent meets the daily recommendation of 60 min of MVPA. The challenge of joining the traditional and mostly reported-based measures that the guidelines are based on with the modern and more precise recordings that are provided by accelerometers is currently being addressed in the field.

Additionally, the accelerometer signal allows estimation of the time spent in sedentary activities and sleep duration for a comprehensive understanding of daily activities. Despite their effectiveness in tracking broad categories of behavior such as PA, sedentary behavior, and sleep, accelerometers encounter challenges in identifying specific types of activities. Although attempts have been made to translate acceleration patterns into different activity types, none have achieved significant success in free-living settings. However, accelerometers excel in recording the time when each acceleration is detected, enabling the estimation of movement intensity. The ability to timestamp accelerations also facilitates the division of the day into various periods. This allows for a detailed understanding of when and at what intensity PA occurs, whether inside or outside of school, during breaks, during PA classes, or during the commute to and from school.

Accelerometers present another significant strength, their capacity to record extensive data, with some brands capturing up to 100 data points per second. However, this wealth of data requires processing to yield meaningful insights into PA. Traditionally, accelerometers process data by providing a measurement of "counts" per minute [7]. The controversy lies in the fact that each accelerometer brand calculates counts differently. Nonetheless, the fundamental concept remains: the more counts accumulated in a specific period of time, the greater the intensity of PA. Modern methods for processing raw accelerations attempt to measure movement in gravitational units, giving a unit of measurement and a meaning to what it is being recorded and collaterally increasing comparability across brands and reproducibility of the measurement.

A limitation that is usually raised when talking about accelerometers is the difficulty of handling the raw data. Researchers should make many decisions that would affect the final measurement, such as the epoch length at which the signal is aggregated, how to identify and handle the nonwear time, and how to select the cutoff points to classify the intensity or algorithm to define the activity types. All of these decisions have been demonstrated to largely affect the estimates of PA, and there are no clear guidelines for making these decisions. In this moment, there are many efforts in form of software tools to help researchers in this decision-making process, such as the R package GGIR [8], that tries to facilitate open-source methods for quality checking the data and providing measures of PA and sleep.

In contrast, a major advantage of processing accelerometer raw signals is the resolution of the measure, allowing for the detection of very short bouts of PA, such as those that characterize children's and adolescents' PA patterns. If we think of vigorous intensity PA, such as jumping or fast running, it often occurs for only a few seconds in children and adolescents. As a general rule, it is recommended to summarize data in periods of 1–15 s to estimate PA in children and adolescents [6].

Accelerometers are usually categorized as research or consumer grade, depending on the targeted end users. The internal sensors and the technology behind both types of accelerometers are virtually identical; therefore, their limitations and strengths are similar. However, there is a distinction that is noteworthy. Most consumer grade accelerometers (or activity or fitness trackers) do not allow access of the user to the raw data that have been collected. The user would only have access to the estimates that are provided by the companies after applying their proprietary closed-source algorithms. This is a major concern, as there is no guarantee that the algorithms that they are using are valid or reliable or even that they are using the same algorithms over time. Thus, their use should be carefully considered in longitudinal study designs.

4.2.8 Other Sensors

In the field of PA measurement, other sensors are used for the measurement of PA either on their own or in combination with accelerometers. The most popular sensors in this category are *GPSs (global positioning systems)* and gyroscopes.

GPS A global positioning system (GPS) is widely utilized for measuring PA, particularly in outdoor settings. GPS technology relies on a network of satellites to provide accurate location information, and when integrated into wearable devices or smartphones, it has become a powerful tool for tracking various aspects of PA and assisting accelerometer-based estimations of PA.

GPSs are highly effective at monitoring outdoor activities such as running, cycling, hiking, and walking. It provides real-time location data, allowing users to track their routes, distances covered, and speeds. This information is valuable for assessing the overall intensity and performance of an activity. Routes are useful for providing context for PA, which may increase the richness of the data by providing information related to walkability or the security of the place where PA is taking place. Additionally, position identification may help to establish the domain of PA, household, occupational or transport, which are easily identifiable by GPS. Moreover, GPS-derived speeds might help to establish the type of activity being performed, with special sensitivity to identifying walking, running, cycling, public transport, or cars. As the relationship between movement (measured by accelerometers) and energy expenditure (determinant of the intensity of the activity) varies across activity types, the combination of GPS with accelerometers has the potential to improve the accuracy of determining PA intensity during daily life in children and adolescents.

It is important to note that while GPSs are highly effective for outdoor activities, they may have limitations in indoor environments or areas with poor satellite visibility. In such cases, accelerometers or gyroscopes are more reliable. GPS may be a good complement for providing a more comprehensive picture of overall PA patterns.

Gyroscopes Gyroscopes may play a crucial role in measuring PA, especially in devices such as accelerometers and inertial measurement units (IMUs). Gyroscopes are able to measure the angular rate (i.e., the rate of rotation or angular velocity around a specific axis). In the context of PA, gyroscopes can detect changes in orientation and movement. They provide information about how fast an object (such as a person's limb or the device itself) rotates. Accurate measurements of angular velocity might contribute to the detection of specific movements and gestures, such as recognizing whether a person is walking, running, or performing specific exercises, and this might then help to improve the quantification of PA intensity, as explained in the previous section.

4.2.9 Smartphones

The potential of smartphones for measuring PA is noteworthy. Like activity wristbands, smartphones feature accelerometers as motion sensors; additionally, they house various other sensors, such as gyroscopes and GPS devices, that could provide diverse insights into PA [9]. However, despite their multitude of sensors, smartphones have predominantly been utilized for quantifying steps and distances, resembling the functionality of a pedometer [9].

A key advantage lies in the widespread use of smartphones globally, enabling large-scale data collection and facilitating big data analyses. For instance, a notable study published in the prestigious journal *Nature* analyzed global PA inequality between countries using step data from a specific mobile application (http://activityinequality.stanford.edu/) [9].

Nevertheless, smartphones have limitations, including variability in how they are carried or worn, affecting the accuracy of PA measurements. Differences between sensors in various devices can also impact the results. Additionally, in populations where smartphone usage is infrequent, such as certain children, using smartphones for PA measurement may be compromised. Otherwise, those populations in which smartphones are popular might benefit from not only measuring their PA patterns but also promoting their PA habits through the use of game-based approaches.

4.3 Method of Choice

The choice of instruments for assessing PA substantially depends on the specific characteristics one seeks to identify within the activity patterns. For instance, if the goal is to assess PA during a particular time frame (such as within a training session or PA lesson), direct observation could be used as a fitting method, or device-based methods that provide a timestamp to isolate such a time frame could also be used as an alternative. Otherwise, pedometers and accelerometers are ideal for ambulatory activities. If the focus is on capturing overall movement, device measures such as accelerometers or their combination with GPS might yield valuable insights. Notably, the most economical alternative among these methods lies in report-based approaches. While offering information with less precision in terms of parameters such as intensity or volume, these methods remain valuable at large scales. The specific outcomes desired, and the level of accuracy required will vary in different settings (clinical, research, or public health). This main decision requires the user to have a clear understanding of the dimensions of PA that need to be measured to capture the desired outcome. Combinations of multiple PA assessments are recommended; however, multiple measurements may not be necessary if an investigator or practitioner is interested in only one facet of PA.

4.4 Decision Factors

Despite the many tools available for assessing PA, recent emphasis has been placed on the reproducibility, comparability, and reliability of the instruments. Elements such as validity (the accuracy of measurement) and reliability (the consistency of measures when the instrument is used repeatedly), together with purpose of the evaluation, cost-effectiveness, strengths, and limitations, should be considered in the decision-making process.

Instruments provide distinct types of information regarding PA, such as its type, timing, location, or purpose. Reporting-based methods can offer insights into these aspects, while device-based methods yield more precise information about the quantity of PA, including intensity, frequency, volume, or the number of steps taken. Importantly, it has been underscored that defining the context and measurement model of a questionnaire is pivotal for scrutinizing the instrument's properties accurately. This involves a meticulous consideration of factors such as the type of activity, the time of day, and the intended purpose. Such clarity is indispensable for establishing robust associations between PA patterns and health indicators, ultimately enabling more targeted and effective interventions in the realm of child and adolescent health.

4.4.1 Selecting Tool

Traditionally, validity and feasibility have been the two major determinants considered when selecting the tool to assess PA. Classifying the feasibility versus validity of the different instruments is very common in the field of PA measurement and has been the cornerstone of the seminars on this topic in recent decades.

However, this is an oversimplified answer to a complex dilemma. Putting aside the obvious characteristics that the selected tool should have demonstrated, e.g., validity and reliability, and of course, the feasibility of the tool, there are still a handful of tools that might be selected; thus, what is the next step in the decision-making process? The major decision factors we should focus our attention on are the purpose of the evaluation and the setting in which the measurement takes place. Similarly, five key characteristics have been described that should be recognized when selecting a PA measure [9, 10]:

(a) Purpose of the assessment
(b) Objectivity of the tool
(c) Participants and administrator burden
(d) Strengths and limitations of each instrument
(e) Population characteristics

4.4.1.1 Purpose of the Assessment

The first crucial step in this process involves defining the dimensions and domains that one aims to measure, ensuring a comprehensive understanding of the facets of PA that are pertinent to the assessment. Identifying these dimensions provides a conceptual framework for selecting appropriate tools that can be used to effectively measure them. For example, when the goal is to measure PA at the group level and with minimal resources, employing questionnaires emerges as a viable and efficient option. Questionnaires provide self-reported data from individuals within a population, offering insights into their activity levels or even preferences and perceived barriers. This method is particularly useful for obtaining a broad overview and identifying trends within a community or in the school context.

For a more in-depth exploration of motivations and promotion strategies related to PA, interviews become an invaluable tool. Conducting interviews allows us to determine the subjective experiences, personal motivations, and potential hindrances faced by individuals in maintaining an active lifestyle.

In cases where an objective and precise measurement of PA at an individual level is needed, leveraging technology through device-based methods such as accelerometers, fitness trackers, or smartwatches becomes essential. These tools offer accurate information on an individual's movement patterns, capturing steps, volume, and even the intensity of PA. The choice of device depends on the specific requirements of the assessment, ranging from consumer-grade devices or smartphones for promoting PA in settings such as schools to research-grade devices for rigorous scientific investigations.

Consumer-grade devices and smartphones, with their user-friendly interfaces and accessibility, are particularly effective at promoting PA, especially in environments such as schools.

Researchers utilizing these tools can generate robust and nuanced data, facilitating a deeper understanding of the physiological, psychological, and sociodemographic factors influencing PA patterns. This level of detail is invaluable for informing evidence-based interventions and policies aimed at promoting PA on a broader scale.

In conclusion, the purpose of assessing PA determines the choice of tools and methodologies employed. Defining the dimensions and domains of interest is the initial step in guiding the selection of appropriate assessment tools. Whether questionnaires are used for group-level insights, interviews are used for detailed motivations, or devices are used for objective individual measurements, each method serves a unique purpose. Moreover, tailoring the choice of tools to the specific context, be it consumer-grade devices for promotional initiatives or research-grade instruments for scientific inquiries, ensures that the assessment aligns with its intended objectives, contributing to a more comprehensive understanding of PA and its impact on health and well-being.

4.4.1.2 Objectivity of the Tool

When evaluating the objectivity of tools used to measure PA, it is important to recognize that no method is entirely free from subjectivity. The objectivity of different tools varies, and understanding this spectrum is essential for accurate and meaningful assessments. Here, we present a subjective-to-objective scale that includes common tools: interviews, questionnaires, activity diaries, and wearable devices.

Interviews Heavily rely on verbal communication. While they allow for in-depth exploration, they introduce subjectivity through interpretation. Responses may be influenced by recall bias, personal perception, or the respondent's understanding of the questions.

Questionnaires Provide a structured framework aiming to standardize information collection. However, subjectivity can still arise due to self-reports, as individuals may interpret questions differently or may have difficulty recalling important specific details of daily PA.

Activity Diaries Involve participants in recording their activities over a specified period. This method introduces a temporal component, potentially reducing recall bias. Nevertheless, subjectivity persists, as individuals may not record every detail or may alter entries based on their perception of the desired response.

Device-Based Methods Positioned on the more objective side of the scale, wearable devices, such as accelerometers, offer real-time, quantifiable data. These tools minimize reliance on self-reports, providing an objective measure of PA. While wearable devices enhance objectivity, processing decisions during their use introduce some subjectivity. For instance, setting sleep schedules or establishing activity intensity thresholds involves subjective decisions. Assumptions about what constitutes a meaningful level of PA may vary between individuals and populations.

The objectivity of PA measurement tools exists on a spectrum. While interviews, questionnaires, and activity diaries introduce subjectivity, wearable devices enhance objectivity but are not immune to subjectivity, particularly in decision-making processes. Recognizing the inherent subjectivity of each tool is crucial for researchers and practitioners to make informed decisions and draw accurate conclusions from PA data.

4.4.1.3 Participant and Administrator Burden

Another essential consideration in the choice of adequate PA assessment is the burden imposed on both participants and administrators when selecting assessment instruments. Assessing PA in youth involves soliciting information directly from the participants. The burden placed on them can vary significantly depending on the chosen assessment tool. Additionally, understanding the burden on administrators is crucial for optimizing the efficiency of data collection processes. For example, digital tools can alleviate some of these burdens, but the selection of an assessment method remains a critical consideration. The following is an overview of the participant and administrator burdens associated with different instruments:

Questionnaires are simple methods that impose low levels of demand on participants. The structured nature of the questions allows for straightforward and relatively quick responses. Administrators, while still experiencing a moderate burden, primarily deal with tasks related to data entry and digitalization of information. The process becomes more streamlined when questionnaires are conducted digitally.

The interviews are in the middle of the burden spectrum, offering a more interactive approach than questionnaires. However, they require participants to engage in conversation, making them somewhat more demanding. Administrators face a substantial burden from interviews involving tasks such as transcribing, interpreting language nuances, and making judgments about responses, which adds to the overall complexity of the population.

Diaries carry a notably high burden, requiring a substantial commitment from participants. Maintaining a daily record of activities demands discipline and consistent effort. Administrators also encounter a moderate burden with diaries, primarily related to tasks such as data entry and digitalization. However, this burden is less intensive than the challenges involved in transcribing interviews.

Device-based methods introduce a variable burden that can range from low to moderate, depending on the nature of the requirements. Simply wearing a device may impose a low burden, but if participants need to log daily sleep or activity details, the burden could increase. The level of engagement and the specific tasks assigned to participants play crucial roles in determining the overall burden associated with using devices in research methodologies. Importantly, administrators may encounter various burdens related to device management and data processing. The administrator burden encompasses tasks such as device setup, troubleshooting, and ensuring participants' compliance with device usage. The processing burden arises from the need to manage and analyze the data collected from devices. Depending on the complexity and volume of the data, administrators may face challenges in terms of data entry, storage, and organization. The decision-making burden is another aspect to consider, especially when devices generate large amounts of data with varying degrees of relevance. Administrators may need to make decisions about data filtering, prioritization, and interpretation. This burden is heightened if the devices provide real-time data, requiring timely decisions on how to manage and analyze the information effectively.

Understanding and carefully considering participant and administrator burdens are essential when choosing PA assessment tools for children and adolescents. Balancing the need for accurate data with the practicalities of implementation ensures that assessments are both reliable and feasible, especially given the complexity of the movement behaviors of children and adolescents.

4.4.1.4 Population Characteristics

One notable challenge is encountered when evaluating PA in young children, as they may face difficulties in accurately recalling and assessing their activity levels. Understanding the diverse characteristics of the population is fundamental to designing effective PA measures. Age, developmental stage, and cognitive ability are critical factors that influence how individuals perceive their PA levels. Young children may have difficulties reporting their activities accurately due to limitations in their memory development. This challenge can lead to underestimation or overestimation of their actual activity. Expressing PA verbally can be challenging for children, especially those in the early stages of language development. Subjectivity in interpreting the intensity and duration of activities compounds these challenges, making standardization difficult. This may result in incomplete or inaccurate descriptions of their activities. The subjective interpretation of activities may differ from an adult's perspective, making it difficult to standardize assessments.

To address these issues, various solutions can be implemented. Observational methods, where trained observers directly assess children's PA, offer a more accurate alternative to self-reports. The inclusion of parents or caregivers of children under 10 years of age in the assessment process can provide valuable supplementary information, contributing to a more comprehensive understanding of children's movement behaviors, although the limited validity of these reports should be kept in mind. Device-based methods, such as accelerometers or wearable devices, offer real-time data, eliminating the need for self-reports and providing a more quantifiable assessment. Additionally, incorporating visual aids or game-based approaches can increase the level of engagement in the assessment process for young children, potentially improving their ability to recall and report activities accurately. At this stage, a combined approach of device-based and report-based measures may allow a more accurate characterization of PA behavior.

4.5 Final Considerations

The assessment of PA in children and adolescents emerges as a multifaceted challenge, necessitating the consideration of various factors in comprehending the intricacies associated with their movement lifestyles [11]. Reporting-based methods offer insights into the contextual, objective, and qualitative dimensions of PA. However, their efficacy is constrained by a lack of precision in gauging the volume and intensity of the activities undertaken. While device-based methods, such as movement sensors, provide a broader perspective on activity patterns, integrating them with report-based methods is critical for understanding the complexity of movement patterns [11].

The integration of new technologies emerges as a potent tool, presenting a valuable opportunity for continuous monitoring of PA, both within and outside the school environment. Initiatives are needed to address the mounting volume of data and the escalating use of devices, particularly smartphones, among adolescent demographic issues. The impending era of "big data" promises sophisticated tools that will illuminate the complexity of patterns of PA among children and adolescents throughout the day. This approach holds substantial promise for clinical practice, as it offers a precise and comprehensive understanding of PA in this population and of its correlations with health markers.

The accurate determination of PA assumes pivotal significance, as it not only serves as a diagnostic compass but also directs interventions toward areas that can most effectively enhance different facets of health [11]. As we explore the complex relationships among technology, data, and PA, there is growing potential to enhance interventions and promote healthier lifestyles among younger generations [12].

References

1. Caspersen CJ, Powell KE, Christenson GM. Physical activity, exercise, and physical fitness: definitions and distinctions for health-related research. Public Health Rep. 1985;100(2):126.
2. Bull FC, Al-Ansari SS, Biddle S, Borodulin K, Buman MP, Cardon G, et al. World Health Organization 2020 guidelines on physical activity and sedentary behaviour. Br J Sports Med. 2020;54(24):1451–62.
3. Janz KF, Lutuchy EM, Wenthe P, Levy SM. Measuring activity in children and adolescents using self-report: PAQ-C and PAQ-A. Med Sci Sports Exerc. 2008;40(4):767–72.

4. Tudor-Locke C, Williams JE, Reis JP, Pluto D. Utility of pedometers for assessing physical activity. Sports Med. 2004;34(5):281–91.
5. Tudor-Locke C, Lutes L. Why do pedometers work? Sports Med. 2009;39(12):981–93.
6. Migueles JH, Cadenas-Sanchez C, Ekelund U, Delisle Nyström C, Mora-Gonzalez J, Löf M, et al. Accelerometer data collection and processing criteria to assess physical activity and other outcomes: a systematic review and practical considerations. Sports Med. 2017;47(9):1821–45.
7. Keadle SK, Lyden KA, Strath SJ, Staudenmayer JW, Freedson PS. A framework to evaluate devices that assess physical behavior. Exerc Sport Sci Rev. 2019;47(4):206–14.
8. Migueles JH, Rowlands AV, Huber F, Sabia S, van Hees VT. GGIR: a research community–driven open source R package for generating physical activity and sleep outcomes from multi-day raw accelerometer data. J Meas Phys Behav. 2019;2(3):188–96.
9. Althoff T, Sosič R, Hicks JL, King AC, Delp SL, Leskovec J. Large-scale physical activity data reveal worldwide activity inequality. Nature. 2017;547(7663):336–9.
10. Sylvia LG, Bernstein EE, Hubbard JL, Keating L, Anderson EJ. Practical guide to measuring physical activity. J Acad Nutr Diet. 2013;114(2):199–208.
11. Barnett L, Hinkley T, Okely AD, Salmon J. Child, family and environmental correlates of children's motor skill proficiency. J Sci Med Sport. 2012;16(4):332–6.
12. Tremblay MS. Challenges in global surveillance of physical activity. Lancet Child Adolesc Health. 2020;4(1):2–3.

Chapter 5
Health-Related Physical Fitness Assessment in School Settings

Kai Zhang, Cristina Cadenas-Sanchez, Brooklyn Fraser, and Justin J. Lang

5.1 Introduction

Physical fitness comprises multiple components that collectively demonstrate an individual's ability to perform physical activity (PA) [1]. These components are divided into two categories, depending on whether they relate more to public health

---

K. Zhang
Healthy Active Living and Obesity Research Group, Children's Hospital of Eastern Ontario Research Institute, Ottawa, ON, Canada

School of Human Kinetics, University of Ottawa, Ottawa, ON, Canada

C. Cadenas-Sanchez
Department of Cardiology, Stanford University, Stanford, CA, USA

Veterans Affairs Palo Alto Health Care System, Palo Alto, CA, USA

Department of Physical Education and Sports, Faculty of Sports Science, Sport and Health University Research Institute (iMUDS), Granada, Spain

B. Fraser
Menzies Institute for Medical Research, University of Tasmania, Hobart, TAS, Australia

Alliance for Research in Exercise, Nutrition and Activity (ARENA), University of South Australia, Adelaide, SA, Australia

J. J. Lang (✉)
Alliance for Research in Exercise, Nutrition and Activity (ARENA), University of South Australia, Adelaide, SA, Australia

Centre for Surveillance and Applied Research, Public Health Agency of Canada, Ottawa, ON, Canada

School of Epidemiology and Public Health, Faculty of Medicine, University of Ottawa, Ottawa, ON, Canada
e-mail: justin.lang@phac-aspc.gc.ca

© The Author(s), under exclusive license to Springer Nature Switzerland AG 2024
A. García-Hermoso (ed.), *Promotion of Physical Activity and Health in the School Setting*, https://doi.org/10.1007/978-3-031-65595-1_5

or athletic ability: (a) health-related fitness: cardiorespiratory fitness (CRF), musculoskeletal fitness (MF), flexibility, and body composition and (b) skill-related fitness: agility, balance, coordination, power, speed, and reaction time [2]. The classification of fitness components has been debated for decades [3, 4]. For instance, muscular power was historically recognized as a skill-related component, whereas contemporary evidence highlights its greater relevance to health than flexibility [4, 5]. Despite these constant discussions, scientists unanimously recognize that achieving an adequate level of physical fitness is important for the health and well-being of children and adolescents (collectively referred to as youth hereinafter), particularly the components related to health. Cross-sectional studies suggest that high health-related fitness levels among youth are associated with a range of health benefits, such as better cardiovascular, skeletal, and mental health [6–8]. Longitudinal studies have shown that fitness levels track across the lifespan, and the levels during childhood or adolescence strongly predict cardiovascular profile, disability, and premature mortality in adulthood [9–11]. This is especially important for population health planning and thus strengthens the rationale for early detection of fitness levels and trends among generations. In addition, the youth's physical fitness measures can be considered a facilitator for the essential skills needed to achieve PA goals [12]. Further, evaluating fitness levels in youth, especially CRF, summarizing the physiological response to an individual's PA, can objectively indicate youths' recent PA levels [13]. Thus, the measures of health-related fitness can help identify who may be at risk for health issues or lack adequate PA.

Assessing health-related fitness through laboratory methods is often impractical for large populations due to resource, technical, and time limitations. There is a growing interest in using field-based physical fitness measurements for population health surveillance [14]. Evidence suggests that these measures are scalable for large population settings, especially within school environments for students [15]. The school system has recently become a favorable location to implement national fitness surveillance for youth, such as in Korea and Slovenia [16]. Over 15 published physical fitness test batteries exist worldwide for preschoolers and youth; the FitnessGram, Eurofit, and ALPHA are the most widely used internationally. Nevertheless, considerable deviations are evident in the measures, protocols, and data reporting of fitness assessment, creating a need for more work in fitness assessments in the school context to avoid the potential for negative outcomes [17]. Hence, several considerations may be undertaken, including pedagogical meaning, supportive feedback, and safety requirements.

This chapter introduces health-related physical fitness components and identifies reliable, valid, and feasible fitness assessments in school settings. This chapter will also explore the challenges encountered during the assessment process within school settings, followed by the proposal of strategies to facilitate successful implementation. Lastly, emerging issues and areas of future research will be outlined.

5.2 Overview of Health-Related Physical Fitness

5.2.1 Introducing Health-Related Physical Fitness Components

This section concisely presents the definitions, health implications, and common laboratory-based assessments for each component of health-related physical fitness.

5.2.1.1 Cardiorespiratory Fitness

CRF reflects an individual's ability to transport oxygen from the atmosphere to the mitochondria to support energy production during muscular activity [18]. International trends indicate a decline in CRF among youth since the 1980s. Despite a mild resurgence in the 2010s, a significant downward trend persists [19]. Promoting regular PA that target increased CRF among youth is crucial for effective health promotion. Improved CRF is not only a result of vigorous PA but also an indicator of enhanced overall health [20]. CRF is meaningfully associated with multiple cardiovascular risk factors among youth [16]. Evidence also indicates that high CRF levels are associated with better academic achievement and cognition among youth [21]. Furthermore, a large body of evidence supports CRF levels in youth being inversely related to metabolic and cardiovascular health in adulthood [18]. More importantly, among adults, CRF is a strong predictor of cardiovascular diseases (CVD), all-cause mortality, and mortality attributable to various cancers [22]. In 2020, the American Heart Association published a statement underscoring the critical role of CRF in youth health, advocating for its integration into clinical practice [23]. While lab-based measures of CRF with indirect calorimetry, also known as maximal cardiopulmonary exercise testing (CPX), are widely considered the gold standard for assessing peak oxygen uptake (VO_{2max}), their practicality in school settings is limited due to costly equipment, a lack of technicians, and time constraints. CPX also requires participants to attain maximal exertion until exhaustion on a graded treadmill or cycle ergometer, which poses risks and is unsuitable for some young children.

5.2.1.2 Musculoskeletal Fitness

MF is defined as a multidimensional concept: muscular strength (i.e., the ability to exert a maximal force on one occasion); endurance (i.e., the ability to continue to perform successive exertions or repetitions against a submaximal load); and power (i.e., the ability to exert force per unit of time) [24]. Improved MF is a marker and a benefit of vigorous-intensity physical activities, including those that strengthen muscle and bone, which are strongly recommended by the World Health Organization (WHO) PA and sedentary behavior guidelines for youth [25]. Published studies present mixed findings on the secular trends of youth MF across different countries, year spans, and tests [19]. These inconsistencies are particularly concerning regarding the significance of MF for health. Existing systematic reviews corroborate a prospective negative association between MF in childhood and adiposity and cardiometabolic parameters later in life, with a positive association for future bone health [26] and positive cross-sectional associations for self-esteem and perceived competence [5]. Moreover, recent evidence highlights muscular strength as a reliable predictor of all-cause mortality in adults [27, 28], underscoring the importance of assessing MF in schools, given its robustness to track from youth into mid-adulthood [10]. The lab-based standard measurement of MF employs dynamometry, examining specifically by isometric, isokinetic, and single-repetition maximal isotonic tests (1-RM, typically regarded as the gold-standard measure of muscular strength) on specific muscles or muscle groups [29].

5.2.1.3 Flexibility

Flexibility is described as the ability of body tissues to move a single or a series of joints through their maximal range of motion (ROM) without causing injury [30]. It is an important fitness component because insufficient flexibility can hinder the performance of daily tasks, especially motor activities [31]. Flexibility activities, such as yoga and stretching, are exclusively recommended for youth in PA guidelines [25]. In youth, hamstring flexibility is associated with motor competence [32]. In addition, the lack of flexibility during this stage may contribute to current and future episodes of low-back pain [33], which has become a costly medical issue globally [34]. There is ongoing debate regarding whether flexibility should continue as a major fitness component, as it lacks predictive and concurrent validity to meaningful health and performance outcomes than other fitness components [30]. However, some highlight the robust cardiovascular, metabolic, and skeletal muscle adaptations that can occur due to stretching and flexibility training [30, 35]. The gold-standard flexibility assessment involves using a goniometer to measure a specific joint's ROM [36], such as cervical spine flexion or hip abduction.

5.2.1.4 Body Composition

Body composition refers to the different body tissue types, mainly muscle, fat, and bone, that are related to health [37]. More often, the components are limited to fat-free mass (FFM), body mass index (BMI), and body fat percentage (BF%), reflecting the energy balance between diet and physical activities [38]. As a result of the high prevalence of childhood obesity, body composition assessment has been emphasized in youth since the health hazards of overweight and obesity are well-accepted in public health and clinical settings [39]. However, obesity is not the only concern because too low body fat levels also merit recognition for its associated health risks. This is particularly relevant in certain areas where children are at greater risk for developing undernutrition or eating disorders [40]. Body composition is also a modifier that affects fitness performance, thereby offering valuable insights into the overall health condition of youth [4]. Body composition changes constantly throughout childhood [41], and there are several methods used to quantify a living individual's total body composition in the laboratory [31]. Underwater (hydrostatic) weighing has traditionally been considered a gold standard for BF% [31]. Other lab-based methods, including densitometry, air displacement plethysmography, and dual-energy X-ray absorptiometry (DXA), have been widely used in youth research [42].

5.2.2 Measuring Health-Related Physical Fitness Among Youth in School Settings

This section highlights the most common field-based measures of physical fitness while discussing their reliability, validity, feasibility, and secular performance among youth.

5.2.2.1 Cardiorespiratory Fitness

Field-based measures of CRF, many of which are reliable, valid, and feasible, allow many participants to be tested simultaneously.

(a) 20-m shuttle run test (20mSRT), was first introduced by Professor Luc Léger in the 1980s [43]. It has become the primary global field-based assessment of CRF in youth, implemented in over 50 countries [16]. As a progressive test, the 20mSRT requires participants to run between two lines 20 m apart, paced by an audio recording that usually starts at 8.5 km/h, increasing by 0.5 km/h per minute. Participants continue until they cannot synchronize with the audio pace for two consecutive laps, at which point their score (e.g., laps, stages, time) is recorded [43]. The 20mSRT has well-documented high reliability [44] and moderate to high criterion validity [45, 46], which means personal VO_{2max} can be estimated from the test score using validated equations [43, 47]. Further, it is applicable in population-based surveillance as it is time- and cost-effective, allowing multiple participants to test simultaneously with minimal equipment and flexible locations [48]. Although youth's motivations and performance can impact the results of CRF tests [49], the protocol of 20mSRT incorporating a progressive pace with audio signals alleviates this concern. While assessors (e.g., schoolteachers) may encounter difficulties recording those who fail to reach the end lines in a large testing group, implementing practical training could mitigate this issue. Synthesizing 20mSRT performance data, [14] identified Northern European and sub-Saharan African youths as exhibiting the

highest global CRF levels. However, they observed a decline exceeding 7% from 1981 to 2014, followed by decelerated and stable changes since 2000.
(b) Run tests have long been used in school-based fitness surveys in different countries [50, 51]. During run tests, participants are assigned a specific distance or time, and they are instructed to complete the race in the shortest possible time or cover the longest possible distance [23]. Among the run tests, the 1.5-mile distance and 12-min time exhibit high reliability [44, 52] and the highest criterion validity, ranging from moderate to high [53]. Despite their longstanding usage in schools, run tests pose challenges, including a preference for distance runs over timed ones for quicker record-keeping [54], impracticality in schools without adequate infrastructure and space (e.g., playgrounds), and variability of test results affected by individual motivation, pace ability, and external factors like weather. Asian countries have largely used distance run tests (e.g., Japan, Korea), with Japanese youth notably outperforming their peers before the 2000s [55]. However, temporal analysis of run tests from five continents signals a considerable decline (4–5% per decade) from the mid-1970s [51]. Nonetheless, these comparative data and trends warrant updates.

5.2.2.2 Musculoskeletal Fitness

Unlike CRF, no universal measure represents total MF levels, a characteristic also observed in field-based tests [31]. Field tests often correspond to distinct body parts (e.g., hand, leg) and different MF components (i.e., strength, endurance, and power), suggesting that MF assessments from one region (e.g., hands) cannot represent MF in another (e.g., legs) [56]. Furthermore, superior leg power (long jump performance) does not imply equivalent leg endurance (prolonged squats). As a result, a small subset of assessments is usually used in test batteries to extrapolate the "whole body" MF, although the validity of this approach has been questioned [57].

(a) Handgrip strength (HGS), characterized as a maximal isometric grip force task [58], is a practical, scalable, and feasible method for assessing overall strength for clinical and population screening and surveillance [56]. When testing HGS, the youth squeeze the handgrip dynamometer as hard as possible for 5 s, and the instructors record the scores, usually in kilograms [59]. It has high to very high test-retest reliability in youth [44] and high to very high construct validity with upper body, lower body, and overall strength [58, 60]. Nonetheless, careful consideration of protocol differences (e.g., elbow flexed or extended, both hands or the dominant hand, seated or standing) and device variations (e.g., grip size, calibration, brand) is necessary to ensure validity [61, 62]. Furthermore, the HGS is a test safe for youth and requires little tester expertise. Due to its brief duration (about 2 min per person) and minimal participant effort, it limits the need for participant motivation and boasts a high completion rate. The National Academy of Medicine (NAM) recommends it as an acceptable measure for school-based settings [4]. A recent review examined global trends in youth

HGS, indicating a general improvement between 1967 and 2017. However, these trends varied across countries, with noticeable declines among youth from Australia, Estonia, Canada, England, Spain, and Turkey within different age spans [56]. Cross-country comparisons are largely absent in the literature, and existing data needs to be updated [55].

(b) The standing long jump (SLJ) is another widely used test for assessing lower-body muscular power in most batteries [63]. It is a practical, feasible, and scalable measurement of functional explosive strength for population screening and surveillance. During the SLJ, youth are asked to stand behind the starting line, push off vigorously, and jump as far as possible [64]. The process takes approximately 5 min per participant and is easily administered by untrained schoolteachers [65]. SLJ shows near-perfect reliability in youth, with reliability coefficients improving with age [66]. It also shows strong construct validity when compared with other lower- and upper-body (e.g., basketball throw and push-ups) explosive strength tests (e.g., vertical jump, squat jump, and countermovement jump) [64, 67]. Like HGS, SLJ has minimal participant fatigue effects and is generally safe, which is also recommended by NAM for school-based testing [4]. Tomkinson et al.'s recent review (2021) examining the latest global temporal trends in SLJ performance in youth showed an initial steady increase from the 1960s to the 1980s, followed by a slowdown in the 1990s and a subsequent decline since 2000 [68]. The overall improvement observed over the analyzed period was negligible (1.73 cm). Similar to HGS, international comparisons in SLJ are limited, and updates are warranted [55].

(c) Field-based tests assessing core muscular endurance are also widely used in fitness test batteries [57]. Common tests such as curl-ups, push-ups, sit-ups, and pull-ups demonstrate acceptable reliability and validity and are currently employed in youth assessments [20]. However, there is limited evidence linking muscular endurance to health in youth [26], although some evidence exists for adults [69, 70]. Temporal changes in muscular endurance show mixed findings, with consistent declines observed in arm hang tests across Europe [15]. However, increases have been reported in Greece, New Zealand, and Portugal, while decreases were observed in England and Poland for curl-ups/sit-ups tests [65].

5.2.2.3 Flexibility

Given the numerous joints in the human body, it is not feasible for a single test to comprehensively evaluate an individual's overall flexibility. Sit-and-reach test (SRT), initially designed by Wells and Dillon [71], and its modified versions (e.g., back-saver SRT [72] have been primarily included in fitness test batteries for estimating hamstring and lumbar spine flexibility. The SRT records the fingertips-to-tangent feet distance while youth sit on the floor with legs fully extended and feet against a marked testing box [73]. The SRT demonstrates high reliability among youth [74], but low to moderate and low criterion validity for estimating hamstring and lumbar flexibility, respectively [75]. Unlike angular tests such as knee extension, the SRT is a linear test with simple procedures that are easy to administer. It requires minimal skills training to conduct, and the equipment necessary for the test is affordable. The cross-country comparisons of SRT still need to be present in the literature, while the reported secular trends of SRT from different countries are mixed (Table 5.1).

5.2.2.4 Body Composition

(a) BMI, based on height and weight (weight (kg)/height (m)^2), is the most common and practical method to estimate body fat worldwide. Unlike adults with definite BMI cut-points for weight status (e.g., normal and overweight) recommended by WHO, youth have no fixed threshold since their BMIs change with age and vary between sexes [76]. As such, the weight status thresholds are defined using z-scores, which indicate the number of standard deviations by which a given BMI deviates from the median BMI for a specific age and sex population published by WHO [77]. Available evidence shows high intra- and inter-observer reliability in measuring BMI in children [78]. While BMI generally indicates moderate validity compared to BF% in youth [79], it has long been criticized for its lack of differentiation between FFM and fat mass [80]. However, despite this limitation, youth's BMI shows strong validity in predicting future cardiovascular profiles and risk of death, outperforming even more accurate and complex measures (e.g., hydrostatic weighing). As a result, it is generally well-accepted in population surveillance and clinical settings [81]. Validation studies have reported that schoolteachers or staff can conduct highly accurate anthropometric measurements in school settings [82, 83]. However, ethical debates surrounding confidentiality and privacy, school-to-parent notifi-

Table 5.1 International secular trends of sit-and-reach test and waist circumference among youth

Country	Citation(s)	SRT	WC
Brazil	[95, 96]	↓ (2008–2014)	≈ (2002–2007)
Canada	[97]	? (2007–2017)	↘ (2007–2017)
China	[98–100]	≈ (1985–2014)	↗ (1993–2015)
Croatia	[101]	? (1999–2013)	
Hong Kong	[102]	? (1998–2015)	
Japan	[103]		↑ (1978–1994)
Korea	[104]		≈ (2005–2015)
Lithuania	[105]	↓ (1992–2012)	
Mozambique	[106]	↓ (1992–2012)	
Spain	[107]		↑ (1995–2002)
US	[108]		↑ (1998–2004)

Note: *SRT* sit-and-reach test, *WC* waist circumference, ↑ increasing, ↓ decreasing, ↗ general increasing with few mixed findings, ↘ general decreasing with few mixed findings, ≈ no significant change, ? fluctuations across years or mixed findings between age and sex subgroups

cation policy, and students' discomfort with BMI measurements remain unresolved and warrant attention [84]. International increases in BMI trends have recently plateaued after four decades in many high-income European countries and Asia-Pacific regions since 2000, while accelerating in East and South Asia [85]. However, despite the overall rise in BMI, more youth continue to experience moderate to severe underweight, especially in Central, East, and West Africa [85].

(b) WC measurement identifies those with the abdominal type of obesity, which is widely used to assess body composition in fitness assessments. Importantly, WC is the essential component of the metabolic syndrome definition endorsed by the International Diabetes Federation (IDF) [86]. It is typically measured in the horizontal plane midway between the lowest ribs and the iliac crest using an inelastic measuring tape [87]. Like BMI, cut-points of WC to define central obesity in adults have been proposed by the IDF [88] and WHO [87]. Recommendations for youth generally reflect the age- and sex-specific 90th percentile developed by country-specific samples [89–92] or international pooled data [93]. WC shows high intra- and inter-observer reliability [44] and criterion-related validity compared to abdominal adipose tissues [79]. Moreover, WC may better predict the risk of CVD and mortality than BMI [94] and is often recommended for clinical practice. However, although WC can be taken reasonably quickly in school settings, it is not free of self-esteem influence. For this reason, and to protect youth privacy during exposure of the trunk, WC should be assessed in an appropriate space (e.g., a nurse's office) instead of in group settings [4]. There is a lack of international trends or cross-country comparisons regarding WC, while the reported secular trends from different countries yield mixed findings (Table 5.1).

5.2.3 Measuring Health-Related Physical Fitness in Preschool Children

This section introduces the most common fitness measures among preschoolers and briefly compares them with those among youth.

5.2.3.1 Common Field-Based Fitness Tests

(a) For CRF, the 20mSRT, the 0.5-mile run/walk, and the 3-min run seem to be the dominant field-based measures in preschoolers, showing acceptable reliability [109]. A preschooler-adapted version of the 20mSRT beginning at a running speed of 6.5 km/h developed for the PREFIT (Assessing FITness in PREschool children) test battery is likely the most practical. The protocol recommends that

two assessors concurrently run with a small group of preschoolers to remove the cognitive aspect of pacing, which is difficult for some preschoolers [110].
(b) For MF, the HGS and SLJ are reliable measures in preschoolers [109]. When choosing a dynamometer for HGS in preschoolers, it's crucial to consider factors such as reliability [62, 111], the ability to detect lower values (e.g., <5 kg), and an adjustable grip span, which seems to enhance reliability when set at 4 cm [112]. To improve the feasibility of SLJ, [110] suggested using footprints to replace a line to provide preschoolers with a clear starting point for their jump.
(c) For flexibility, the SRT is a reliable method for preschoolers [109]. It also shows fair criterion-related validity for estimating hamstring flexibility measured by the passive straight-leg raise test [113]. It's important to note that using an adapted sit-and-reach box, which has a lower height, enabling preschoolers to position their palms parallel to the floor rather than being elevated unnaturally, could enhance the reliability and validity of the test [113].
(d) For body composition, measures (i.e., height, weight, WC) show high reliability in preschoolers [109]. Data from the current study indicate that BMI and WC are valid measures for assessing body composition, as confirmed by DXA and magnetic resonance imaging (MRI) in preschoolers [114].

5.2.3.2 Comparisons in Fitness Tests Between Preschool Children and Youth

Measuring physical fitness in preschool children is a nascent and burgeoning area of research. It enables early detection of child developmental delays or deficiencies and sets a benchmark for future health tracking. Physical fitness tests for youth and preschool children share commonalities: a unified goal of assessing fitness levels, parallel testing methods for evaluating accordant fitness components, and the feasibility of conducting tests in school settings. Nevertheless, differences also exist. Tests tailored for preschoolers tend to be more playful, concise, and less physically demanding. They prioritize successful task completion rather than quantifiable performance, often observed in tests for youth. While there is substantial evidence among youth, future research should validate the above-mentioned fitness tests in preschool children and investigate the correlations between test performance and health indicators within this age group.

5.3 Fitness Surveillance

This section showcases the national health surveys that include fitness assessments and highlights widely used physical fitness test batteries for both preschoolers and youth.

5.3.1 National Health Surveys

National health surveys are large-scale assessments governments conduct to gather health-related information, such as blood tests, chronic disease, and PA from their populations. Some national health surveys incorporate physical fitness assessments, such as the Canadian Health Measures Survey (CHMS) and the National Health and Nutrition Examination Survey (NHANES). Despite their costs, these surveys provide valuable national fitness estimates and aid in developing norm-referenced standards [115]. Several countries, including Korea and Slovenia [20], implement youth fitness surveillance within their school systems. This strategy yields benefits for students, including tracking physical fitness and disease risk, providing feedback, and informing the design of health-promotion interventions.

5.3.2 Physical Fitness Test Batteries

Physical fitness test batteries constitute comprehensive collections of field-based tests that assess each fitness component, offering a thorough understanding of an individual's physical fitness [65]. Notable examples include FitnessGram, prevalent across the US [116] and Hungary [117]; Eurofit and the recently developed ALPHA, both extensively used throughout Europe [46, 118]. In addition, PREFIT, the first battery specially designed for preschoolers, is broadly implemented in Spain [119]. Upon concisely reviewing the health-related fitness assessments, we have suggested scalable tests for each physical fitness component implemented in school settings (Fig. 5.1).

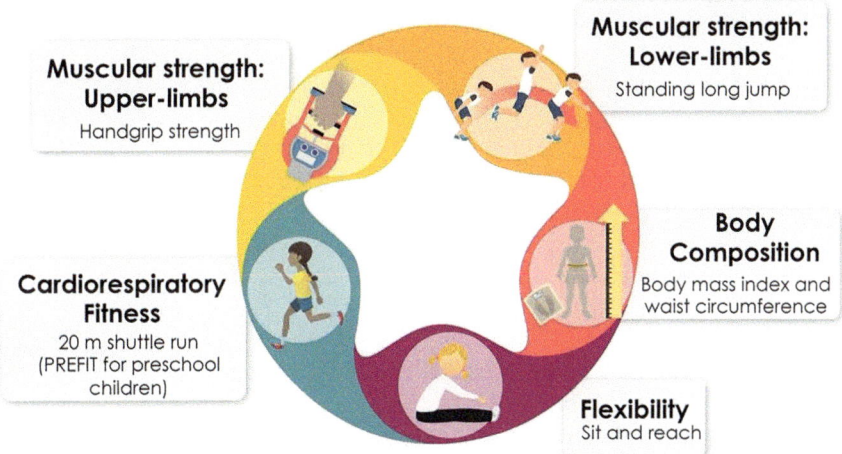

Fig. 5.1 Suggested health-related physical fitness assessment battery

5.4 Implementation of Fitness Assessment in School Settings

5.4.1 Challenges and Considerations

Most youths spend a substantial part of their day at school or in the school environment. Therefore, the school setting provides a unique opportunity to measure and monitor youth physical fitness levels. However, there are challenges and considerations that should be acknowledged and overcome before fitness testing in schools can be implemented, many of which have been discussed by the NAM [120].

5.4.1.1 Time and Resource Constraints

Although the school setting is one of the most promising locations to assess the physical fitness of school-aged youth, it is also a time-restricted setting as students must engage in all elements of the broader school curriculum [121]. Therefore, time and resource constraints are major considerations and potential challenges in introducing regular assessments of physical fitness in schools. To facilitate the school-based fitness assessment, it is crucial to engage with educators and the broader school community and to clearly convey the benefits and the need to measure, monitor, and develop childhood physical fitness levels [122]. The assessment of physical fitness should be integrated into the curriculum in a considered way to prevent any major distractions or resource reallocations and to minimize teacher and participant burden [120]. The workload of school staff is another critical consideration. If regular fitness assessments were to be implemented in school settings, testing needs to be resourced appropriately and conducted by well-trained staff.

5.4.1.2 The Precision of the Assessment Procedure

Another key consideration is ensuring a precise assessment of physical fitness. Effective school-based professional development is required to ensure educators and assessors are well-trained in implementing fitness tests safely, confidently, and reliably, with minimal bias [120]. Building and maintaining a positive and encouraging testing atmosphere is also important. It enables the youth of all performance levels to showcase their true levels without quitting or even cheating on tests, which helps bolster precision.

5.4.1.3 Interpretation and Communication of Results

As part of the professional development educators and assessors receive, training should be provided on how to interpret fitness results appropriately. Norm- and criterion-referenced fitness standards are two evaluation approaches commonly used to interpret the fitness levels of youth and discern individuals and populations that may be at risk based on fitness performance. (a) Norm-referenced standards rank youth's performance relative to peers of the same age and sex. Specifically, these individual test outcomes can be standardized into percentile ranks or z-scores within a specified population. This method enables youth to gauge their performance against others and enables comparisons between countries. Published normative values for various fitness reference points among youth are accessible from different continents [123, 124], countries [97, 125, 126], and even consolidated international datasets [93]. In preschoolers aged 3–6 years, Chile [127], Poland [128], and Spain [119] report national normative values in several physical fitness components. However, the norm-referenced approach cannot provide information on whether an individual's performance is sufficient for maintaining health [120]. Additionally, norm standards are time- and population-dependent. The temporal aspect necessitates frequent updates, which can be resource-intensive or render previous standards obsolete and invalid. (b) Criterion-referenced standards provide an absolute threshold related to health status, which a youth must attain to be considered healthy. An example is identifying cut-points in CRF that discriminate between groups of youth who have or do not have reduced cardiovascular disease risk [15, 129]. FITNESSGRAM established criterion-referenced standards in its fifth version and updated them in 2011 [130]. Two recent reviews have summarized the criterion-referenced cut-points for CRF and MF among youth [131, 132]. Assessors could use the standards above to interpret and determine if testing scores are valid or vary too far from expectations, necessitating adjusting the measures [82, 133].

Communicating results to participants and their parents/guardians consistently, with a focus on providing positive and supportive feedback, also matters [134]. Factors known to influence test performance (e.g., age, sex, pubertal status) should be considered before communicating fitness results to ensure greater context is provided (e.g., how each participant is faring to others of similar age, sex, and body size). Furthermore, consistent communication with all students is required, with a need to be equally supportive of students from a range of ability levels [84]. That said, communication and reporting techniques may need to be tailored to participants and families from a range of sociodemographic backgrounds with varying health literacy skills, for example [135].

5.4.1.4 Ethical Considerations

Ethical considerations are important and should be factored into any communication strategy related to the dissemination of fitness test results. Ensuring confidentiality is critical to maintaining the trust of the participant engaging in the testing [136]. Appropriate data storage should also be considered, whereby all fitness test results should be stored securely to ensure data are not lost and the privacy of results maintained.

5.4.1.5 Practical and Pedagogical Considerations

Before the assessment of fitness levels can be introduced in the school setting, there are practical considerations that should be overcome. For example, access to test equipment, adequate space to perform fitness tests, and appropriate class management techniques during fitness test sessions are required to ensure quality fitness testing can be conducted safely and effectively in a range of different school settings. Furthermore, to successfully implement fitness tests into the curriculum, positive pedagogical approaches to fitness testing must be considered. Key recommendations emphasize that fitness testing should be integral to fitness instruction, teachers should use test results to evaluate their instruction and student progress, and there should be an overarching expectation that all children can achieve basic health-related fitness standards [137]. Others have proposed similar recommendations, including assessing fitness as part of a year-long curriculum, ensuring students understand why they are participating in fitness assessments, and using criterion-referenced assessments instead of norm-referenced assessments [138].

5.4.2 Strategies for Successful Implementation

5.4.2.1 Training and Professional Development for Teachers

Successful fitness assessments in school settings require adequate training and support for schoolteachers. Based on the potential challenges, this procedure may comprise (a) Understanding assessment protocols. The protocols include the purpose and procedure of each assessment, ensuring that teachers are knowledgeable about the administration techniques, and maintaining consistency across assessments [139]. (b) Data collection techniques. This may include training from a fitness expert to ensure the proper use of assessment tools, along with guidance on recording and organizing assessment data. (c) Result interpretation. The aforementioned published reference standards will greatly help identify areas of improvement for individual students or groups and make informed decisions regarding promoting intervention strategies.

Overall, by prioritizing teachers' training and professional development, schools can guarantee that fitness assessments are conducted accurately, meaningfully, and in alignment with the educational goals of promoting student health and well-being.

5.4.2.2 Collaborative Approaches

Implementing fitness assessment programs in school settings requires collaboration among various stakeholders [121, 140]: (a) School administrators. Collaborating with school administrators is essential to gain their support and raise awareness regarding the role of fitness assessments within the school curriculum. It is relevant to share with them the benefits of fitness assessment in promoting student health and academic achievement and discuss how it aligns with the school's missions and goals. Administrators can help to provide resources, allocate time for assessment, and help establish a supportive environment for implementation [141]. (b) Physical education teachers. Their role is of utmost importance. They need to work closely to ensure their active involvement in the implementation process. They are in charge of the assessment protocols, data collection, and result interpretation. They collaborate to develop a shared vision and goals for fitness assessment through the different school stages (from preschool to adolescence) and provide ongoing support and guidance throughout the process [139, 142]. Moreover, fostering collaboration between physical education teachers and other teachers across disciplines would be interesting. For instance, after collecting their fitness data, the physical education teacher can coordinate with the mathematics teacher to help them analyze the data and understand their results in percentiles. (c) Parents or legal guardians. It is crucial to engage parents and legal guardians in the process by sharing information about the purpose, benefits, and procedures [143]. It is important to communicate with them through the school news (e.g., blog, app, website, etc.), parent-teacher meetings, or a specific session dedicated to doubts or questions. Also, giving information about the results of the fitness tests to the parents through a fitness report will be of great value. (d) Students. It is important to engage students (especially those older than 6 years) by involving them in the fitness assessment process and giving them the feeling of being part of the evaluation. As for students, we need to educate them about the purpose, benefits, and procedures of fitness assessment and explain how it can help them understand their own health and fitness levels. This would help encourage students to set their personal goals (e.g., improve CRF this school year) and track their progress [120].

In general, by fostering collaboration between these stakeholders, schools can create a supportive ecosystem for the successful implementation of fitness assessments. This collaborative approach ensures that all stakeholders are involved, motivated, and working towards the common goal of promoting student health and well-being.

5.4.2.3 Innovative Testing Method

Incorporating innovative approaches to fitness assessment poses a challenge, particularly when evaluating young children like preschoolers. In recent years, the implementation of various methods aimed at enhancing the attractiveness of physical education classes has become notable. These methods can also be employed in the context of fitness testing.

Utilizing gamification in fitness assessment holds particular interest as it can transform the evaluation process into an interactive and engaging experience for students [144]. To implement gamification, teachers can design fitness-related games or challenges that foster students to participate in various fitness tests while tracking their progress. For example, understanding students' preferences, such as their favorite movie, book, or TV program, can guide teachers in tailoring the games to assess fitness effectively. This approach serves as a powerful tool to keep the students engaged in fitness tests and increase their overall involvement in the assessment process.

An alternative approach for young children involves creating fairy tale or story-based fitness assessments. This strategy is particularly effective for preschoolers aged three to five, as they are familiar with listening to fairy tales. Teachers can design or adapt popular children's stories to align with fitness tests, making the assessment process more imaginative and enjoyable. For example, the PREFIT project implemented this approach successfully, where preschoolers were engaged in assisting characters like Cofito or Cofita in overcoming various adventures. In one scenario, Cofito found himself on a lipid island, seeking to escape from "grasito" (representing small deposits of adipose tissue), necessitating a fast-paced run to complete the PREFIT 4x10m shuttle run test. More details can be found elsewhere [110]. This interactive and story-driven method gives children an element of excitement and motivation to the fitness assessment experience.

5.4.2.4 Using a Common Result Metric to Report Performance

Implementing regular and consistent international/national fitness surveys using common measures is identified as a top priority when it comes to assessing and reporting the fitness of youth. This crucial aspect was ranked as the third top priority in an expert consensus derived from a Delphi Study [65]. Such emphasis calls for the need for standardized protocols and measurement practices across countries. Currently, there is a lack of standardized protocols and measurement practices across countries, leading to challenges in comparing and evaluating fitness levels on a global scale. For example, CRF is measured using a submaximal step test in Canada, a treadmill test in the USA, and various field-based tests (e.g., 20mSRT, distance runs) [120].

To provide a comprehensive understanding of the global health status of youth, it is imperative to establish regular and consistent international and national fitness surveys [65]. Standardizing measurement protocols and adopting common result metrics would facilitate accurate comparisons and enable researchers, policymakers, and professionals to gain valuable insights into the fitness levels of young populations worldwide [145, 146]. Such insights are crucial to inform evidence-based decision-making for interventions and public health initiatives targeting the well-being of young populations.

5.5 Priorities for Future Fitness Research

The abovementioned Delphi study [65], which included 46 fitness research experts from six continents, identified the top 10 international priorities for physical fitness research and surveillance among youth. Addressing these priorities is key to progressing the research field forward, with a handful pertinent to enable widespread standardized fitness assessment in school settings. Below are recommended key priorities.

5.5.1 Standardized Protocols, Common Measures, Universal Test Batteries

The identified priorities in this Delphi study were the need to implement regular and consistent international/national fitness surveys using common measures (third priority) and to develop a common/universal international field-based fitness test battery (eighth priority) [65]. Most countries do not regularly assess the physical fitness levels of youth, and in those countries that do, there are notable differences in measurement protocols [65, 147]. Thus, developing a field-based fitness test battery that includes a set of scalable, valid, reliable, and cost-effective standardized fitness measures that can be easily implemented in a school setting is essential in future fitness research.

5.5.2 Reliability and Validity of Fitness Measures

The seventh priority identified in the Delphi study was the need to continue to assess the reliability and validity of fitness measures [65]. The reliability and criterion validity of field-based fitness tests of youth have been systematically reviewed [44, 79], with findings helping determine widely used test batteries such as ALPHA [148]. However, the Delphi study [65] outlined limited reliability and validity evidence that exists on fitness tests for preschoolers and youth from low- and middle-income countries. It is also required to understand better the reliability and validity of different tests of MF and motor fitness.

5.5.3 Developing Universal Health-Related Fitness Cut-Points

The need to establish universal health-related fitness cut-points for youth was identified as the fifth priority [65] and would be instrumental in physical fitness assessment in school settings. However, the above-mentioned two recent reviews [131, 132] have concluded that data remain insufficient to establish health-related criterion-referenced cut-points for CRF and MF among youth. The variability of current evidence was driven predominantly by the lack of standardized physical fitness measures and no consensus on how best to account for body size, age, and sex. As such, the absence of universal health-related physical fitness cut-points means there is no accepted way to identify children with low fitness and is a major barrier to the interpretation and communication of physical fitness for population health. Developing universal health-related fitness cut-points would enable a more accurate understanding of the current state of youth levels, ensure consistent reporting within and between schools and countries, identify potentially unhealthy or "at risk" groups of youth, and allow trends in childhood health and fitness to be monitored.

5.6 Conclusions

Health-related physical fitness is an important aspect of maturation and development among youth because of the strong connection with not only current health status but also future health status in adulthood. There remain many ways to measure the components that help describe an individual's fitness level. Selecting an existing fitness test battery that incorporates multiple assessments is probably the best approach to ensure the use of a comprehensive assessment. When measuring fitness among youth, it is important to select standardized tests and that the protocols for these tests are followed closely. The school environment remains the most promising area to engage youth in regular and consistent fitness monitoring to help identify those in need of PA interventions. Internationally, regular fitness surveillance has been a core feature for some countries. Data from these efforts have been integral to support the interpretation of fitness data through norm-referenced values. However, there remain many areas of future research to help advance the field of fitness surveillance and measurement. An important step forward is through international collaborative research to help tackle common research objectives.

References

1. Ortega FB, Ruiz JR, Castillo MJ, Sjöström M. Physical fitness in childhood and adolescence: a powerful marker of health. Int J Obes. 2008;32(1):1–11.
2. Corbin C, Pangrazi RP, Franks D. Definitions: health, fitness, and physical activity. Washington, DC: President's Council on Physical Fitness and Sports; 2000. Available from: https://files.eric.ed.gov/fulltext/ED470696.pdf.
3. Fleishman E. The structure and measurement of physical fitness, vol. 1. 1st ed. Englewood Cliffs: Prentice-Hall; 1964. 207 p.
4. Pate RR. The evolving definition of physical fitness. Quest. 1988;40(3):174–9.
5. Smith SR, O'Neil PM, Astrup A, Finer N, Sanchez-Kam M, Fraher K, et al. Early weight loss while on lorcaserin, diet and exercise as a predictor of week 52 weight-loss outcomes. Obesity. 2014;22(10):2137–46.
6. Fraser BJ, Blizzard L, Schmidt MD, Juonala M, Dwyer T, Venn AJ, et al. Childhood cardiorespiratory fitness, muscular fitness and adult measures of glucose homeostasis. J Sci Med Sport. 2018;21(9):935–40.
7. García-Hermoso A, Ramírez-Vélez R, García-Alonso Y, Alonso-Martínez AM, Izquierdo M. Association of cardiorespiratory fitness levels during youth with health risk later in life: a systematic review and meta-analysis. JAMA Pediatr. 2020;174(10):952.

8. Henriksson H, Henriksson P, Tynelius P, Ortega FB. Muscular weakness in adolescence is associated with disability 30 years later: a population-based cohort study of 1.2 million men. Br J Sports Med. 2019;53(19):1221–30.
9. Fraser BJ, Rollo S, Sampson M, Magnussen CG, Lang JJ, Tremblay MS, et al. Health-related criterion-referenced cut-points for musculoskeletal fitness among youth: a systematic review. Sports Med. 2021;51(12):2629–46.
10. García-Hermoso A, Izquierdo M, Ramírez-Vélez R. Tracking of physical fitness levels from childhood and adolescence to adulthood: a systematic review and meta-analysis. Transl Pediatr. 2022;11(4):474–86.
11. Matton L, Thomis M, Wijndaele K, Duvigneaud N, Beunen G, Claessens AL, et al. Tracking of physical fitness and physical activity from youth to adulthood in females. Med Sci Sports Exerc. 2006;38(6):1114–20.
12. Ceschia A, Giacomini S, Santarossa S, Rugo M, Salvadego D, Da Ponte A, et al. Deleterious effects of obesity on physical fitness in pre-pubertal children. Eur J Sport Sci. 2016;16(2):271–8.
13. Ruiz JR, Rizzo NS, Hurtig-Wennlöf A, Ortega FB, Àrnberg WJ, Sjöström M. Relations of total physical activity and intensity to fitness and fatness in children: the European Youth Heart Study. Am J Clin Nutr. 2006;84(2):299–303.
14. Lang JJ, Tremblay MS, Léger L, Olds T, Tomkinson GR. International variability in 20 m shuttle run performance in children and youth: who are the fittest from a 50-country comparison? A systematic literature review with pooling of aggregate results. Br J Sports Med. 2018;52(4):276.
15. Lang JJ, Tremblay MS, Ortega FB, Ruiz JR, Tomkinson GR. Review of criterion-referenced standards for cardiorespiratory fitness: what percentage of 1 142 026 international children and youth are apparently healthy? Br J Sports Med. 2019;53(15):953–8.
16. Lang JJ. Exploring the utility of cardiorespiratory fitness as a population health surveillance indicator for children and youth: an international analysis of results from the 20-m shuttle run test. Appl Physiol Nutr Metab. 2018;43(2):211.
17. Whitehead M. Physical literacy. Unpublished paper given at IAPESWG Congress, Melbourne. 1993.
18. Ross R, Blair SN, Arena R, Church TS, Després JP, Franklin BA, et al. Importance of assessing cardiorespiratory fitness in clinical practice: a case for fitness as a clinical vital sign: a scientific statement from the American Heart Association. Circulation. 2016;134(24):e653–99. Available from: https://www.ahajournals.org/doi/10.1161/CIR.0000000000000461.
19. Tomkinson GR, Lang JJ, Tremblay MS. Temporal trends in the cardiorespiratory fitness of children and adolescents representing 19 high-income and upper middle-income countries between 1981 and 2014. Br J Sports Med. 2019;53(8):478–86.
20. Lang JJ, Tomkinson GR, Janssen I, Ruiz JR, Ortega FB, Léger L, et al. Making a case for cardiorespiratory fitness surveillance among children and youth. Exerc Sport Sci Rev. 2018;46(2):66–75.
21. Marques A, Santos DA, Hillman CH, Sardinha LB. How does academic achievement relate to cardiorespiratory fitness, self-reported physical activity and objectively reported physical activity: a systematic review in children and adolescents aged 6–18 years. Br J Sports Med. 2018;52(16):1039.
22. Han M, Qie R, Shi X, Yang Y, Lu J, Hu F, et al. Cardiorespiratory fitness and mortality from all causes, cardiovascular disease and cancer: dose–response meta-analysis of cohort studies. Br J Sports Med. 2022;56(13):733–9.
23. Raghuveer G, Hartz J, Lubans DR, Takken T, Wiltz JL, Mietus-Snyder M, et al. Cardiorespiratory fitness in youth: an important marker of health: a scientific statement from the American Heart Association. Circulation. 2020;142(7):e101–18. Available from: https://www.ahajournals.org/doi/10.1161/CIR.0000000000000866.
24. Caspersen CJ, Powell KE, Christenson GM. Physical activity, exercise, and physical fitness: definitions and distinctions for health-related research. Public Health Rep. 1985;100(2):126–31.

25. Bull FC, Al-Ansari SS, Biddle S, Borodulin K, Buman MP, Cardon G, et al. World Health Organization 2020 guidelines on physical activity and sedentary behaviour. Br J Sports Med. 2020;54(24):1451–62.
26. García-Hermoso A, Ramírez-Campillo R, Izquierdo M. Is muscular fitness associated with future health benefits in children and adolescents? A systematic review and meta-analysis of longitudinal studies. Sports Med. 2019;49(7):1079–94.
27. García-Hermoso A, Cavero-Redondo I, Ramírez-Vélez R, Ruiz JR, Ortega FB, Lee DC, et al. Muscular strength as a predictor of all-cause mortality in an apparently healthy population: a systematic review and meta-analysis of data from approximately 2 million men and women. Arch Phys Med Rehabil. 2018;99(10):2100–13.e5.
28. Hillsdon M, Foster C. What are the health benefits of muscle and bone strengthening and balance activities across life stages and specific health outcomes? J Frailty Sarcopenia Falls. 2018;03(02):66–73.
29. Fernandez R. One repetition maximum clarified. J Orthop Sports Phys Ther. 2001;31(5):264.
30. Nuzzo JL. The case for retiring flexibility as a major component of physical fitness. Sports Med. 2020;50(5):853–70.
31. American College of Sports Medicine. In: Liguori G, Feito Y, Fountaine CJ, Roy B, editors. ACSM's guidelines for exercise testing and prescription. 11th ed. Philadelphia: Wolters Kluwer; 2022. 513 p.
32. Lopes L, Póvoas S, Mota J, Okely AD, Coelho-e-Silva MJ, Cliff DP, et al. Flexibility is associated with motor competence in schoolchildren. Scand J Med Sci Sports. 2017;27(12):1806–13.
33. Sadler SG, Spink MJ, Ho A, De Jonge XJ, Chuter VH. Restriction in lateral bending range of motion, lumbar lordosis, and hamstring flexibility predicts the development of low back pain: a systematic review of prospective cohort studies. BMC Musculoskelet Disord. 2017;18(1):179.
34. Mutubuki EN, Beljon Y, Maas ET, Huygen FJPM, Ostelo RWJG, Van Tulder MW, et al. The longitudinal relationships between pain severity and disability versus health-related quality of life and costs among chronic low back pain patients. Qual Life Res. 2020;29(1):275–87.
35. Mota J, Martins J, Onofre M. Portuguese Physical Literacy Assessment Questionnaire (PPLA-Q) for adolescents (15–18 years) from grades 10–12: development, content validation and pilot testing. BMC Public Health. 2021;21(1):2183.
36. Norkin CC, White DJ. Measurement of joint motion: a guide to goniometry. 5th ed. Philadelphia: F.A. Davis Company; 2016. 571 p.
37. Thibault R, Genton L, Pichard C. Body composition: why, when and for who? Clin Nutr. 2012;31(4):435–47.
38. Wells JCK. Measuring body composition. Arch Dis Child. 2005;91(7):612–7.
39. Hills AP, Andersen LB, Byrne NM. Physical activity and obesity in children. Br J Sports Med. 2011;45(11):866–70.
40. Wells JCK. Body composition of children with moderate and severe undernutrition and after treatment: a narrative review. BMC Med. 2019;17(1):215.
41. Lohman TG. Applicability of body composition techniques and constants for children and youths. Exerc Sport Sci Rev. 1986;14:325–57.
42. García-Hermoso A. Health-related fitness during early years, childhood, and adolescence. In: Matson JL, editor. Handbook of clinical child psychology, Autism and Child Psychopathology Series. Cham: Springer International Publishing; 2023. p. 763–88. Available from: https://link.springer.com/10.1007/978-3-031-24926-6_35.
43. Léger LA, Mercier D, Gadoury C, Lambert J. The multistage 20 metre shuttle run test for aerobic fitness. J Sports Sci. 1988;6(2):93–101.
44. Artero EG, España-Romero V, Castro-Piñero J, Ortega FB, Suni J, Castillo-Garzon MJ, et al. Reliability of field-based fitness tests in youth. Int J Sports Med. 2011;32(03):159–69.
45. Mayorga-Vega D, Aguilar-Soto P, Viciana J. Criterion-related validity of the 20-m shuttle run test for estimating cardiorespiratory fitness: a meta-analysis. J Sports Sci Med. 2015;14(3):536–47.

46. Ruiz JR, Castro-Pinero J, Artero EG, Ortega FB, Sjostrom M, Suni J, et al. Predictive validity of health-related fitness in youth: a systematic review. Br J Sports Med. 2009;43(12):909–23.
47. Paradisis GP, Zacharogiannis E, Mandila D, Smirtiotou A, Argeitaki P, Cooke CB. Multi-stage 20-m shuttle run fitness test, maximal oxygen uptake and velocity at maximal oxygen uptake. J Hum Kinet. 2014;41(1):81–7.
48. Brusseau TA, Fairclough SJ, Lubans DR, editors. The routledge handbook of youth physical activity. New York: Routledge, Taylor & Francis Group; 2020. 1 p.
49. Tomkinson GR, Lang JJ, Blanchard J, Léger LA, Tremblay MS. The 20-m shuttle run: assessment and interpretation of data in relation to youth aerobic fitness and health. Pediatr Exerc Sci. 2019;31(2):152–63.
50. Catley MJ, Tomkinson GR. Normative health-related fitness values for children: analysis of 85347 test results on 9–17-year-old Australians since 1985. Br J Sports Med. 2013;47(2):98–108.
51. Tomkinson GR, Macfarlane D, Noi S, Kim DY, Wang Z, Hong R. Temporal changes in long-distance running performance of Asian children between 1964 and 2009. Sports Med. 2012;42(4):267–79.
52. Safrit MJ. The validity and reliability of fitness tests for children: a review. Pediatr Exerc Sci. 1990;2(1):9–28.
53. Mayorga-Vega D, Bocanegra-Parrilla R, Ornelas M, Viciana J. Criterion-related validity of the distance- and time-based walk/run field tests for estimating cardiorespiratory fitness: a systematic review and meta-analysis. PLoS One. 2016;11(3):e0151671.
54. Cooper CB, Storer TW. Exercise testing and interpretation a practical approach. Cambridge: Cambridge University Press; 2004.
55. Macfarlane DJ, Tomkinson GR. Evolution and variability in fitness test performance of Asian children and adolescents. In: Tomkinson GR, Olds TS, editors. Medicine and sport science. Basel: Karger; 2007. p. 143–67. Available from: https://www.karger.com/Article/FullText/101358.
56. Dooley FL, Kaster T, Fitzgerald JS, Walch TJ, Annandale M, Ferrar K, et al. A systematic analysis of temporal trends in the handgrip strength of 2,216,320 children and adolescents between 1967 and 2017. Sports Med. 2020;50(6):1129–44.
57. Plowman SA. Top 10 research questions related to musculoskeletal physical fitness testing in children and adolescents. Res Q Exerc Sport. 2014;85(2):174–87.
58. Milliken LA, Faigenbaum AD, Loud RL, Westcott WL. Correlates of upper and lower body muscular strength in children. J Strength Cond Res. 2008;22(4):1339–46.
59. Feito Y, Magal M, American College of Sports Medicine, editors. Fitness assessment manual. 6th ed. Philadelphia: Wolters Kluwer; 2022. 193 p.
60. Wind AE, Takken T, Helders PJM, Engelbert RHH. Is grip strength a predictor for total muscle strength in healthy children, adolescents, and young adults? Eur J Pediatr. 2010;169(3):281–7.
61. España-Romero V, Artero EG, Santaliestra-Pasias AM, Gutierrez A, Castillo MJ, Ruiz JR. Hand span influences optimal grip span in boys and girls aged 6 to 12 years. J Hand Surg. 2008;33(3):378–84.
62. España-Romero V, Ortega FB, Vicente-Rodríguez G, Artero EG, Rey JP, Ruiz JR. Elbow position affects handgrip strength in adolescents: validity and reliability of Jamar, DynEx, and TKK dynamometers. J Strength Cond Res. 2010;24(1):272–7.
63. Bianco A, Jemni M, Thomas E, Patti A, Paoli A, Ramos Roque J, et al. A systematic review to determine reliability and usefulness of the field-based test batteries for the assessment of physical fitness in adolescents – the ASSO project. Int J Occup Med Environ Health. 2015;28(3):445–78.
64. Castro-Piñero J, Ortega FB, Artero EG, Girela-Rejón MJ, Mora J, Sjöström M, et al. Assessing muscular strength in youth: usefulness of standing long jump as a general index of muscular fitness. J Strength Cond Res. 2010;24(7):1810–7.

65. Lang JJ, Zhang K, Agostinis-Sobrinho C, Andersen LB, Basterfield L, Berglind D, et al. Top 10 international priorities for physical fitness research and surveillance among children and adolescents: a Twin-Panel Delphi study. Sports Med. 2023;53(2):549–64.
66. Docherty D, editor. Measurement in pediatric exercise science: published for the Canadian Society for Exercise Physiology. Champaign: Human Kinetics; 1996. 344 p.
67. Holm I, Fredriksen P, Fosdahl M, Vøllestad N. A normative sample of isotonic and isokinetic muscle strength measurements in children 7 to 12 years of age. Acta Paediatr. 2008;97(5):602–7.
68. Tomkinson GR, Kaster T, Dooley FL, Fitzgerald JS, Annandale M, Ferrar K, et al. Temporal trends in the standing broad jump performance of 10,940,801 children and adolescents between 1960 and 2017. Sports Med. 2021;51(3):531–48.
69. Fujita Y, Nakamura Y, Hiraoka J, Kobayashi K, Sakata K, Nagai M, et al. Physical-strength tests and mortality among visitors to health-promotion centers in Japan. J Clin Epidemiol. 1995;48(11):1349–59.
70. Katzmarzyk PT, Craig CL. Musculoskeletal fitness and risk of mortality. Med Sci Sports Exerc. 2002;34(5):740–4.
71. Wells KF, Dillon EK. The sit and reach—a test of back and leg flexibility. Res Q Am Assoc Health Phys Educ Recreat. 1952;23(1):115–8.
72. López-Miñarro PA, de Andújar PSB, Rodrñguez-Garcña PL. A comparison of the sit-and-reach test and the back-saver sit-and-reach test in university students. J Sports Sci Med. 2009;8(1):116–22.
73. Castro-Piñero J, Chillón P, Ortega FB, Montesinos JL, Sjöström M, Ruiz JR. Criterion-related validity of sit-and-reach and modified sit-and-reach test for estimating hamstring flexibility in children and adolescents aged 6–17 years. Int J Sports Med. 2009;30(09):658–62.
74. Ramirez-Velez R, Bustamante J, Czerniczyniec A, Aguilar de Plata AC, Lores-Arnaiz S. Effect of exercise training on Enos expression, NO production and oxygen metabolism in human placenta. PLoS One. 2013;8(11):e80225.
75. Mayorga-Vega D, Merino-Marban R, Viciana J. Criterion-related validity of sit-and-reach tests for estimating hamstring and lumbar extensibility: a meta-analysis. J Sports Sci Med. 2014;13(1):1–14.
76. Weir CB, Jan A. BMI classification percentile and cut off points. In: StatPearls. Treasure Island: StatPearls Publishing; 2024. Available from: http://www.ncbi.nlm.nih.gov/books/NBK541070/.
77. De Onis M. Development of a WHO growth reference for school-aged children and adolescents. Bull World Health Organ. 2007;85(09):660–7.
78. Stomfai S, Ahrens W, Bammann K, Kovács É, Mårild S, on behalf of the IDEFICS Consortium, et al. Intra- and inter-observer reliability in anthropometric measurements in children. Int J Obes. 2011;35(S1):S45–51.
79. Castro-Pinero J, Artero EG, Espana-Romero V, Ortega FB, Sjostrom M, Suni J, et al. Criterion-related validity of field-based fitness tests in youth: a systematic review. Br J Sports Med. 2010;44(13):934–43.
80. Prentice AM, Jebb SA. Beyond body mass index. Obes Rev. 2001;2(3):141–7.
81. Ortega FB, Sui X, Lavie CJ, Blair SN. Body mass index, the most widely used but also widely criticized index. Mayo Clin Proc. 2016;91(4):443–55.
82. Morrow JR, Martin SB, Jackson AW. Reliability and validity of the FITNESSGRAM®: quality of teacher-collected health-related fitness surveillance data. Res Q Exerc Sport. 2010;81(sup3):S24–30.
83. Thompson HR, Linchey JK, King B, Himes JH, Madsen KA. Accuracy of school staff-measured height and weight used for body mass index screening and reporting. J Sch Health. 2019;89(8):629–35.
84. Ruggieri DG, Bass SB. A comprehensive review of school-based body mass index screening programs and their implications for school health: do the controversies accurately reflect the research? J Sch Health. 2015;85(1):61–72.

85. Abarca-Gómez L, Abdeen ZA, Hamid ZA, Abu-Rmeileh NM, Acosta-Cazares B, Acuin C, et al. Worldwide trends in body-mass index, underweight, overweight, and obesity from 1975 to 2016: a pooled analysis of 2416 population-based measurement studies in 128·9 million children, adolescents, and adults. Lancet. 2017;390(10113):2627–42.
86. Zimmet P, Alberti G, Kaufman F, Tajima N, Silink M, Arslanian S, et al. The metabolic syndrome in children and adolescents. Lancet. 2007;369(9579):2059–61.
87. Nishida C, Ko GT, Kumanyika S. Body fat distribution and noncommunicable diseases in populations: overview of the 2008 WHO Expert Consultation on Waist Circumference and Waist–Hip Ratio. Eur J Clin Nutr. 2010;64(1):2–5.
88. Lear SA, James PT, Ko GT, Kumanyika S. Appropriateness of waist circumference and waist-to-hip ratio cutoffs for different ethnic groups. Eur J Clin Nutr. 2010;64(1):42–61.
89. Aeberli I, Gut-Knabenhans M, Kusche-Ammann R, Molinari L, Zimmermann M. Waist circumference and waist-to-height ratio percentiles in a nationally representative sample of 6-13 year old children in Switzerland. Swiss Med Wkly. 2011;141:w13227. Available from: https://smw.ch/index.php/smw/article/view/1307.
90. Khadilkar A, Ekbote V, Chiplonkar S, Khadilkar V, Kajale N, Kulkarni S, et al. Waist circumference percentiles in 2–18 year old Indian children. J Pediatr. 2014;164(6):1358–62.e2.
91. Ma GS, Ji CY, Ma J, Mi J, Sung RY, Xiong F, et al. Waist circumference reference values for screening cardiovascular risk factors in Chinese children and adolescents. Biomed Environ Sci. 2010;23(1):21–31.
92. Poh BK, Jannah AN, Chong LK, Ruzita Abd T, Ismail Mohd N, McCarthy D. Waist circumference percentile curves for Malaysian children and adolescents aged 6.0–16.9 years. Int J Pediatr Obes. 2011;6(3–4):229–35.
93. Xi B, Zong X, Kelishadi R, Litwin M, Hong YM, Poh BK, et al. International waist circumference percentile cutoffs for central obesity in children and adolescents aged 6 to 18 years. J Clin Endocrinol Metab. 2020;105(4):e1569–83.
94. Van Dijk SB, Takken T, Prinsen EC, Wittink H. Different anthropometric adiposity measures and their association with cardiovascular disease risk factors: a meta-analysis. Neth Heart J. 2012;20(5):208–18.
95. Gaya AR, Mello JB, Dias AF, Brand C, Cardoso VD, Nagorny GAK, et al. Temporal trends in physical fitness and obesity among Brazilian children and adolescents between 2008 and 2014. J Hum Sport Exerc. 2019;15(3):549–58. Available from: http://hdl.handle.net/10045/97090.
96. Leal DB, De Assis MAA, González-Chica DA, Da Costa FF. Trends in adiposity in Brazilian 7–10-year-old schoolchildren: evidence for increasing overweight but not obesity between 2002 and 2007. Ann Hum Biol. 2014;41(3):255–62.
97. Colley R, Wong S, Hoffmann MD, Doyon CY, Lang JJ, Tomkinson GR. Normative-referenced percentile values for physical fitness among Canadians. Health Rep. 2019;30(10):3–11.
98. Dong Y, Lau PWC, Dong B, Zou Z, Yang Y, Wen B, et al. Trends in physical fitness, growth, and nutritional status of Chinese children and adolescents: a retrospective analysis of 1.5 million students from six successive national surveys between 1985 and 2014. Lancet Child Adolesc Health. 2019;3(12):871–80.
99. Liang Y, Xi B, Song A, Liu J, Mi J. Trends in general and abdominal obesity among Chinese children and adolescents 1993–2009. Pediatr Obes. 2012;7(5):355–64.
100. Ma S, Hou D, Zhang Y, Yang L, Sun J, Zhao M, et al. Trends in abdominal obesity among Chinese children and adolescents, 1993–2015. J Pediatr Endocrinol Metab. 2021;34(2):163–9.
101. Kasović M, Štefan L, Petrić V. Secular trends in health-related physical fitness among 11–14-year-old Croatian children and adolescents from 1999 to 2014. Sci Rep. 2021;11(1):11039.
102. Poon ETC, Tomkinson GR, Huang WY, Wong SHS. Temporal trends in the physical fitness of Hong Kong adolescents between 1998 and 2015. Int J Sports Med. 2023;44(10):728–35.

103. Anzo M, Inokuchi M, Matsuo N, Takayama JI, Hasegawa T. Waist circumference centiles by age and sex for Japanese children based on the 1978–1981 cross-sectional national survey data. Ann Hum Biol. 2015;42(1):56–61.
104. Kim C, Miller RS, Braffett BH, Pan Y, Arends VL, Saenger AK, et al. Ovarian markers and irregular menses among women with type 1 diabetes in the Epidemiology of Diabetes Interventions and Complications study. Clin Endocrinol. 2018;88(3):453–9.
105. Venckunas T, Emeljanovas A, Mieziene B, Volbekiene V. Secular trends in physical fitness and body size in Lithuanian children and adolescents between 1992 and 2012. J Epidemiol Community Health. 2017;71(2):181–7.
106. Dos Santos FK, Prista A, Gomes TNQF, Daca T, Madeira A, Katzmarzyk PT, et al. Secular trends in physical fitness of Mozambican school-aged children and adolescents. Am J Hum Biol. 2015;27(2):201–6.
107. Moreno LA, Sarría A, Fleta J, Marcos A, Bueno M. Secular trends in waist circumference in Spanish adolescents, 1995 to 2000-02. Arch Dis Child. 2005;90(8):818–9.
108. Li C, Ford ES, Mokdad AH, Cook S. Recent trends in waist circumference and waist-height ratio among US children and adolescents. Pediatrics. 2006;118(5):e1390–8.
109. Ortega FB, Cadenas-Sánchez C, Sánchez-Delgado G, Mora-González J, Martínez-Téllez B, Artero EG, et al. Systematic review and proposal of a field-based physical fitness-test battery in preschool children: the PREFIT battery. Sports Med. 2015;45(4):533–55.
110. Cadenas-Sanchez C, Martinez-Tellez B, Sanchez-Delgado G, Mora-Gonzalez J, Castro-Piñero J, Löf M, et al. Assessing physical fitness in preschool children: feasibility, reliability and practical recommendations for the PREFIT battery. J Sci Med Sport. 2016;19(11):910–5.
111. Molenaar HMT, Zuidam JM, Selles RW, Stam HJ, SER H. Age-specific reliability of two grip-strength dynamometers when used by children. J Bone Joint Surg Am. 2008;90(5):1053–9.
112. Sanchez-Delgado G, Cadenas-Sanchez C, Mora-Gonzalez J, Martinez-Tellez B, Chillón P, Löf M, et al. Assessment of handgrip strength in preschool children aged 3 to 5 years. J Hand Surg Eur Vol. 2015;40(9):966–72.
113. Ayán Pérez C, Álvarez Pérez S, González Baamonde S, Martínez De Quel Ó. Influence of the box dimensions on the reliability and validity of the sit and reach in preschoolers. J Strength Cond Res. 2020;34(9):2683–92.
114. Karlsson A, Kullberg J, Stokland E, Allvin K, Gronowitz E, Svensson P, et al. Measurements of total and regional body composition in preschool children: a comparison of MRI, DXA, and anthropometric data. Obesity. 2013;21(5):1018–24.
115. Laurson KR, Saint-Maurice PF, Welk GJ, Eisenmann JC. Reference curves for field tests of musculoskeletal fitness in U.S. children and adolescents: the 2012 NHANES National Youth Fitness Survey. J Strength Cond Res. 2017;31(8):2075–82.
116. Bai Y, Saint-Maurice PF, Welk GJ, Allums-Featherston K, Candelaria N, Anderson K. Prevalence of youth fitness in the United States: baseline results from the NFL PLAY 60 FITNESSGRAM partnership project. J Pediatr. 2015;167(3):662–8.
117. Welk GJ, Saint-Maurice PF, Csányi T. Health-related physical fitness in Hungarian youth: age, sex, and regional profiles. Res Q Exerc Sport. 2015;86(sup1):S45–57.
118. Tomkinson GR, Carver KD, Atkinson F, Daniell ND, Lewis LK, Fitzgerald JS, et al. European normative values for physical fitness in children and adolescents aged 9–17 years: results from 2 779 165 Eurofit performances representing 30 countries. Br J Sports Med. 2018;52(22):1445–56.
119. Cadenas-Sanchez C, Intemann T, Labayen I, Peinado AB, Vidal-Conti J, Sanchis-Moysi J, et al. Physical fitness reference standards for preschool children: the PREFIT project. J Sci Med Sport. 2019;22(4):430–7.
120. Institute of Medicine. Fitness measures and health outcomes in youth. Washington, DC: National Academies Press; 2012. Available from: http://www.nap.edu/catalog/13483.
121. Drenowatz C, Hinterkörner F, Greier K. Physical fitness and motor competence in upper Austrian elementary school children—study protocol and preliminary findings of a state-wide fitness testing program. Front Sports Act Living. 2021;22(3):635478.

122. Krochmal P, Cooper DM, Radom-Aizik S, Lu KD. US school-based physical fitness assessments and data dissemination. J Sch Health. 2021;91(9):722–9.
123. Ortega FB, Leskošek B, Blagus R, Gil-Cosano JJ, Mäestu J, Tomkinson GR, et al. European fitness landscape for children and adolescents: updated reference values, fitness maps and country rankings based on nearly 8 million test results from 34 countries gathered by the FitBack network. Br J Sports Med. 2023;57(5):299–310.
124. Ramírez-Vélez R, Rodrigues-Bezerra D, Correa-Bautista JE, Izquierdo M, Lobelo F. Reliability of health-related physical fitness tests among Colombian children and adolescents: the FUPRECOL study. PLoS One. 2015;10(10):e0140875.
125. García-Hermoso A, Ramírez-Vélez R, Lubans DR, Izquierdo M. Effects of physical education interventions on cognition and academic performance outcomes in children and adolescents: a systematic review and meta-analysis. Br J Sports Med. 2021;55(21):1224–32.
126. Sagat P, Štefan L, Petrić V, Štemberger V, Blažević I. Normative values of cardiorespiratory fitness in Croatian children and adolescents. PLoS One. 2023;18(4):e0284410.
127. Godoy-Cumillaf A, Bruneau-Chávez J, Fuentes-Merino P, Vásquez-Gómez J, Sánchez-López M, Alvárez-Bueno C, et al. Reference values for fitness level and gross motor skills of 4–6-year-old chilean children. Int J Environ Res Public Health. 2020;17(3):797.
128. Przednowek KH, Niewczas M, Wójcik Ł, Paśko W, Iskra J, Przednowek K. Physical fitness percentiles of Polish children aged 4–7 years. Sci Rep. 2021;11(1):7367.
129. Ruiz JR, Cavero-Redondo I, Ortega FB, Welk GJ, Andersen LB, Martinez-Vizcaino V. Cardiorespiratory fitness cut points to avoid cardiovascular disease risk in children and adolescents; what level of fitness should raise a red flag? A systematic review and meta-analysis. Br J Sports Med. 2016;50(23):1451–8.
130. Welk GJ, De Saint-Maurice Maduro PF, Laurson KR, Brown DD. Field evaluation of the new FITNESSGRAM® criterion-referenced standards. Am J Prev Med. 2011;41(4):S131–42.
131. Fraser BJ, Blizzard L, Buscot MJ, Schmidt MD, Dwyer T, Venn AJ, et al. Muscular strength across the life course: the tracking and trajectory patterns of muscular strength between childhood and mid-adulthood in an Australian cohort. J Sci Med Sport. 2021;24(7):696–701.
132. Rollo S, Fraser BJ, Seguin N, Sampson M, Lang JJ, Tomkinson GR, et al. Health-related criterion-referenced cut-points for cardiorespiratory fitness among youth: a systematic review. Sports Med. 2022;52(1):101–22.
133. Berkson SS, Espinola J, Corso KA, Cabral H, McGowan R, Chomitz VR. Reliability of height and weight measurements collected by physical education teachers for a school-based body mass index surveillance and screening system. J Sch Health. 2013;83(1):21–7.
134. Jones MM, Carnes MC, Adams T, Bryant LG, Church B, Stillwell JL. Parents' perceptions and use of school-based body mass index report cards. J Sch Health. 2018;88(11):787–793. https://doi.org/10.1111/josh.12685.
135. Mor-Anavy S, Lev-Ari S, Levin-Zamir D. Health literacy, primary care health care providers, and communication. Health Lit Res Pract. 2021;5(3):e194–200. Available from: https://journals.healio.com/doi/10.3928/24748307-20210529-01.
136. Altman E, Linchey J, Santamaria G, Thompson HR, Madsen KA. Weight measurements in school: setting and student comfort. J Nutr Educ Behav. 2022;54(3):249–54.
137. Silverman S, Keating XD, Phillips SR. A lasting impression: a pedagogical perspective on youth fitness testing. Meas Phys Educ Exerc Sci. 2008;12(3):146–66.
138. Phillips SR, Marttinen R, Mercier K. Fitness assessment: recommendations for an enjoyable student experience. Strategies. 2017;30(5):19–24.
139. Myers ND, Lee S, Chun H, Zhu W. Measurement in physical education and exercise science (MPEES): a summary of MPEES-related activities in 2022. Meas Phys Educ Exerc Sci. 2023;27(2):85–96.
140. Bogataj Š, Trajković N, Cadenas-Sanchez C, Sember V. Effects of school-based exercise and nutrition intervention on body composition and physical fitness in overweight adolescent girls. Nutrients. 2021;13(1):238.

141. Langford R, Bonell CP, Jones HE, Pouliou T, Murphy SM, Waters E, et al. The WHO Health Promoting School framework for improving the health and well-being of students and their academic achievement. Cochrane Database Syst Rev. 2014;2014(4):CD008958. Available from: https://doi.wiley.com/10.1002/14651858.CD008958.pub2.
142. Marques A, Balsa D, Domingos M, Cavalheiro R, Carreira T, Moreira T, et al. The attitude of Portuguese physical education teachers toward physical fitness. Children. 2022;9(7):1005.
143. Stanford FC, Taveras EM. The Massachusetts school-based body mass index experiment—gleaning implementation lessons for future childhood obesity reduction efforts. Obesity. 2014;22(4):973–5.
144. Cocca A, Espino Verdugo F, Ródenas Cuenca LT, Cocca M. Effect of a game-based physical education program on physical fitness and mental health in elementary school children. Int J Environ Res Public Health. 2020;17(13):4883.
145. Domone S, Mann S, Sandercock G, Wade M, Beedie C. A method by which to assess the scalability of field-based fitness tests of cardiorespiratory fitness among schoolchildren. Sports Med. 2016;46(12):1819–31.
146. Ortega FB, Ruiz JR. Fitness in youth: methodological issues and understanding of its clinical value. Am J Lifestyle Med. 2015;9(6):403–8.
147. McGrath R, Cawthon PM, Clark BC, Fielding RA, Lang JJ, Tomkinson GR. Recommendations for reducing heterogeneity in handgrip strength protocols. J Frailty Aging. 2022;11(2):143–50. Available from: https://link.springer.com/article/10.14283/jfa.2022.21.
148. Ruíz JR, España Romero V, Castro Piñero J, Artero EG, Ortega FB, Cuenca García M, Jiménez Pavón D, Chillón P, Girela Rejón M, Mora J, Gutiérrez A, Suni J, Sjöstrom M, Castillo MJ. Batería ALPHA-Fitness: test de campo para la evaluación de la condición física relacionada con la salud en niños y adolescentes. Nutr Hosp. 2011;26(6):1210–4.

Chapter 6
Motor Skill Assessment in Children and Adolescents

Nadia Cristina Valentini

6.1 Motor Development and Assessment Across Childhood and Adolescence: The Role of Motor Assessment and the Relevance of Cross-Cultural Evidence

Children's motor skill proficiency has been recognized as an essential factor related to their health outcomes, such as physical activity (PA), fitness, and healthy weight status [1–5], and it is also a predictor of engagement in PA later in adolescence or adulthood [1]. Youth motor proficiency has also been described to be moderately relevant to individuals' perceptions of competence [4–7]; longitudinal evidence has suggested that being motor proficient at young ages (5–7 years) predicts how competent individuals perceive themselves in adolescence (16 years old) [8]. In addition, experimental evidence, although not very robust, supports the role of motor skill proficiency in longitudinally moderating the influence of cognitively enriched PA on working memory and social–emotional skills in school-aged children [9].

On the other hand, poor motor skills often lead children to avoid PA [4, 5, 10–12] and perceive themselves as less capable of completing motor tasks and being accepted by their peers [13]. Although fundamental motor skill proficiency is expected to be attained during childhood through direct and indirect-oriented activities such as recreational games, recess play, after-school sports, or daily motor challenge activities, research has shown that individual constraints and poor environmental opportunities for participation and practice lead to motor delays [2, 5]. Furthermore, although motor impairments are detected in the first years of life, mild deficits are usually detected later, at preschool and school age, as the complexity of the tasks increases and due to peer comparisons [14, 15]. Consequently,

---

N. C. Valentini (✉)
Universidade Federal do Rio Grande do Sul, Porto Alegre, Brazil
e-mail: nadiacv@esef.ufrgs.br

appropriate opportunities to learn new motor skills are critical beginning at an early age, whether the focus is to foster a skilled child or compensate for motor delays in a child with motor impairments. Appropriate motor programs can improve children's motor competence [2, 5], self-perceptions [2, 5], and quality of life [16–18], and the first step in implementing an effective program is accurately assessing children's difficulties and potentialities.

Assessing children's motor proficiency is essential for (a) establishing a baseline for clinical or educational intervention, (b) specifying the extent of motor deficits and how those deficits impact children's function in different contexts, (c) complementing the diagnosis of disabilities and identifying motor difficulties or impairments, (d) defining children's levels of motor proficiency to plan and implement interventions, providing children with adequate opportunities to nurture development, optimize function, prevent undesired outcomes, and strengthen individual potential, (e) evaluating the effectiveness of the intervention in promoting the acquisition of motor skills and decreasing impairments, and (f) supporting families and teachers in caring for a child at home or school. All these goals may be accomplished if motor assessments have several attributes, namely, purpose, validity, reliability, and value, to obtain strong and trustworthy information that could help researchers and clinicians build knowledge and support professional actions (Fig. 6.1).

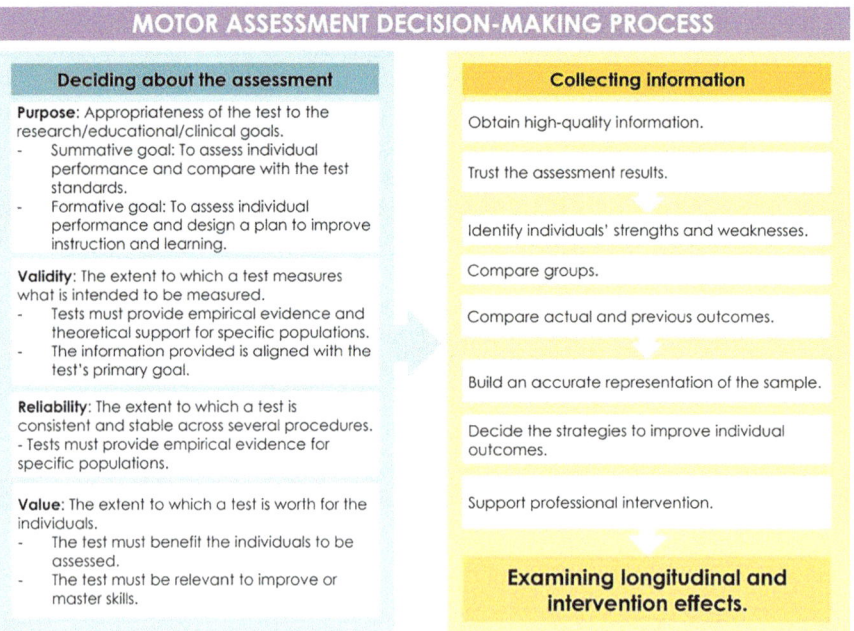

Fig. 6.1 The motor assessment decision process, the attributes of a functional assessment, and its implications for professional practice

Several valid and reliable motor assessments have been extensively used in research, education, and clinical settings to assess motor proficiency in children and adolescents. Some of those assessments have robust psychometric evidence in the original samples and across different cultures, which are essential features of a trustworthy assessment. Cross-cultural validity is critical—psychometrics should be appropriately examined for individuals in different socioeconomic and cultural contexts. Assessments with strong and rigorous cross-cultural psychometric evidence are applicable, suitable, and meaningful in other cultures, allowing researchers to trust the results without cultural biases, compare outcomes, and reasonably understand the factors that affect cross-cultural differences.

Robust cross-cultural adaptation of motor assessment and the investigation of its validity involve several essential procedures [10, 19, 21–27]. The first step is to enroll several independent translators in the translation and back-translation of the assessment and the meeting of those professionals on a committee to review the translation and language adequacy and solve possible concerns. The second step is time-consuming and involves the implementation of an empirical investigation of the translated and adapted versions of the scale, starting with (a) examining expert content validity regarding the clarity and pertinence of the items, (b) revising items if experts point out a lack of clarity or pertinence, (c) implementing face validity by professionals who use the assessment, (d) determining the nationally representative sample (i.e., regarding ethnicity, socioeconomic status, sex, geographic regions), (e) conducting a pilot study with the target population, (f) examining content, construct, and criterion validity, (g) examining interrater and intrarater reliability, (h) examining the results of a specific culture relating to the original data reported for the culture where the test was developed, and (i) adapting the scores to the cultural context and developing new standards if necessary. Each step covers the necessary procedures for examining the validity of the assessments cross-culturally, and different statistical procedures have been used to achieve those goals; these choices should be aligned with the research's objectives and test specificity; each step has advantages and weaknesses, highlighting the relevance of considering covering all steps in the cross-cultural validity process. Despite the well-known relevance of robust psychometrics, it is essential to note that although several motor assessments are used worldwide, some have very restricted psychometric evidence in several countries. The restricted cross-cultural psychometric evidence is probably due to the complex process involved and the substantial economic and time constraints, which limit the understanding of motor status in specific cultures and populations (Table 6.1).

Consequently, when choosing a motor assessment, it is essential to consider its worldwide established psychometrics and ability to discriminate, predict, and evaluate motor performance. Discrimination is related to the motor assessment capability to determine an individual's functional status, to discriminate between individuals with different levels of motor performance, or to sort individuals' performance into

Table 6.1 Several procedures and statistical analyses used to determine cross-cultural motor validity

Translation, back-translation and cross-cultural adaptation: • Translate to new language, provide a synthesis, back to the original language and provide a prefinal version	Qualitative approach • Review and rewrite items for language and semantic, conceptual, experiential, and idiomatic equivalence
Translated and adapted version: Initial empirical evidence • Examine expert content validity: Items clarity and pertinence • Examine face validity by target population and by professionals who will use the test • Determine the national representative sample • Conduct a pilot study with a target-population	Qualitative and quantitative approach: • Examine content validity: CVC, Gweet's AC1/AC2, Kappa, Percentage Agreement, Brenann-Prediger, Scott's Pi, Krippendorff's Alpha • Revise, improve, or delete items with low scores and reexamine experts' agreement • Choose a representative sample (i.e., sex, age, region, SES, ethnicity) using national data • Examine the target population characteristics regarding to clarity, relevance, difficulty, and sensitivity
Conduct the empirical study with the target population: • Examine content, internal structure, criterion-related validity • Examine consistency and measurement agreement among raters • Temporal stability: Test–retest reliability	Quantitative approach: • Examine Internal Structure, Criterion-Related Validity (Relationship to Other Variables), response processes • Cronbach alpha, Omega, McDonald's, and Gutmann's tests • EFA (LMP-95% CI; Bartlett's Sphericity test; OIPA; WRMR) CFA, ML, WLSMV, WLS, AVE • Fit indices (GFI, CFI, RNI, TLI, RMSEA, SMSR, Chi2 ratio, ECVI) • Model invariance: Multigroup analysis, MIMIC • Discriminant validity: HTMT ratio of correlations, correlations... • Concurrent and criterion validity: Pearson correlations, Kendall's tau coefficient, discriminant analysis, ANOVA, Chi2, t tests • Predictive validity: Correlations, ICC, Chi2, ANOVA, regression • Item-developmental level validity: ANOVA, correlations • Item' difficulty, discrimination, variance, hierarchic order, and separation; IRT, Rasch model (dichotomous and polytomous items, Infit and outfit indices)
Conduct the empirical study with the target population: • Examine consistency and agreement among raters • Temporal stability: test–retest stability	Quantitative approach: • Examine reliability: Interrater, intrarater reliability and test reliability • ICC, pared t test, Gweet's AC1/AC2, Kappa, weighted kappa, percentage agreement Composite reliability, Pearson correlations, ICC, pared t test

(continued)

Table 6.1 (continued)

Motor trajectories, cross-cultural comparisons, and norms: • Examine motor development trajectories • Adapt the scores to the specific cultural context • Development of normative standards, if necessary	Quantitative approach: • Developmental trajectories: GEE, ANOVA, percentiles for each age group, time series • Cross-cultural comparison: One sample t test, independent t test, ANOVA, generalized linear models, structural equation models, multigroup analyses, MIMIC • Standard deviations, percentile ranks, Scaled score, T scores, QI scores, GAMLSS, Bayesian GAMLSS

CVC Content validity coefficient, *AC1* Gweet's agreement coefficient, *KMO-95% CI* Kaiser–Meyer–Olkin with bootstrap 95% confident interval, *OIPA* Optimal Implementation of Parallel Analysis, *ECA* Exploratory Factor Analysis, *WRMR* Weighted Root-Mean Square residual, *CFA* Confirmatory Factor Analysis, *ML* Maximum Likelihood, *WLSMV* Weighted Least Square Mean, *WLS* Weighted Least Squares, *AVE* Average variance extracted, *GEE* Generalized Estimating Equations, *GFI* Goodness-of-Fit Index, *CFI* Comparative Fit Index, *RNI* Relative Noncentrality Index, *TLI* Tucker Lewis Index, *RMSEA* Root Mean Square Error of Approximation, *SRMSR* Standardized Root Mean Square Residual, chi^2 *ratio* Chi-square Ratio, *ECVI* Expected Cross-Validation Index, *MIMIC* Multiple-indicator/multiple cause, *HTMT* Heterotrait–Monotrait, *ICC* Intraclass correlation coefficient, *IRT* Item response theory, *GAMLSS* Generalized additive models for location scale and shape

predefined categories. The assessment has proprieties that ensure that clinicians, educators, or researchers can identify meaningful differences in individuals' functions or groups of individuals at a specific time. Consequently, the test must involve complex and easy tasks requiring a particular level of skillfulness; as such, the discriminator role at the top and the end of the test must be understood, separating individuals with different performance levels. Prediction is related to the ability of a motor assessment to predict an outcome or to establish a prognosis. The assessment has proprieties that ensure clinicians, educators, or researchers that the likelihood of a specific observed outcome occurring at an early age might be exhibited in the future. This predictability of assessment enables professionals to select the appropriate treatment and set goals for individual programs to anticipate the need for school, clinical, or home adjustments to support children's development. Evaluation is related to the motor assessment capability to monitor individual progress, assess individual longitudinal changes, and provide information on overall intervention program evaluation. The NRS-2002 reveals motor assessment responsiveness to detect meaningful changes in motor function over time. Detecting the magnitude of motor changes over time for an individual or group is a critical quality of a motor assessment; it will be a relevant attribute used to deliberate about the outcomes of an intervention program. Examining motor assessments' discriminative, predictive, and evaluative attributes is critical to ensure that the assessments are appropriately used in research, clinical, or educational settings.

6.2 Valid and Reliable Motor Skill Assessments for Children and Adolescents

6.2.1 Bayley Scale of Infant and Toddler Development— BSITD-III and IV

The BSITD III [28] and IV [29] are recognized as valid and reliable assessments with norms established within large national samples across different geographical regions in the last 50 years. The scale's primary goals are to determine developmental cognitive, motor, and language functioning; detect developmental delays; monitor children's progress over time; and plan for individualized intervention in clinical and research settings in early childhood (from 1 to 42 months of life). The BSITD social–emotional and adaptive behavior domains have been investigated less worldwide, although they provide intriguing information for understanding a child's strengths and weaknesses through indirect observation.

Several versions of the TSVR have been used worldwide for decades. The third version, published in 2006 [28], is still in use and is one of the most widely used standardized tools for assessing neurodevelopment in early childhood [30]. The use of the new version (BSITD-IV) [29], published in 2019, is increasing gradually; both editions will be discussed in this chapter. The BSITD-III and IV are standardized and have established norms for representative samples of North American children [28, 29]. The BSIDT III and IV normative samples used information from the 2017 US census to include information from culturally and linguistically diverse backgrounds (i.e., age, sex, race/ethnicity, parents' education, and geographic regions); children with disabilities (i.e., Down syndrome, autism spectrum disorder, language delay, language impairment, developmental delay, and motor impairment); children born prematurely (moderate/late premature and very/extremely); children with prenatal alcohol and drug exposure; and bilingual children, improving the evaluative capacity of the assessment to create a representative sample.

The assessment involved observation and interaction between the child and examiner for several items. The cognitive scale (91 items BSITD-III and 81 BSITD-IV) measures the child's ability to pretend-play, explore objects, attend to object relationships, show concept formation, and perform other cognitive processing tasks. The language scale (97 items BSITD-III and 79 BSITD-IV) assesses receptive and expressive communication, measuring the child's ability to understand instructions, respond to spoken language, label objects, recognize objects based on spoken descriptions, produce preverbal language, and use vocabulary. The motor scale (138 items BSITD-III and 104 BSITD-IV) assesses fine and gross motor skills; measures the child's ability to complete prehension, perceptual-motor integration, motor planning, and motor speed; coordinates limb and trunk movements; and shows control of static and dynamic movements. The raw score is obtained by the sum of all the items the child received credit for (BSITD

III—dichotomic scores: yes or no; BSITD IV—polytomous scores from 0–2: 0 = not present, 1 = emerging, 2 = mastery) and the sum of items from previous ages in BSITD III); scaled and composite scores (i.e., standardized scores) are also provided. The performance was classified using a composite score: very superior (>130), superior [116–125], above average [106–115], average [22, 87–105], below average [26, 78–86], borderline [68–77] or extremely low (<69). For the BSITD IV, the authors recommended adjustment for prematurity to age 3 for language and motor composite scores, regardless of the degree of prematurity; however, for cognitive composite, correction for prematurity is generally recommended over the first 24 months (extreme level of prematurity until three years of age) and whenever the uncorrected cognitive score is 0.33–0.47 SD below the baseline score [31].

The BSITD test is completed in 30–90 min, depending on the examiner's practice, the child's age, and the BSITD version (III or IV) used. The IV has fewer items than does the third version, and parents can now assess some of the items, decreasing the duration of the intervention. The BSITDs (III and IV) have digital training available. BSITD IV provides online training opportunities for beginners and more experienced professionals; online training is freely available when acquiring the Bayley Complete Kit. It is also possible to pay separately for an online independent study program. Online programs provide detailed guidance for administering and scoring BSITD and are also helpful for more experienced researchers.

Regarding the BSITD III score, the psychometrics for the original sample validity were examined for internal consistency and reliability, with interrater agreement and test–retest stability for both normative and clinical samples; the results confirm the acceptable degree of precision in the several psychometric procedures adopted. The BSITD III has been translated into the Arabic, Chinese, Czech, Danish, Dutch, Finnish, French, German, Italian, Nepali, Norwegian, Persian, Portuguese, Russian, Spanish, Swahili, Swedish, and Vietnamese languages [32] and is available to professionals. The third version of the scale also has robust cross-cultural validity in several countries: Australia [33], Belgium [34], Brazil [35], Denmark [36], Egypt [37], Ethiopia [38], Germany [39], Italy [40], Iran [41], Malawi [42], the Netherlands [34, 43], Nepal [44, 45], Russia [46], Sri Lanka [47], South Africa [48], Suriname [32, 49], Taiwan [50], and Vietnam [51]. Although adaptations and deletions of items are necessary in some countries, overall, these studies support the validity and reliability of these items with adequate indices. It is essential to note that some cross-cultural studies were not conducted with representative samples, limiting the ability to generalize the results and review norms. For example, the translation and cultural adaptation conducted in Brazil [35] included a small ($N = 207$) and restricted sample regarding age (12–42 months of age) and geographical region (Sao Paulo); the authors reported adequate evidence of construct validity regarding the factor model and internal consistency and convergent validity with the Peabody Developmental Motor Scale second edition.

Several studies have shown significant differences in motor function between children of various ages from the norm-referenced American sample and children from Australia [52], Belgium [34], Denmark [36], Europe [34, 43], Egypt [37], Germany [53], Italy [40], Iran [41], Kenya [45], Malawi [42], Nepal [45], the Netherlands [34], Sri Lanka [47], South Africa [54], Taiwan [50], the UK, and Ireland [28]; in many countries, these differences did not affect clinical diagnosis. However, reference values were adjusted for Dutch children [43], and specific norm-reference values have been recommended to avoid over- and underestimating children's development [43]. For example, no differences were found in other countries, such as China [33], and no need for Chinese norms was established.

Regarding the BSITD IV psychometrics for the original sample, the assessment showed adequate to excellent subscales and total score interrater reliability, excellent internal consistency, appropriate concurrent validity with the BSITD III, and adequate to excellent convergent validity with the Wechsler Preschool and Primary Scale of Intelligence (fourth edition). However, the convergent validity results with the Peabody Developmental Motor Scales second edition had mixed results ranging from poor to excellent [31]. Overall, research on the validity and reliability of this new version of the scale is still scarce worldwide. Several studies have provided some evidence; for example, discriminant validity analysis (DVA) suggests that the BSITD can detect global deficits in children who are diagnosed with autism spectrum disorder at a very young age, distinguishing those children from other groups who exhibit more targeted delays [55].

To conclude, considering that the incidence of developmental delay is greater in children with disabilities, preterm children, and children suffering from adverse neonatal outcomes (i.e., leukomalacia, periventricular hemorrhage, and encephalopathy), identifying the risk of delays is critical considering that intervention programs are most effective early in life. Both versions of the Bayley scale provided psychometric evidence that was sensitive to changes in those populations; therefore, it could be incorporated into routine assessments among high-risk populations. In addition, the BSITD IV Social-Emotional and Adaptive Behavior Questionnaire has been under-investigated, and it provides interesting information that can support professionals in interventions or researchers in understanding the factors underlying motor development; therefore, it may be relevant for advancing knowledge in the area further; it can be administered remotely. It is also important to highlight that the design and content of most BSITD cognitive, motor, and language tasks focused on child-friendly and child-familiar themes. This factor increases its ecological validity; therefore, it can be generalized to real-life situations and facilitate child assessment. Another substantial advance in the use of the BSITD scale is that psychometric tests were also conducted on subsamples of children with disabilities or children with risk factors. Therefore, this assessment is also recommended for those populations. These factors combined to make the BSITD a robust assessment for children with unique contributions to the motor development area with strong discriminative, predictive, and evaluative attributes.

6.2.2 Peabody Developmental Motor Scales-Second Edition—PDMS-2

The PDMS-2 is a standardized assessment of children's gross and fine motor skills from the first month of life to 72 months of age used in clinical and research settings [56]. The *PDMS-2* is an inclusive assessment of motor skills with the primary objective of (a) establishing the child's motor proficiency relative to standard norms, (b) identifying relative differences in fine and gross motor development among children, (c) establishing individual goals in clinical and educational interventions, (d) monitoring the child's progress, (e) remediating gross and fine motor difficulties, and (f) providing information to develop and implement intervention strategies for families in homes [56].

The PDMS-2 has two subscales for the fine motor component: visuomotor integration and grasping. The visuomotor integration test included 72 tasks assessing visual tracking, hand position related to body line, intention to reach, reaching, transference and manipulation of objects with intention, motor precision, and cutting and folding. The grasping subscale included 26 tasks assessing grasping, manipulating, holding, and releasing objects and manual agility.

The PDMS-2 has four subscales for the gross motor component—stationary, locomotor skills, and object manipulation—for children aged 12 months and older and a reflexes subscale (walking, asymmetrical tonic neck, Landau reaction, protecting reaction forward, protection reaction sideways, right reaction forward, protecting reaction backward) for children under 11 months. The stationary subscale has 30 tasks assessing the children's head and trunk support, changes in positions when sitting, from lying down to sitting, and from sitting to standing, and body support in standing positions. The locomotor skill subscale included 89 tasks assessing limb coordination, position changes, body weight transference, pivoting, walking, running, body support, and jumps. The object manipulation subscale included 24 tasks assessing children's ability to catch, throw, and kick in sitting and standing positions [56].

The assessment took approximately 40–60 min. The administration begins in each subscale, considering the child's age. However, the baseline age was defined based on child compliance with the first baseline level. The motor tasks were scored on three levels of performance. If the child performed the task correctly, the score was two. If the child performed the tasks partially, the score was one. If the child did not perform correctly, the score was zero. The sum of the points comprises the raw score for each subscale. Raw scores, age equivalents, percentile ranks, subtest-scaled scores, and composite index scores (gross motor index, fine motor index, total motor index) were obtained for the PDMS-2. The categorization of motor performance in each subscale has seven levels [56]: very superior [17–20]; superior [15, 16]; above average [13, 14]; average [8–12]; below average [6, 7]; poor [4, 5]; and very poor [1–3].

Regarding the psychometrics in the original sample, the PDMS-2 standards were established with a representative sample ($n = 2.003$) from 46 American states and one Canadian province (2000). The original sample comprised a representative sample regarding sex, ethnicity (e.g., European Americans, African Americans, and Hispanic Americans), physical and intellectual disabilities from the U.S., and other Canadian children and showed good internal consistency. All the subscales and motor quotients were assessed, and the test-retest reliability was acceptable; moreover, the interrater reliability was high for all the subscales and motor quotients [56]. The two-factor model (fine and gross motor skills) showed acceptable indices of fit, confirming its construct validity. The criterion and construct validity have also shown acceptable indices [56].

The psychometric properties of the PDMS-2, which includes different indices and adjustments, have been confirmed in several countries for different age groups of children. In Brazil, the validation study covered the total age range of the PDMS-2 ($n = 635$ children), with results showing high internal consistency [57]; adequate fit indices for construct [57], concurrent [19], predictive [19], and developmental validity [19]; and discriminant item criterion validity [19]. In Portugal [58], the validity of the PDMS-2 was investigated with a sample of 540 preschool children (3–6 years old), with the results indicating its accuracy in detecting delays, and the fit indices confirmed the validity of the instrument for assessing Portuguese preschool children's gross and fine motor skills. In China [59], for children aged 3–6 years, excellent internal consistency, content, and structural validity have been reported. Fair external consistency was found in Taiwan for children aged 3–6 years [60]. Good reliability of the PDMS-2 was confirmed for children aged 4 and 5 years in the Netherlands [61], for newborn children in Iran [62], for 3- to 6-year-old children in China [59] and Taiwan [60], and for children aged zero to 71 months in Brazil [57]. These combined results ensure the validity and reliability of the use of PDMS-2 for early diagnosis. Professionals in several countries can safely plan specifically the implementation of intervention programs for children with motor delays or enhance motor acquisition in children who present adequate development.

One of the strengths of the PMDS is the acceptability of the test among the clinical community due to its multidimensional structure (i.e., reflexes, visuomotor integration, grasping, stationary balance, locomotor skills, and object manipulation), which allows for a broad view of motor development and specific insights into setting goals for intervention. Monitoring and ensuring development opportunities in which children can successfully engage are fundamental to achieving short-, medium-, and long-term benefits in promoting early childhood education, a challenge for teachers in which the PMDS-2 can be an essential ally.

Moreover, it evaluates the effectiveness of pedagogical and clinical intervention programs, as it measures proficiency in tasks that are part of everyday school life and can be applied playfully within the school context. Motor tasks are part of a child's daily life and make it easy to comprehend. The tasks are attractive and use playful materials easily found in schools, daycare centers, and child intervention centers; therefore, they are also familiar to children. With the PDMS-2, it is possible to monitor children's development in the first five years of life; it also covers an age with only a few motor assessments (from 2 to 3 years old).

Another advantage of PDMS-2 is that it is easy to apply.

The length of the assessment may be a high demand for a child. For children, such as children with attention deficits, language problems, cognitive delays, and cerebral palsy, the demand for an extended test can lead to the child becoming intolerant of the test or even refusing to participate; in these cases, the PDMS-2 is a suitable tool since the assessment can be stopped and continued within five days. It is important to note that training with the scale is essential before use. However, no specific certification is required to apply the test, nor is it professional-specific; knowledge about a child's developmental trajectories and typical and atypical development is beneficial for understanding assessment. Therefore, PDMS-2 is a robust assessment tool with discriminative, predictive, and evaluative features.

6.2.3 Movement Assessment Battery for Children—Second Edition—MABC-2

The MABC-2 [63] is an observational, valid, reliable, and norm-referenced assessment used in research, educational, and clinical settings worldwide to identify overall motor impairments and motor impairment in specific domains: fine or gross motor skills, static or dynamic, and balance. The MABC-2 is designed to identify children and adolescents (3–16 years and 11 months) with motor impairments. Moreover, we aimed to measure motor changes as a result of the intervention. The battery has several examples of clinical cases and an intervention manual to support intervention program planning. Nonetheless, the primary use of this battery has been associated with identifying developmental coordination disorders.

The MABC-2 comprises three tests to assess manual dexterity: static and dynamic balance; aiming and catching; a total of eight different tasks (i.e., posting coins, threading beads or lace, placing or turning pegs, building a triangle using screws and nuts; drawing trails; catching beanbags; throwing bean bags; balancing one or two legs; walking on lines; jumping or hopping on mats) according to individuals' age (Age Band 1: children 3:0 to 6:11 years old; Age Band 2: children from 7:0 to 10:11 years old; Age Band 3: children from 11:0 to 16:11). The MABC-2 motor behavior screening tool includes daily tasks to assess how children and adolescents (with norms ranging from 5:0 to 12:11 years old) perform in predictable (section A) and dynamic and unpredictable (section B) contexts (self-care, classroom skills, and physical education or recreational skills); it also includes a section regarding teacher perceptions about the nonmotor factors that may influence movement function, such as impulsivity, distractibility, and anxiety (section C). In addition, an intervention manual is also part of the battery. The test administration takes 20–30 min for each child; the checklist may be administered during the classroom routine or at home without a constrained time [63].

The raw scores, standardized scores, percentiles, and independent performance classifications for manual dexterity, aiming and catching, balance, and total score are provided. The classification of performance was performed using percentiles.

The 5th percentile (total score in the test at and included 56) is the standard measure of severe motor coordination difficulties. Children with performance above the 5th and 15th percentiles (total scores in the test from 57 to and including 67) are considered *at risk* of motor difficulties, requiring monitoring and further assessment. A score above the 15th percentile (above 67) indicated that the child's performance was within the range of typical development [63, 64].

Different cutoff values have been used in related research since the MABC-2 is a well-recognized tool for identifying the likelihood of developmental coordination disorder. A score less than or equal to the 5th percentile is a clear indication of the disorder (Criteria A) when combined with the recommended DSM-5 guidelines [65]; motor delays meaningfully interfere with children's daily activities at home and during school tasks (Criterion B); motor skill deficits are not better explained by intellectual disability or are not attributable to neurological or sensory conditions affecting movement (Criterion D); and delays are observed early in life during children's motor milestone acquisition (Criterion C). Children are considered at risk of developmental coordination disorder when the percentiles are above the 5th to and including the 15th percentile [64, 66]. The DCD international clinical guidelines recommend that children with performance below the 15th percentile benefit from intervention [66].

The MABC-2 Checklist screen [63], organized into three sections, uses *a* Likert scale (zero = very well, 1 = just ok, 2 = almost, 3 = not close) to describe how well the child deals with the tasks in sections A and B. The examiner decides whether the child can or cannot do it and how she does it. The total scores of sections A and B were used to categorize motor performance by age. If the scores are in the Red Zone, the child has definite movement difficulties; in the Amber Zone, the child is 'at-risk' or needs further investigation; in both cases, the use of the MABC-2 test is recommended. If the child's scores are in the Checklist Green Zone, the child has no apparent motor difficulties.

Across countries, the MABC-2 has shown good psychometric reliability mainly for Brazilian [27], British [63], Chinese [59, 67], Greek [68], Norwegian [69], Taiwanese [60, 70], and Thai children [71]. However, for Belgian children aged 3–4 years, the reliability of the scale was poor [72]. Fair to excellent internal consistency was reported for Brazilian [27], Chinese [59], Greek [68], Japanese [73], Taiwanese [67], and Norwegian [69] children at different age bands. However, poor internal consistency has been reported for Belgian children aged 3–4 [68] and for Taiwanese children aged 6–12 years old with DCD [60]. The content and structural validity of the scale were excellent for Chinese children [59] and excellent and good for UK [74] and Thai [71] children; for Brazilian children, these indices were fair [27]. Regarding norms, the MABC-2 UK normative data were accepted for use in Germany [75]; however, in the Netherlands and Flanders [76], norms were adjusted since the standard scores deviated from the UK reference values.

MABC-2 administration and scoring require training. The lack of training is inappropriate since several tasks of the MABC-2 include a subjective component; examiners must have sufficient training and knowledge about movement disorders [78]; and with training, the test can be conducted by different professionals in health and educational settings. In addition, the need for specific equipment limits the use of these devices by professionals with fewer economic resources available. The restricted number of motor tasks—only eight in each age band—and the use of only the best performance trial—have been noted as weaknesses since overlooking the individual variance and ceiling effect [79] in the test are potential limitations of the MABC-2. Another limitation is that the norms have been established only for the UK population, although they have been used worldwide.

The MABC-2 has the potential to screen children with disorders and motor difficulties. Although the test provides the overall score, scores on each subtest are provided, including percentiles, consequently allowing the researchers or clinicians to indicate the domains in which poor performance is observed (e.g., manual dexterity, balance, aiming, and catching); therefore, specific strategies may be designed for each child in a specific domain. These tests are easy to apply and require only a short time to conduct, which increases their feasibility for extensive studies. Currently, motor function is assessed in many studies on diverse cultures, appropriate psychometrics, allowing for international comparisons and monitoring of disorder prevalence. The MABC-2 checklist can screen children with soft-to-potential signs of motor impairments [77], allowing practitioners to refer the child to further assessment with the MABC-2 test or another assessment tool. The MABC-2 can be used at school; teachers may observe children with poor performance in predictable and unpredictable contexts (checklist sections A and B); and if their scores fail in zones for poor performance or at risk, the MABC-2 test should be used. To conclude, although the MABC-2 was designed with the primary purpose of discriminative and evaluative assessment, its discriminant attributes have also received strong support in the literature.

6.2.4 Test of Gross Motor Development, Third Edition—TGMD-3

One of the current assessments of children's motor proficiency is the TGMD-3 [80]; these two versions have been widely used worldwide. The TGMD-3 is a process-oriented observational assessment, referenced by norms and criteria, designed to assess children's (3–10 years old) motor proficiency in fundamental motor skills. The primary goals of the assessment are to identify motor proficiency levels, screen motor delays among children, assess motor changes over time and individual progress, and guide and evaluate the effects of instructional intervention programs.

Each subtest included locomotor skills (i.e., run, gallop, hop, skip, jump, and slide) and ball skills (i.e., strike with one or two hands, dribble, catch, kick, overhand and underhand throw); each skill has three to five performance criteria that need to be observed portraying the skill's appropriate movement pattern; the child must demonstrate the criteria to score 1— no half credits are allocated for the performance (dichotomous items). The sum of the observed criteria for each subscale comprises the total raw score; raw scores can be converted into percentile and scaled scores. Categorization of motor performance and age equivalence is also provided. The test administration and performance coding take approximately 20–30 min per child and require systematic observation of the performance criteria and assessor training [80].

Regarding TGMD-3 psychometrics, the original validation and posterior norms were conducted with a representative sample of the U.S. population concerning children's socioeconomic status, sex, disability status, race, ethnicity, age, geographic region, and parental education level; therefore, bias toward those factors seems to be minimal [80]. The original validation study showed an overall very high internal consistency for the composite scores and subtests (locomotor and ball skills), and it remained exclusive across age, sex, and all racial and ethnic groups. The TGMD-3 also has above-acceptable item difficulty and item discrimination values. Test–retest reliability showed high agreement for locomotor and ball skills and total TGMD-3 scores. The construct validity analysis supported a one-factor [81] and two-factor structure [82] of gross motor skill competence for the TGMD-3.

It is one of the most common tools examined worldwide across different countries. Adequate evidence for the validity of the TGMD-3 has been provided across several countries, including Brazil [26], France-Canada [83], Germany [84], Iran [85–87], Italy [88], Iraq [89], and Spain [90]. Adequate internal consistency has been reported for Brazilian [26] and German [84] children. Good fit indices for the construct validity of the two-factor model were reported for Brazilian [26], Spanish [90], German [84], Iranian [85, 86], and Iraqi [89] children. For Spanish [90] and Iranian [85] children, an adequate fit was also reported for the one-factor model, similar to the original data in the U.S [80–82]. For German children, concurrent validity was found between the TGMD-3 and German youth games [84]. The validity of the items has been reported for Australia [91] in a longitudinal sample and for Brazil [26] and Spain [90] in cross-sectional samples, providing further support for the predictive validity of the TGMD-3. For Brazilian and Spanish children, evidence was also provided for differential functioning for age in nine locomotor and ten ball skills items, suggesting that the TGMD-3 has items with different difficulty levels capable of differential functioning across age groups [92]. In addition, a recent longitudinal study suggested that TGMD-3 scores predict physical fitness six months later [93]. A short version to screen children and recommend further assessment has been proposed for Brazilian children [22] and Irish children [94], with appropriate evidence of internal consistency, validity, and reliability. Cross-cultural developmental trajectory validity has also been assessed to better understand the influence of culture, economics, resources, and opportunities for children in different countries [95].

Regarding TGMD-3 reliability, the original data have shown adequate-to-high test–retest reliability for American children [81, 82]. Robust results for reliability have also been provided for Brazilian (i.e., intrarater, interrater, test–retest) [26], French-Canadian speaking [83], Spanish [90], German (i.e., test–retest, interrater, interrater) [84], Italian [87], and Iranian [85] children and the two versions short version, Brazilian [22] and Irish [94]. Recently, reliability studies examining experienced raters [96], experienced versus novice raters [97, 98], the use of different strategies for rater training, such as consensus-building processes among raters regarding performance criteria [98] and the use of video records [97–99], and the impact of online and live rater training on scoring accuracy [96, 98] have shown that different strategies could be used to improve raters with different experience levels and background accuracies.

Although validity and reliability studies are more common in children with typical development, TGMD-3 psychometrics have also been examined in children with disabilities with adequate psychometric evidence. The TGMD-3 has demonstrated sensitivity for detecting deficits and differentiating the motor performance of children with disabilities (i.e., intellectual disability, attention deficit hyperactivity disorder, and language disorders) [100], Down syndrome [101], and autism spectrum disorder [81]. Acceptable internal consistency and reliability for children with intellectual disabilities [102] and developmental coordination disorders [103] have been reported. For children with visual impairments, the original TGMD-3 revealed adequate internal consistency, interrater reliability, and fit indices for the two-factor model [104]; short versions have also shown acceptable validity for this population [105]. Good reliability and feasibility results, as well as confirmation of the two-factor model, have been reported for children with mental and behavioral disorders [87]. In addition, for children with autism spectrum disorder [106, 107], excellent levels of internal consistency and test–retest, interrater and interrater reliability were also achieved for assessing TGMD-3 scores through the use of visual support (i.e., a combination of picture cards, short verbal prompts, and physical demonstrations) [106], and adequate content and developmental criterion validity were achieved through the use of TGMD-3 animations in an app as pedagogical visual support [107].

The TGMD-3 has several strengths and several weaknesses. The TGMD-3 is a norm- and criterion-referenced assessment of gross motor skills covering many skills ($n = 13$) and different age bands—from preschool to school-age children—used worldwide. The current studies investigating the TGMD-3 two-factor model supported the TGMD-3 subtests (i.e., locomotor and ball skills) and the overall motor quotient, suggesting that the TGMD-3 covers most skills related to children's gross motor function. The test has shown little ceiling or floor effect since, in this new version, more demanding motor criteria were added to the skills; slopes are provided for the subtests, as well as locomotor and ball skills, helping professionals interpret the results. Its core comprises skills that children usually do when playing and practice in several games at school; the fundamental motor skills assessed are part of the general school curriculum, which supports the ecological validity of the TGMD-3. Although some bias may be related to cultural differences (i.e., striking with two hands using a bat), the current version also incorporated the strike with one hand using the paddle—diminishing the bias of a skill more practiced by Americans.

The TGMD-3 is easy to administer, requires little equipment and can be conducted in open and closed physical spaces. However, TGMD-3 is time-consuming for teachers to use with the whole group in the school setting, but shorter forms have now been proposed with valid and reliable results. Several strategies may improve the feasibility of its use in schools. First, the use of the short form is recommended in countries with established valid versions; currently, it is recommended for Brazilian and Irish children. Second, the protocol for administering the TGMD-3 may be adapted by using stations for each skill and by the teacher assessing a small group of children or conducting the TGMD-3 subtests on different days. Third, specific skills may be the focus of the PE curriculum at a specific grade and time (e.g., month, trimester, semester); the teacher may elect only those skills to be assessed—although no standard scores would be obtained—and the teacher will have insights into what motor criteria in each skill need more practice for a child or a group of children.

Another interesting feature is that the TGMD-3 can be used to assess children with disabilities; valid and reliable evidence supports its use. The literature has also provided strategies for adapting or using technological support to assess these populations. It is a test that accurately discriminates performance levels, a relevant clinical and educational practice feature. Validity and reliability are vital within the original sample and across different countries, allowing researchers to compare data and investigate cultural differences in children's motor proficiency. In addition, evidence of the ability of the TGMD-3 to predict PA in children reinforces its ecological and predictive validity. Therefore, the TGMD-3 is currently recognized worldwide as an effective discriminative, predictive, and evaluative assessment tool.

6.2.5 *Bruininks-Oseretsky Test of Motor Proficiency Second Edition—BOT-2*

The BOT-2 [108] is a valid, reliable, and norm-referenced product-oriented assessment design for assessing gross and fine motor proficiency in children, adolescents, and young adults (aged 4:0 to 21:11 years). The main goals of the BOT-2 include screening and detecting motor impairments, supporting the referral of children to intervention programs, making decisions about program goals, and evaluating motor intervention effectiveness. The BOT-2 included several subtests assessing children's motor function domains. Body coordination subtests assess the control and coordination of the large musculature used to maintain posture and balance. The strength and agility subtest assesses fitness and coordination in casual play, competitive sports, and PA. The fine manual control subtest assesses control and the coordination of the muscles of the hands and fingers. The manual coordination subtests assess the control and coordination of the arms and hands. Therefore, four subtests were used to assess gross motor skills (i.e., bilateral coordination, balance, running speed/agility, and strength) and four fine-motor skills (i.e., fine-motor precision, fine-motor integration, manual dexterity, and upper-extremity coordination) [108].

The BOT-2 has 53 items in the long form and 14 in the short form; these items were obtained from the long form. The BOT-2 short-form was designed to be a briefer screen of motor proficiency and has often been used to determine children's need for further assessment. The BOT-2 provided raw scores, age-based standard scores, percentile ranks, and descriptive categorization of motor performance. The administration of the long form is time-consuming and requires 45–60 min, whereas the administration of the short form takes approximately 15–20 min. The BOT-2 has been used by practitioners and researchers in educational and clinical contexts [108, 109].

Regarding the psychometric qualities of the original sample from the U.S., internal consistency was reported to be good for the long-form and acceptable for the short-form [108]. The authors also reported good to excellent content, structural, and criterion validity for the long form [108]; fair responsiveness was also reported in the original sample [108]. Regarding reliability, for the long and short forms, good to excellent interrater reliability [108, 109] and moderate to substantial test–retest reliability for the short and long forms across all ages (4:0 to 21:11 years old) were reported for the original U.S. sample [108, 109]. However, for the subtests independently, the test–retest reliability was generally weak except for the strength and agility subtest; the coefficients for the three age groups assessed in the original sample (i.e., strength and agility with knee push-ups and strength and agility with full push-ups) were good; this subtest is one in which professionals can have more confidence in the stability of scores over time [109].

Regarding psychometric studies worldwide, the evidence is very limited for the long and short forms. For the long form, the unidimensionality of the model, good internal consistency, and adequate reliability have been reported for Taiwanese children aged 3–6 years [110]; excellent indices have been reported for children aged 4–12 years [111]. Both Taiwanese samples were moderately large (nearly 500 children) and composed of children with intellectual disabilities [110, 111]. For a small sample of Brazilian children ($n = 187$), the dimensionality of the BOT-2 was not supported, and poor fit indices were found [112]; caution is recommended in the interpretation of those results since the sample was small and not representative of the Brazilian population. In addition, a trajectory of change in motor percentiles for children aged 6–10 years with typical development in a cross-sectional Brazilian study further supported the developmental validity of the BOT-2 long-form [113].

For the short form, cross-cultural support for the unidimensionality of the BOT-2 has been reported for Belgian children aged 6–8 years in a large sample (nearly 2500 children). However, in this Belgian sample, ceiling effects were found for children aged 9–11 years, and a 12-item model, instead of 14, showed a better fit [114]. The results provided support for the use of the BOT-2 for assessing 6- to 8-year-old children whose performance was below average to above average, and the suitability of the BOT-2 for assessing competence decreased as the competence level increased; moreover, the BOT-2 was a less reliable measurement for more motor-competent nine 11-year-old children [114]. Furthermore, in Australia, the results of a study with eight 12-year-old children suggested that the short form lacked strong structural validity evidence; from the 14 proposed items, nine showed misfits and must be removed to improve the short-form indices of fit [115]. It is crucial to note that the Australian sample was small ($n = 123$) and not representative of the population.

The BOT-2 has several limitations. The length of the long form is time-consuming and quite demanding for young children. Although there is a straightforward scoring process, this process is also time-consuming. Overall, the psychometric evidence for children aged 4 and 5 years is still weak. There is a lack of robust evidence to support the temporal stability (test–retest reliability) of the BOT-2 for the independent subtest and the bidimensionality of the model (i.e., fine and gross motor domains), and it still lacks predictive validity since its publication. In addition, norms are not current since the last version was published in 2005.

The BOT-2 has several strengths and weaknesses. The possibility of assessing several domains of childhood behavior, fine manual control and coordination, body coordination, strength and agility provides a comprehensive understanding of children's and adolescents' strengths and weaknesses, which are essential features for practitioners. All the items assessed in the BOT-2 reflect the real-world childhood context and support the ecological validity of the BOT-2. The long form of BOT-2 is very time-consuming. However, the BOT-2 provides a short form that can be easily used to screen children in larger sample studies and school settings due to teacher time constraints. In addition, if the long form is the teacher's choice, the subtest may be conducted on different days, and the teacher may choose those aligned with the PE curriculum.

The BOT-2 manual provides comprehensive information with pictures that help the assessors understand the tasks. Currently, video training that complements manual information is available. The validity, reliability, and norms provided for a representative national sample are adequate; the normative sample included children with disabilities (11.4%), and the BOT-2 also has adequate support for discriminating between the scores of children with and without disabilities. In addition, examples of clinical cases are provided for children with cognitive impairments, developmental coordination disorders and autism spectrum disorders. Professionals use the complete form to determine which children are eligible for special education services, physical therapy, or occupational therapy. It has been used in several countries to complement the diagnoses of developmental coordination disorders. Although not extensive, some validity and reliability of the scale have been reported across countries, ensuring its usage in other cultures with caution. Therefore, the BOT-2 is a discriminative and evaluative assessment, and some evidence of its predictive validity has been provided. However, overall, more robust evidence is still scarce.

6.2.6 Körperkoordination Für Kinder—KTK

The KTK (Motor Coordination Battery for Children) [116, 117] is a reliable product-oriented assessment designed to assess motor coordination in children and adolescents aged 5–14 years with and without disabilities; the original data are from

Germany. The KTK's primary goals are to screen children and adolescents with poor motor coordination, to detect subtle signs of motor impairment in children with brain injuries or behavioral disorders and to guide school curricular decisions and program implementation to foster children's improvement in motor coordination.

The KTK consists of four subtests: (a) walking backward along a balance beam with decreasing width (from 6 to 4.5 to 3 cm); (b) hopping high over a foam obstacle with an increasing height in consecutive 5 cm; (c) jumping sideways over a slat for 15 s; (d) moving sideways from one wooden platform to another for 20 s. The raw scores obtained in each subtest were compared to the original normative data and transformed into motor quotients for each task; percentiles are also provided. The sum of the four standardized item scores was calculated as the overall motor quotient (MQ) of the KTK [116]. The KTK tasks are the same for the different age bands. The KTK is easy to apply and has little time demand; test administration generally lasts 10–20 min. These characteristics combined make the KTK a simple and low-cost test [118] that is easy to administer and potentially useful for physical education teachers in school settings [119] and researchers with large sample sizes to screen children with poor motor coordination.

The KTK psychometrics, related to validity (i.e., content and construct), reliability, and norms, were established with an original sample of 1228 German children and adolescents aged 5–14 years. The sample was composed of children and adolescents without and with disabilities (i.e., confirmed and suspected intellectual disabilities, behavioral disorders, and speech disorders). The KTK internal consistency of the four tasks in children (i.e., 6–9 years) was high, and the factor analysis confirmed the unidimensionality of the KTK—body coordination. The discriminant validity indicated that the KTK could differentiate between children with typical and those with atypical development or disability. High test–retest reliability coefficients were reported for the four tasks [116, 117].

KTK psychometrics worldwide are still restricted. The construct validity was examined for Australian [120] and Brazilian [119] children; in both studies, the confirmatory factor analysis indicated an adequate fit for a unidimensional model, body coordination, similar to the original data [116, 117]. Adequate internal consistency was found for the KTK in studies of Brazilian [119], Chinese [121], Spanish [122], Finnish [123], Portuguese [123], and Belgian [123] children. Adequate concurrent validity was reported for the KTK and TGMD-3 for Chinese children (9–10 years old) [121]. Fair convergent validity was found between the KTK and BOT-2 Short Form [124] and between the KTK and the Motor Proficiency [125] Test for Belgian children aged 6 to 1 year and 5 to 6 years, respectively. Convergent validity was also examined for KTK and MABC for Dutch children in a randomized sample of 134 children with typical development (5–13 years old) and a referred sample of 74 children with disabilities (5–12 years old) [126]. Fair discriminant power was observed for KTK for Dutch 130 and Belgian 128 children, although the KTK tends to detect a high prevalence of motor impairments compared to the MABC [126] and short BOT-2 versions [124].

Cross-cultural validity was examined in one study enrolling children from Finland, Portugal, and Belgium, and significant differences between countries were found as children's age increased; Finnish children demonstrated greater performance than did Portuguese and Belgian children [123]. The ability of the KTK to longitudinally predict PA and fitness in Portuguese (6–10 years old) [11] and Brazilian (6–13 years old) [127] children was reported in two longitudinal studies. Regarding reliability, moderate to high KTK reliability coefficients were reported among Spanish [122] and Portuguese [11, 128] children. High interrater reliability is reported for Australian [120] and Spanish [122] children, and high test–retest reliability is reported for Spanish [122] children.

The KTK has several weaknesses. The original normative values of KTK were established more than four decades ago in Germany and are still in use today, lacking addressed diversity and worldwide changes in economic, social, and cultural factors. Most studies using KTK were conducted in Europe; therefore, regarding validity, the world representation of children is poor, constraining the possibility of comparing data around the world. Another weakness of the KTK is related to the sample size and representativeness of the samples. Several validation studies were conducted with small and nonrepresentative samples [120–122, 126], and the psychometrics were quite limited—none of the current studies examined all the validity and reliability procedures in one representative sample. Therefore, caution is recommended when interpreting KTK psychometrics. The evidence of its validity and reliability for children with disabilities is not robust, and further studies are necessary to investigate the feasibility and sensitivity of its use for those populations. The KTK also has several strengths: the KTK is easy to administer and takes little time; consequently, it seems suitable for school settings or large screening studies [119]. In addition, since motor coordination is the core of these tasks, it is suitable for assessing children in different fields, such as physical education, sports, health sciences, medicine, and biomechanics [129]. These combined factors suggest that the KTK is an evaluative assessment tool with some evidence of its ability to discriminate children with different performances, and some evidence of its predictive validity has been provided. However, overall, more robust evidence is still scarce.

6.3 Motor Assessment Use in Education and Clinical Settings and Research

The assessments presented in this chapter are commonly used in education, clinical practice, and research. However, although several assessments may have similar goals, it is essential to consider the adequacy of an assessment related to the research's theoretical conceptualization and objectives, the clinical or educational cases to be assessed, the individual-specific levels of motor proficiency, and how the assessment will be aligned with the research conceptual and operational model [130]. Motor assessments administered in school and clinical settings are usually part of administration programs to determine children's eligibility for special services, the program goals, and the program's effectiveness on children's performance. When teachers and clinicians search for an assessment, selecting those with robust, valid, and reliable evidence for their working population is crucial. BSITD-III and IV, PDMS-2, TGMD-3, MABC-2, BOT-2, PDMS-2, and KTK have the potential for use in schools and clinical settings; however, professionals must consider several constraints, such as the time to administer the test, the availability of the required equipment, the high amount of training to administer and interpret the scores, and the goals of using it.

Professionals must be knowledgeable about the assessments, the assessment's intended goals, how these goals are aligned with the intervention program or school curriculum, and the educational and clinical benefits of assessing a child or a specific group of children. Assessments must complement the educational and clinical purpose of a specific individual or group. In addition, to achieve the goal of complementing professional intervention plans, assessments related to the frequency with which they will be applied, the length of assessment, the required training and retraining of professionals, the resources available in schools or clinics, the target individual domains to be measured, the specificity of the tasks to be designed to improve individuals' movement, and how the results will be used to improve children's and adolescents' development and health need to be considered. Another essential feature is that reflecting on how the assessment results may help families understand the child's development and joining the professional intervention force is also essential; a clear understanding of the assessment goals and possibilities by families should be a practitioner's target.

Regarding research, as the study protocol is established, researchers must plan the assessor's training since it takes time to understand the test protocol, coding, and scoring system. Assessor training may be conducted individually and in groups, coding performance from video records and in person. Team meetings to ensure that the assessor's team carefully understands the application protocol and the behavior codification are also crucial. Appropriate reliability is usually reached after several hours of assessor training, especially if the assessment is process-oriented and requires codifying behaviors (i.e., TGMD-3). It is important to note that after assessors achieved above 80% agreement, they could start coding the children's performance to achieve high interrater reliability. For high interrater reliability, it is recommended that the same assessor reassess the video records or the same child within 15-day intervals to diminish the possibility of individual motor performance changes. The time reported in previous assessments or published research methods may be used to estimate the time the assessor needs to complete the test, code the child, and score the performance. Assessors in educational and clinical settings and researchers still need effective training protocols to overcome the differences in instructions for the tests and in interpreting the qualitative features of several motor assessment codes.

Although several assessments discussed in the chapter are well recognized worldwide, comprehensive evidence of motor assessment psychometrics is still needed even in the population where norms were established. In countries where the assessments were developed and validated and norms were established, follow-up psychometric studies must be conducted to ensure that the responsiveness of the motor assessment is appropriate for distinct subgroups (i.e., sex, ethnicity, cultural background, disabilities). In addition, even in those countries, the specificity and sensitivity of motor assessments are somewhat overlooked by researchers. Furthermore, ecological validity may be assessed depending on the researcher's or clinician's goals. Children and adolescents are engaged daily in several activities involving several motor demands, from playing games, dancing, and playing sports to doing homework at school or at home; the extension of the assessment goals is aligned with those activities that need further support. For some assessments, norms were established several decades ago (i.e., KTK), so a revision is needed.

Furthermore, in several countries, especially in low- and middle-income countries, where most children and adolescents live, the reliability and validity of motor assessments still need to be investigated since the psychometrics of the original samples may be inappropriate for individuals developing under different socioeconomic and cultural contexts. In addition, even within a country, families' cultural backgrounds may provide distinct childcare opportunities for motor development; research still needs to examine the discrimination and responsiveness of motor assessments for specific populations. In addition, motor assessment prediction in longitudinal studies is still under examination, limiting the understanding of developmental trajectories and the mechanism behind changes across childhood and adolescence.

6.4 Conclusions

This chapter reviews various assessments that aid in observing a child's performance in diverse motor tasks, predominantly focusing on gross motor skills. Some assessments also consider fine motor skills. These recognized tools are effective at identifying behavioral characteristics exhibited by children during motor tasks in different settings, such as at home, at school, during recreation, and during sports. This relevance extends to children's participation in various childhood activities.

Motor *assessment* is vital *for providing* appropriate care for children and adolescents, *compensating* for adverse outcomes, and *optimizing* their capabilities. Proper motor assessment is crucial *for* understanding motor development within a specific context and setting interventional goals. *In addition*, motor development is related to cognitive, language, social–emotional, and physical health. These *intricate* developmental relationships emphasize the relevance of selecting the appropriate assessment via an integrative approach to promote children's and adolescents' well-being. In addition, to make decisions and design programs to improve children's competence, professionals need motor assessments that are practical to administer and code, relevant to the child and their families, sensitive to children's changes, specific for a diverse population, discriminant of soft and robust signs of disorders, predictive of *children's* achievement, and responsive to *children's* needs.

It is essential to recognize that in the last two decades, unambiguous and objective improvements in motor assessments *have* occurred worldwide; however, several potential challenges are still faced by health professionals and researchers, namely, (a) improving the access and training of valid and normalized assessments for researchers living in low- and moderate-income countries, as the economic cost for acquiring and training is generally too high; (b) extending motor assessment psychometric studies across different populations and cultures within and between countries, as several assessments still lack robust evidence specifically for cross-cultural, concurrent, convergent, predictive, and hypothesis validity; (c) developing new assessments or reducing the number of original long assessments so that the time to complete motor assessments in educational settings becomes feasible for education settings; (d) extending the training of examiners to standardize the instruction and codification of behavior to control bias and allow for adequate cross-cultural studies; (e) including technology to conduct assessments to unify instruction and demonstrations, to improve coding, to allow examiners with a disability to conduct tests, and to enhance children's performance, especially those with a disability; (f) improving ecological validity in assessment and assessment protocols by further studying the different contexts of development that the child lives in; and (g) developing.

References

1. Barnett LM, Webster EK, Hulteen RM, De Meester A, Valentini NC, Lenoir M, et al. Correction to: through the looking glass: a systematic review of longitudinal evidence, providing new insight for motor competence and health. Sports Med. 2022;52(4):921–1. https://doi.org/10.1007/s40279-021-01563-1.
2. Berleze A, Valentini NC. Intervention for children with obesity and overweight and motor delays from low-income families: fostering engagement, motor development, self-perceptions, and playtime. Int J Environ Res Public Health. 2022;19(5):2545. https://www.mdpi.com/1660-4601/19/5/2545
3. Martins C, Romo-Perez V, Webster EK, Duncan M, Lemos LF, Staiano AE, et al. Motor competence and body mass index in the preschool years: a pooled cross-sectional analysis of 5545 children from eight countries. Sports Med. 2023;54:505. https://pubmed.ncbi.nlm.nih.gov/37747664/
4. Spessato BC, Gabbard C, Robinson L, Valentini NC. Body mass index, perceived and actual physical competence: the relationship among young children. Child Care Health Dev. 2013;39(6):845–50. https://pubmed.ncbi.nlm.nih.gov/23199334/
5. Valentini NC, Nobre GC, de Souza MS, Duncan MJ. Are BMI, self-perceptions, motor competence, engagement, and fitness related to physical activity in physical education lessons? J Phys Act Health. 2020;17(5):493–500. https://journals.humankinetics.com/view/journals/jpah/17/5/article-p493.xml
6. De Meester A, Barnett LM, Brian A, Bowe SJ, Jiménez-Díaz J, Van Duyse F, et al. The relationship between actual and perceived motor competence in children, adolescents and young adults: a systematic review and meta-analysis. Sports Med. 2020;50(11):2001–49. https://pubmed.ncbi.nlm.nih.gov/32970291/
7. Gu X, Thomas KT, Chen Y-L. The role of perceived and actual motor competency on children's physical activity and cardiorespiratory fitness during middle childhood. J Teach Phys

Educ. 2017;36(4):388–97. https://journals.humankinetics.com/view/journals/jtpe/36/4/article-p388.xml
8. Lloyd M, Saunders TJ, Bremer E, Tremblay MS. Long-term importance of fundamental motor skills: a 20-year follow-up study. Adapt Phys Act Q. 2014;31(1):67–78. https://pubmed.ncbi.nlm.nih.gov/24385442/
9. Hill PJ, Mcnarry MA, Mackintosh KA, Murray MA, Pesce C, Valentini NC, et al. The influence of motor competence on broader aspects of health: a systematic review of the longitudinal associations between motor competence and cognitive and social-emotional outcomes. Sports Med. 2023;54:375. https://doi.org/10.1007/s40279-023-01939-5.
10. Logan SW, Kipling Webster E, Getchell N, Pfeiffer KA, Robinson LE. Relationship between fundamental motor skill competence and physical activity during childhood and adolescence: a systematic review. Kinesiol Rev (Champaign). 2015;4(4):416–26. https://journals.humankinetics.com/view/journals/krj/4/4/article-p416.xml
11. Lopes VP, Rodrigues LP, Maia JAR, Malina RM. Motor coordination as predictor of physical activity in childhood. Scand J Med Sci Sports. 2011;21(5):663–9. https://doi.org/10.1111/j.1600-0838.2009.01027.x. https://pubmed.ncbi.nlm.nih.gov/21917017/
12. Wagner MO, Kastner J, Petermann F, Bös K. Factorial validity of the movement assessment battery for children-2 (age band 2). Res Dev Disabil. 2011;32(2):674–80. https://www.sciencedirect.com/science/article/pii/S0891422210002891Ekornås
13. Lundervold AJ, Tjus T, Heimann M. Anxiety disorders in 8–11-year-old children: motor skill performance and self-perception of competence. Scand J Psychol. 2010;51(3):271–7. https://doi.org/10.1111/j.1467-9450.2009.00763.x.
14. Magalhães LC, Cardoso AA, Missiuna C. Activities and participation in children with developmental coordination disorder: a systematic review. Res Dev Disabil. 2011;32(4):1309–16. https://www.sciencedirect.com/science/article/pii/S0891422211000308
15. Griffiths A, Morgan P, Anderson PJ, Doyle LW, Lee KJ, Spittle AJ. Predictive value of the movement assessment battery for children—second edition at 4 years, for motor impairment at 8 years in children born preterm. Dev Med Child Neurol. 2017;59(5):490–6. https://doi.org/10.1111/dmcn.13367.
16. Kanitkar A, Szturm T, Parmar S, Gandhi DBC, Rempel GR, Restall G, et al. The effectiveness of a computer game-based rehabilitation platform for children with cerebral palsy: protocol for a randomized clinical trial. JMIR Res Protoc. 2017;6(5):e93. https://www.researchprotocols.org/2017/5/e93/
17. Miller MM, Ray JM, Van Zant RS. The effects of Astym therapy® on a child with spastic diplegic cerebral palsy. Clin Med Insights Case Rep. 2017;10:117954761774699. https://doi.org/10.1177/1179547617746992.
18. Mueller SM, Petersen JA, Jung HH. Exercise in Huntington's disease: current state and clinical significance. Tremor and Other Hyperkinetic Movements. 2019:9. https://doi.org/10.7916/TM9J-F874.
19. Valentini NC, Zanella LW. Peabody Developmental Motor Scales-2: the use of Rasch analysis to examine the model unidimensionality, motor function, and item difficulty. Front Pediatr. 2022;10:10. https://doi.org/10.3389/fped.2022.852732.
20. Zanella LW, Valentini NC, Copetti F, Nobre GC. Peabody Developmental Motor Scales—second edition (PDMS-2): reliability, content and construct validity evidence for Brazilian children. Res Dev Disabil. 2021;111(103871):103871. https://www.sciencedirect.com/science/article/pii/S0891422221000202
21. Valentini N, Pereira K, Nobre G. Content, construct, and criterion validity, reliability, and objectivity for Aquatic Readiness Assessment for Brazilian children. Int J Aquat Res Educ. 2022;13(4):11. https://scholarworks.bgsu.edu/ijare/vol13/iss4/11/
22. Valentini NC, Nobre GC, Zanella LW, Pereira KG, Albuquerque MR, Rudisill ME. Test of Gross Motor Development–3 validity and reliability: a screening form. J Mot Learn Dev. 2021;9(3):438–55. https://doi.org/10.1123/jmld.2020-0061. https://journals.humankinetics.com/view/journals/jmld/9/3/article-p438.xml

23. Chiquetti EM dos S, Valentini NC, Saccani R. Validation and reliability of the test of infant motor performance for Brazilian infants. Phys Occup Ther Pediatr. 2020;40(4):470–85. https://doi.org/10.1080/01942638.2020.1711843.
24. dos Santos Chiquetti EM, Valentini NC. Test of infant motor performance for infants in Brazil: unidimensional model, item difficulty, and motor function. Pediatr Phys Ther. 2020;32(4):390–7. https://www.ingentaconnect.com/content/wk/pep/2020/00000032/00000004/art00024
25. Venetsanou F, Kossyva I, Valentini N, Afthentopoulou A-E, Barnett L. Validity and reliability of the Pictorial Scale of perceived movement skill competence for young Greek children. J Mot Learn Dev. 2018;6(s2):S239–51.
26. Valentini NC, Zanella LW, Webster EK. Test of Gross Motor Development—third edition: establishing content and construct validity for Brazilian children. J Mot Learn Dev. 2017;5(1):15–28.
27. Valentini NC, Ramalho MH, Oliveira MA. Movement assessment battery for children-2: translation, reliability, and validity for Brazilian children. Res Dev Disabil. 2014;35(3):733–40. https://www.sciencedirect.com/science/article/pii/S0891422213004721
28. Bayley N. Bayley scales of infant development and toddler development. 3rd ed. San Antonio: Technical manual. PsychCorp; 2006.
29. Bayley N, Aylward GP. Bayley scales of infant development and toddler development. 4th ed. London: Technical manual. Pearson; 2019.
30. Del Rosario C, Slevin M, Molloy EJ, Quigley J, Nixon E. How to use the Bayley Scales of infant and toddler development. Arch Dis Child Educ Pract Ed. 2021;106(2):108–12. https://pubmed.ncbi.nlm.nih.gov/32859738/
31. Aylward GP. Is it correct to correct for prematurity? Theoretic analysis of the Bayley-4 normative data. J Dev Behav Pediatr. 2020;41(2):128–33. https://doi.org/10.1097/dbp.0000000000000739.
32. Fleurkens-Peeters MJ, Zijlmans WC, Akkermans RP, der Sanden MWGN, Janssen AJ. The United States reference values of the Bayley III motor scale are suitable in Suriname. Infant Behav Dev. 2024;74(101922):101922. https://doi.org/10.1016/j.infbeh.2024.101922.
33. Chinta S, Walker K, Halliday R, Loughran-Fowlds A, Badawi N. A comparison of the performance of healthy Australian 3-year-olds with the standardised norms of the Bayley Scales of infant and toddler development (version-III). Arch Dis Child. 2014;99(7):621–4. https://doi.org/10.1136/archdischild-2013-304834.
34. Hoskens J, Klingels K, Smits-Engelsman B. Validity and cross-cultural differences of the Bayley Scales of infant and toddler development, third edition in typically developing infants. Early Hum Dev. 2018;125:17–25. https://doi.org/10.1016/j.earlhumdev.2018.07.002.
35. Madaschi V, Mecca TP, Macedo EC, Paula CS. Bayley-III Scales of infant and toddler development: transcultural adaptation and psychometric properties. Paid (Ribeirão Preto). 2016;26(64):189–97. https://doi.org/10.1590/1982-43272664201606.
36. Krogh MT, Væver MS. Bayley-III: cultural differences and language scale validity in a Danish sample. Scand J Psychol. 2016;57(6):501–8. https://doi.org/10.1111/sjop.12333.
37. Salah El-Din EM, Monir ZM, Shehata MA, Abouelnaga MW, Abushady MM, Youssef MM, et al. A comparison of the performance of normal middle social class Egyptian infants and toddlers with the reference norms of the Bayley Scales -third edition (Bayley III): a pilot study. PLoS One. 2021;16(12):e0260138. https://doi.org/10.1371/journal.pone.0260138.
38. Hanlon C, Medhin G, Worku B, Tomlinson M, Alem A, Dewey M, et al. Adapting the Bayley Scales of infant and toddler development in Ethiopia: evaluation of reliability and validity. Child Care Health Dev. 2016;42(5):699–708. https://doi.org/10.1111/cch.12371.
39. Fuiko R, Oberleitner-Leeb C, Klebermass-Schrehof K, Berger A, Brandstetter S, Giordano V. The impact of norms on the outcome of children born very-preterm when using the Bayley-III: differences between US and German norms. Neonatology. 2019;116(1):29–36. https://doi.org/10.1159/000497138.

40. Gasparini C, Caravale B, Rea M, Coletti MF, Tonchei V, Bucci S, et al. Neurodevelopmental outcome of Italian preterm children at 1 year of corrected age by Bayley-III scales: an assessment using local norms. Early Hum Dev. 2017;113:1–6. https://doi.org/10.1016/j.earlhumdev.2017.06.007.
41. Hasani Khiabani N, Barzegar M, Raeisi S, Jalalian Chaleshtori M, Heidarabadi S, Bahari GA. Comparison of the performance of Iranian Azeri-speaking children based on Iran and reference Bayley III norms. Iran. J Child Neurol. Spring. 2022 Spring;16(2):39. https://doi.org/10.22037/ijcn.v16i2.32930.
42. Cromwell EA, Dube Q, Cole SR, Chirambo C, Dow AE, Heyderman RS, et al. Validity of US norms for the Bayley Scales of infant development-III in Malawian children. Eur J Paediatr Neurol. 2014;18(2):223–30. https://doi.org/10.1016/j.ejpn.2013.11.011.
43. Steenis LJP, Verhoeven M, Hessen DJ, van Baar AL. Performance of dutch children on the Bayley III: a comparison study of US and dutch norms. PLoS One. 2015;10(8):e0132871. https://doi.org/10.1371/journal.pone.0132871.
44. Kvestad I, Hysing M, Ranjitkar S, Shrestha M, Ulak M, Chandyo RK, et al. The stability of the Bayley scales in early childhood and its relationship with future intellectual abilities in a low to middle income country. Early Hum Dev. 2022;170(105610):105610. https://doi.org/10.1016/j.earlhumdev.2022.105610.
45. Ranjitkar S, Kvestad I, Strand TA, Ulak M, Shrestha M, Chandyo RK, et al. Acceptability and reliability of the Bayley scales of infant and toddler development-III among children in Bhaktapur. Nepal Front Psychol. 2018;9:9. https://doi.org/10.3389/fpsyg.2018.01265.
46. Pavlova P, Maksimov D, Chegodaev D, Kiselev S. A psychometric study of the Russian-language version of the "Bayley Scales of infant and toddler development—third edition": an assessment of reliability and validity. Front Psychol. 2022;13:13. https://doi.org/10.3389/fpsyg.2022.961567.
47. Godamunne P, Liyanage C, Wimaladharmasooriya N, Pathmeswaran A, Wickremasinghe AR, Patterson C, et al. Comparison of performance of Sri Lankan and US children on cognitive and motor scales of the Bayley scales of infant development. BMC Res Notes. 2014;7(1) https://doi.org/10.1186/1756-0500-7-300.
48. Ballot DE, Ramdin T, Rakotsoane D, Agaba F, Davies VA, Chirwa T, et al. Use of the Bayley Scales of infant and toddler development, third edition, to assess developmental outcome in infants and young children in an urban setting in South Africa. Int Sch Res Notices. 2017;2017:1–5. https://doi.org/10.1155/2017/1631760.
49. McLester-Davis LWY, Shankar A, Kataria LA, Hidalgo AG, van Eer ED, Koendjbiharie AP, et al. Validity, reliability, and transcultural adaptations of the Bayley Scales of infant and toddler development (BSID-III-NL) for children in Suriname. Early Hum Dev. 2021;160(105416):105416. https://doi.org/10.1016/j.earlhumdev.2021.105416.
50. Yu Y-T, Hsieh W-S, Hsu C-H, Chen L-C, Lee W-T, Chiu N-C, et al. A psychometric study of the Bayley Scales of infant and toddler development—3rd edition for term and preterm Taiwanese infants. Res Dev Disabil. 2013;34(11):3875–83. https://doi.org/10.1016/j.ridd.2013.07.006.
51. Sun L, Sabanathan S, Thanh PN, Kim A, Doa TTM, Thwaites CL, et al. Bayley III in Vietnamese children: lessons for cross-cultural comparisons. Wellcome Open Res. 2019;4:98. https://doi.org/10.12688/wellcomeopenres.15282.1.
52. Walker K, Badawi N, Halliday R, Laing S. Brief report: performance of Australian children at one year of age on the Bayley scales of infant and toddler development (version III). Aust Educ Dev Psychol. 2010;27(1):54–8. https://doi.org/10.1375/aedp.27.1.54.
53. Kosmann P, Blaeser A, Rochow M, So HY, Ascherl R, Heussinger N, et al. Make Bayley III scores comparable between United States and German norms—development of conversion equations. Neuropediatrics. 2023;54(02):147–52. https://doi.org/10.1055/a-1988-2544.
54. Rademeyer V, Jacklin L. A study to evaluate the performance of black south African urban infants on the Bayley Scales of infant development III. SAJCH. 2013;7(2):54. https://doi.org/10.7196/sajch.547.

55. Dale BA, Caemmerer JM, Winter EL, Kaufman AS. Bayley-4 performance of very young children with autism, developmental delay, and language impairment. Psychol Sch. 2022;59(7):1267–81. https://doi.org/10.1002/pits.22682.
56. Folio R, Fewell RR. Peabody developmental motor Scales-2. Austin: Pro-Ed; 2000.
57. Zanella LZ, Valentini NC, Copetti F, Nobre GC. Peabody Developmental Motor Scales—second edition (PDMS-2): reliability, content and construct validity evidence for Brazilian children. Res Dev Dis. 2021;111. https://pubmed.ncbi.nlm.nih.gov/33571789/:103871.
58. Saraiva LB, Rodrigues LP, Barreiros J. Adaptação e validação da versão portuguesa Peabody Developmental Motor Scales-2: um estudo com crianças pré-escolares. J Phy Edu. 2011;22(4):511–21.
59. Hua J, Gu G, Meng W, Wu Z. Age band 1 of the movement assessment battery for children—second edition: exploring its usefulness in mainland China. Res Dev Disabil. 2013;34(2):801–8. https://doi.org/10.1016/j.ridd.2012.10.012.
60. Wuang Y-P, Su C-Y, Huang M-H. Psychometric comparisons of three measures for assessing motor functions in preschoolers with intellectual disabilities. J Intellect Disabil Res. 2012;56(6):567–78. https://doi.org/10.1111/j.1365-2788.2011.01491.x.
61. van Hartingsveldt MJ, Cup EHC, Oostendorp RAB. Reliability and validity of the fine motor scale of the Peabody Developmental Motor Scales-2. Occup Ther Int. 2005;12(1):1–13. https://doi.org/10.1002/oti.11.
62. Tavasoli A, Azimi P, Montazari A. Reliability and validity of the Peabody developmental motor scales-second edition for assessing motor development of low birth weight preterm infants. Pediatr Neurol. 2014;51(4):522–6. https://doi.org/10.1016/j.pediatrneurol.2014.06.010.
63. Henderson SE, Sugden DA, Barnett A. Movement assessment battery for children—second edition (movement ABC-2). London: The Psychological Corporation; 2007.
64. Geuze RH, Jongmans MJ, Schoemaker MM, Smits-Engelsman BCM. Clinical and research diagnostic criteria for developmental coordination disorder: a review and discussion. Hum Mov Sci. 2001;20(1–2):7–47. https://pubmed.ncbi.nlm.nih.gov/11471398/
65. American Psychiatric Association. Diagnostic and statistical manual of mental disorders (DSM-5 (R)). 5th ed. Arlington: American Psychiatric Association Publishing; 2013.
66. European Academy of Childhood Disability (EACD). Recommendations on the definition, diagnosis and intervention of developmental coordination disorder (pocket version)*: EACD recommendations. Dev Med Child Neurol. 2012;54(11):976–6. https://doi.org/10.1111/j.1469-8749.2011.04175a.x.
67. Chow SMK, Henderson SE. Interrater and test-retest reliability of the movement assessment battery for Chinese preschool children. Am J Occup Ther. 2003;57(5):574–7. https://doi.org/10.5014/ajot.57.5.574.
68. Ellinoudis T, Evaggelinou C, Kourtessis T, Konstantinidou Z, Venetsanou F, Kambas A. Reliability and validity of age band 1 of the movement assessment battery for children—second edition. Res Dev Disabil. 2011;32(3):1046–51. https://pubmed.ncbi.nlm.nih.gov/21333488/
69. Holm I, Tveter AT, Aulie VS, Stuge B. High intra- and inter-rater chance variation of the movement assessment battery for children 2, age band 2. Res Dev Disabil. 2013;34(2):795–800. https://doi.org/10.1016/j.ridd.2012.11.002.
70. Wuang Y-P, Su J-H, Su C-Y. Reliability and responsiveness of the Movement Assessment Battery for children—Second Edition Test in children with developmental coordination disorder. Dev Med Child Neurol. 2012;54(2):160–5. https://doi.org/10.1111/j.1469-8749.2011.04177.x.
71. Jaikaew R, Satiansukpong N. Movement assessment battery for children—second edition (MABC2): cross-cultural validity, content validity, and interrater reliability in Thai children. Occup Ther Int. 2019;2019:1–5. https://www.hindawi.com/journals/oti/2019/4086594

72. Smits-Engelsman BCM, Niemeijer AS, van Waelvelde H. Is the movement assessment battery for children—2nd edition a reliable instrument to measure motor performance in 3 year old children? Res Dev Disabil. 2011;32(4):1370–7. https://doi.org/10.1016/j.ridd.2011.01.031.
73. Kita Y, Suzuki K, Hirata S, Sakihara K, Inagaki M, Nakai A. Applicability of the movement assessment battery for children—second edition to Japanese children: a study of the age band 2. Brain and Development. 2016;38(8):706–13. https://doi.org/10.1016/j.braindev.2016.02.012.
74. Schulz J, Henderson SE, Sugden DA, Barnett AL. Structural validity of the movement ABC-2 test: factor structure comparisons across three age groups. Res Dev Disabil. 2011;32(4):1361–9. https://doi.org/10.1016/j.ridd.2011.01.032.
75. Petermann F. Movement assessment battery for children-2 (movement ABC-2). Editorial comments. Frankfurt: Pearson Assessment; 2009.
76. Niemeijer AS, van Waelvelde H, Smits-Engelsman BCM. Crossing the North Sea seems to make DCD disappear: cross-validation of movement assessment battery for children-2 norms. Hum Mov Sci. 2015;39:177–88. https://www.sciencedirect.com/science/article/pii/S0167945714002000
77. Schoemaker MM, Niemeijer AS, Flapper BCT, Smits-engelsman BCM. Validity and reliability of the movement assessment battery for children-2 checklist for children with and without motor impairments. Dev Med Child Neurol. 2012;54(4):368–75. https://doi.org/10.1111/j.1469-8749.2012.04226.x.
78. Hadwin KJ, Wood G, Payne S, Mackintosh C, Parr JVV. Strengths and weaknesses of the MABC-2 as a diagnostic tool for developmental coordination disorder: an online survey of occupational therapists and physiotherapists. PLoS One. 2023;18(6):e0286751. https://doi.org/10.1371/journal.pone.0286751.
79. French B, Sycamore NJ, McGlashan HL, Blanchard CCV, Holmes NP. Ceiling effects in the movement assessment battery for Children-2 (MABC-2) suggest that non-parametric scoring methods are required. PLoS One. 2018;13(6):e0198426. https://doi.org/10.1371/journal.pone.0198426.
80. Ulrich DA. Test of gross motor development-third edition: examiner's manual. Austin: ProEd; 2019.
81. Webster EK, Ulrich DA. Evaluation of the psychometric properties of the test of gross motor development—third edition. J Mot Learn Dev. 2017;5(1):45–58. https://journals.humankinetics.com/view/journals/jmld/5/1/article-p45.xml
82. Garn AC, Webster EK. Bifactor structure and model reliability of the Test of Gross Motor Development — 3rd edition. J Sci Med Sport 2021;24(1):67–73. https://pubmed.ncbi.nlm.nih.gov/32919885/
83. Maïano C, Morin AJS, April J, Webster EK, Hue O, Dugas C, et al. Psychometric properties of a French-Canadian version of the test of gross motor development—third edition (TGMD-3): a bifactor structural equation modeling approach. Meas Phys Educ Exerc Sci. 2022;26(1):51–62. https://doi.org/10.1080/1091367x.2021.1946541.
84. Wagner MO, Webster EK, Ulrich DA. Psychometric properties of the test of Gross Motor Development, third edition (German translation): results of a pilot study. J Mot Learn Dev. 2017;5(1):29–44. https://doi.org/10.1123/jmld.2016-0006.
85. Mohammadi F, Bahram A, Khalaji H, Ulrich DA, Ghadiri F. Evaluation of the psychometric properties of the Persian version of the test of Gross Motor Development—3rd edition. J Mot Learn Dev. 2019;7(1):106–21. https://doi.org/10.1123/jmld.2017-0045.
86. Mohammadi F, Bahram A, Khalaji H, Ghadiri F. The validity and reliability of test of gross motor development—3rd edition among 3–10 years old children in Ahvaz. Jundishapur Scient Med J. 2017;16(4):379–91.
87. Salami S, Mashhadi M. Validity and reliability of Ulrich Coarse Motor Skills Development Test—third edition in girls and boys aged seven to nine in Tehran. Motor Behavior. 2019;36:127–48. https://jsmdl.ut.ac.ir/article_83746.html?lang=en

88. Magistro D, Piumatti G, Carlevaro F, Sherar LB, Esliger DW, Bardaglio G, et al. Psychometric proprieties of the Test of Gross Motor Development—Third Edition in a large sample of Italian children. J Sci Med Sport. 2020;23(9):860–5. https://doi.org/10.1016/j.jsams.2020.02.014.
89. Al-Hajjaj R, Sohrabi M, Saberi Kakhki A, Hosseini SR. Validity and reliability of the Test of Gross Motor Development—3 in children aged 5 to 9 years in Iraq and a comparison of the development of gross motor skills of Iranian and Iraqi children. J Sports and Motor Dev and Learning. 2021;13(2):219–38. https://doi.org/10.22059/jmlm.2021.327150.1595.
90. Estevan I, Molina-García J, Queralt A, Álvarez O, Castillo I, Barnett L. Validity and reliability of the Spanish version of the Test of Gross Motor Development–3. J Mot Learn Dev. 2017;5(1):69–81. https://doi.org/10.1123/jmld.2016-0045.
91. Temple VA, Foley JT. A peek at the developmental validity of the test of Gross Motor Development–3. J Mot Learn Dev. 2017;5(1):5–14. https://doi.org/10.1123/jmld.2016-0005.
92. Valentini NC, Duarte MG, Zanella LW, Nobre GC. Test of Gross Motor Development-3: item difficulty and item differential functioning by gender and age with Rasch analysis. Int J Environ Res Public Health. 2022;19(14):8667. https://doi.org/10.3390/ijerph19148667.
93. Chen J, Song W, Zhao X, Lou H, Luo D. The relationship between fundamental motor skills and physical fitness in preschoolers: a short-term longitudinal study. Front Psychol. 2023;14:14. https://doi.org/10.3389/fpsyg.2023.1270888.
94. Duncan MJ, Martins C, Ribeiro Bandeira PF, Issartel J, Peers C, Belton S, et al. TGMD-3 short version: evidence of validity and associations with sex in Irish children. J Sports Sci. 2022;40(2):138–45. https://doi.org/10.1080/02640414.2021.1978161.
95. Valentini NC, Nobre GC, Gonçalves DM. Gross motor skills trajectory variation between WEIRD and LMIC countries: a cross-cultural study. PLoS One. 2022;17(5):e0267665. https://doi.org/10.1371/journal.pone.0267665.
96. Maeng H, Webster EK, Pitchford EA, Ulrich DA. Inter- and intrarater reliabilities of the Test of Gross Motor Development—third edition among experienced TGMD-2 raters. Adapt Phys Act Q. 2017;34(4):442–55. https://journals.humankinetics.com/view/journals/apaq/34/4/article-p442.xml
97. Carballo-Fazanes A, Rey E, Valentini NC, Varela-Casal C, Abelairas-Gómez C. Interrater reliability of the test of Gross Motor Development—third edition following raters' agreement on measurement criteria. J Mot Learn Dev. 2023;11(2):225–44. https://doi.org/10.1123/jmld.2022-0068.
98. Carballo-Fazanes A, Rey E, Valentini NC, Rodríguez-Fernández JE, Varela-Casal C, Rico-Díaz J, et al. Intra-rater (live vs. video assessment) and inter-rater (expert vs. Novice) reliability of the Test of Gross Motor Development—third edition. Int J Environ Res Public Health. 2021;18(4):1652. https://doi.org/10.3390/ijerph18041652.
99. Rintala PO, Sääkslahti AK, Iivonen S. Reliability assessment of scores from video-recorded TGMD-3 performances. J Mot Learn Dev. 2017;5(1):59–68. https://doi.org/10.1123/jmld.2016-0007.
100. Pitchford EA, Webster EK. Clinical validity of the Test of Gross Motor Development-3 in children with disabilities from the U.S. national normative sample. Adapt Phys Act Q. 2021;38(1):62–78. https://doi.org/10.1123/apaq.2020-0023.
101. Staples KL, Pitchford EA, Ulrich DA. The instructional sensitivity of the Test of Gross Motor Development-3 to detect changes in performance for young children with and without Down syndrome. Adapt Phys Act Q. 2021;38(1):95–108. https://doi.org/10.1123/apaq.2020-0047.
102. Eyitayo JSG. (n.d.) Aspects of reliability and validity of the TGMD-3 in 7–10 year old children with intellectual disability in Belgium. Psychomotor.gr. https://psychomotor.gr/aspects-of-reliability-and-validity-of-the-tgmd-3-in-7-10-year-old-children-with-intellectual-disability-in-belgium/
103. Wagner MO, Webster E, Urich DA. Reliability and validity of the Test of Gross Motor Development 3 (German version). J Sport Exerc Psychol. 2015;37.
104. Brian A, Taunton S, Lieberman LJ, Haibach-Beach P, Foley J, Santarossa S. Psychometric properties of the Test of Gross Motor Development-3 for children with visual impairments. Adapt Phys Act Q. 2018;35(2):145–58. https://doi.org/10.1123/apaq.2017-0061.

105. Brian AS, Starrett A, Pennell A, Beach PH, Miedema ST, Stribing A, et al. The brief form of the Test of Gross Motor Development-3 for individuals with visual impairments. Int J Environ Res Public Health. 2021;18(15):7962. https://doi.org/10.3390/ijerph18157962.
106. Allen KA, Bredero B, Van Damme T, Ulrich DA, Simons J. Test of gross motor development-3 (TGMD-3) with the use of visual supports for children with autism spectrum disorder: validity and reliability. J Autism Dev Disord. 2017;47(3):813–33. https://pubmed.ncbi.nlm.nih.gov/28091840/
107. Copetti F, Valentini NC, Deslandes AC, Webster EK. Pedagogical support for the Test of Gross Motor Development—3 for children with neurotypical development and with Autism Spectrum Disorder: validity for an animated mobile application. Phys Educ Sport Pedagogy. 2022;27(5):483–501. https://doi.org/10.1080/17408989.2021.1906218.
108. Bruininks BRH, Bruininks BD. Bruininks Bruininks-Oseretsky Test of Motor Proficiency, second edition, manual. Upper Saddle River, NJ: Pearson; 2005.
109. Deitz JC, Kartin D, Kopp K. Review of the Bruininks-oseretsky test of motor proficiency, second edition (BOT-2). Phys Occup Ther Pediatr. 2007;27(4):87–102. https://doi.org/10.1300/j006v27n04_06.
110. Wuang Y-P, Lin Y-H, Su C-Y. Rasch analysis of the Bruininks–Oseretsky Test of Motor Proficiency-Second Edition in intellectual disabilities. Res Dev Disabil. 2009;30(6):1132–44. https://doi.org/10.1016/j.ridd.2009.03.003.
111. Wuang Y-P, Su C-Y. Reliability and responsiveness of the Bruininks–Oseretsky Test of Motor Proficiency-Second Edition in children with intellectual disability. Res Dev Disabil. 2009;30(5):847–55. https://www.sciencedirect.com/science/article/pii/S0891422208001777
112. Okuda PMM, Pangelinan M, Capellini SA, Cogo-Moreira H. Motor skills assessments: support for a general motor factor for the Movement Assessment Battery for children-2 and the Bruininks-Oseretsky Test of Motor Proficiency-2. Trends Psychiatry Psychother. 2019;41(1):51–9. https://pubmed.ncbi.nlm.nih.gov/30994783/
113. Ferreira L, Vieira JLL, Rocha FF da, Silva PN da, Cheuczuk F, Caçola P, et al. Percentile curves for Brazilian children evaluated with the Bruininks-Oseretsky Test of Motor Proficiency, 2nd. Braz J Kinanthropometry Hum Performance 2020; 22:e65027. https://www.scielo.br/j/rbcdh/a/szhb845LK98FH3VTGLV9S4D/?format=html
114. Bardid F, Utesch T, Lenoir M. Investigating the construct of motor competence in middle childhood using the BOT-2 short form: an item response theory perspective. Scand J Med Sci Sports. 2019;29(12):1980–7. https://doi.org/10.1111/sms.13527.
115. Brown T. Structural validity of the Bruininks-Oseretsky test of motor proficiency—second edition brief form (BOT-2-BF). Res Dev Disabil. 2019;85:92–103. https://pubmed.ncbi.nlm.nih.gov/30502549/
116. Kiphard EJ, Schilling F. Körperkoordinationstest für Kinder KTK: Manual. Weinhein: Beltz Test; 1974.
117. Kiphard EJ, Schilling F. Körperkoordinationstest für Kinder 2 KTK: Uberarbeitete und. Ergänzte Auflage ed. Weinhein: Beltz Test; 1974.
118. Cools W, Martelaer KD, Samaey C, Andries C. Movement skill assessment of typically developing preschool children: a review of seven movement skill assessment tools. J Sports Sci Med. 2009;8(2):154–68. https://www.ncbi.nlm.nih.gov/pmc/articles/PMC3761481/
119. Moreira JPA, Lopes MC, Miranda-Júnior MV, Valentini NC, Lage GM, Albuquerque MR. Körperkoordinationstest für kinder (KTK) for Brazilian children and adolescents: factor analysis, invariance and factor score. Front Psychol. 2019;10:480272. https://www.frontiersin.org/articles/10.3389/fpsyg.2019.02524/full
120. Rudd J, Butson ML, Barnett L, Farrow D, Berry J, Borkoles E, et al. A holistic measurement model of movement competency in children. J Sports Sci. 2016;34(5):477–85. https://doi.org/10.1080/02640414.2015.1061202.
121. Li K, Bao R, Kim H, Ma J, Song C, Chen S, et al. Reliability and validity of the Körperkoordinationstest Für Kinder in Chinese children. Peer J. 2023;11(e15447):e15447. https://doi.org/10.7717/peerj.15447.

122. Camacho-Araya T, Woodburn SS, Boschini C. Reliability of the prueba DE coordinación corporal Para niños (Body Coordination Test for children). Percept Mot Skills. 1990;70(3):832–4. https://pubmed.ncbi.nlm.nih.gov/2377417/
123. Laukkanen A, Bardid F, Lenoir M, Lopes VP, Vasankari T, Husu P, et al. Comparison of motor competence in children aged 6–9 years across northern, central, and southern European regions. Scand J Med Sci Sports. 2020;30(2):349–60. https://pubmed.ncbi.nlm.nih.gov/31618478/
124. Fransen J, D'Hondt E, Bourgois J, Vaeyens R, Philippaerts RM, Lenoir M. Motor competence assessment in children: convergent and discriminant validity between the BOT-2 short form and KTK testing batteries. Res Dev Disabil. 2014;35(6):1375–83. https://pubmed.ncbi.nlm.nih.gov/24713517/
125. Bardid F, Huyben F, Deconinck FJA, De Martelaer K, Seghers J, Lenoir M. Convergent and divergent validity between the KTK and MOT 4–6 motor tests in early childhood. Adapt Phys Act Q. 2016;33(1):33–47. https://pubmed.ncbi.nlm.nih.gov/28425769/
126. Smits-Engelsman BCM, Henderson SE, Michels CGJ. The assessment of children with developmental coordination disorders in The Netherlands: the relationship between the movement assessment battery for children and the Körperkoordinations Test für Kinder. Hum Mov Sci. 1998;17(4–5):699–709. https://doi.org/10.1016/s0167-9457(98)00019-0.
127. Lima RA, Bugge A, Ersbøll AK, Stodden DF, Andersen LB. The longitudinal relationship between motor competence and measures of fatness and fitness from childhood into adolescence. J Pediatr. 2019;95(4):482–8. https://doi.org/10.1016/j.jped.2018.02.010.
128. Martins D, Maia J, Seabra A, Garganta R, Lopes V, Katzmarzyk P, et al. Correlates of changes in BMI of children from the Azores islands. Int J Obes. 2010;34(10):1487–93. https://pubmed.ncbi.nlm.nih.gov/20386549/
129. Iivonen S, Kaarina Sääkslahti A, Laukkanen A. A review of studies using the Körperkoordinationstest für Kinder (KTK). Eur J Adapt Phys Act. 2015;8(2):18–36. https://doi.org/10.5507/euj.2015.006.
130. Valentini NC. Motor skills intervention: conceptual and operational model and the determination of fidelity indexes. Phys Educ Sport Pedagogy. 2023:1–17. https://doi.org/10.1080/17408989.2023.2271521.

Part III
Physical Activity During School Hours

Chapter 7
Physical Activity and Health Through Physical Education

Adrià Muntaner-Mas

7.1 Introduction

7.1.1 The Importance of Physical Education

Extensive scientific research substantiates the crucial role of physical education (PE) in promoting lifelong health and well-being in school-aged youth. PE not only encourages youth to be physically active during classes but also motivates them to adopt healthier lifestyles and engage in regular physical activity (PA) outside of school schedules [1]. PE teachers and educational institutions are crucial in this process because they motivate students to practice physical activities regularly, leading to the prevention and combat of various health problems. Importantly, the creation of an environment in PE classes that encourages students to choose active lifestyles is essential for facilitating positive PA patterns that they will carry into adulthood. Thus, it is remarkable that properly conducted PE is closely connected with health and serves as the foundation for developing appropriate habits and knowledge for lifelong health, far beyond the school's walls [2]. It is known that positive PE experiences contribute to positive attitudes toward PA in adulthood and are key drivers of lifetime PA participation [3, 4]. Furthermore, the incorporation of health education strengthens the understanding of the lifelong effects of PE by promoting an informed understanding of the links between PA, physical health, brain health, and general well-being [5]. Students endowed with comprehensive health

---

A. Muntaner-Mas (✉)
GICAFE "Physical Activity and Exercise Sciences Research Group," Faculty of Education, University of Balearic Islands, Palma, Spain

PROFITH "PROmoting FITness and Health Through Physical Activity" Research Group, Sport and Health University Research Institute (iMUDS), Department of Physical Education and Sports, Faculty of Sport Sciences, University of Granada, Granada, Spain
e-mail: adria.muntaner@uib.es

education exhibit enhanced capability in making informed decisions regarding their health status [6].

Investing in comprehensive PE programs is not only an educational priority but also a societal imperative, with far-reaching implications for public health [7, 8]. Over the years, there have been achievements in improving the health impact of PE, including the development of evidence-based programs and the recognition of PE as a public health resource [9]. In their seminal research, Sallis and McKenzie [7] emphasized the significant role that school-based PE can play in enhancing the health of youth. They advocated for a partnership between PE teachers and public health experts in the creation and assessment of PE programs based on empirical evidence. Their paper made a case for a health-centric approach to PE, with a focus on achieving public health objectives. The key goals of such a health-oriented PE, as outlined, were twofold: first, to equip youth with the necessary tools and knowledge for engaging in PA throughout their lives and, second, to ensure that PA is an integral part of the PE curriculum. Building upon this seminal research, an expanding body of evidence has shown the crucial role of PE in nurturing healthy lifestyle habits from childhood through adulthood. For instance, a notable study encompassing data from 65 countries and 222,121 adolescents found that PE attendance is positively connected with adopting future healthy behaviors, with more pronounced benefits observed among those who attend more PE lessons [10]. While significant scientific evidence highlights the importance of PE, ongoing research is indispensable. For instance, this includes implementing and evaluating evidence-based PE programs and experimenting with and assessing the impacts of varying PE programs based on quality and quantity aspects. This book chapter summarizes the myriad health benefits of PE, emphasizing its critical role in promoting physical and brain health from both public health and educational standpoints.

7.1.2 The Connection Between Physical Activity, Physical Education, and Lifelong Health

The critical importance of PA and PE in determining the lifelong health trajectory of young people is more pronounced than ever, particularly in light of the modern challenges posed by sedentary lifestyles and their associated health consequences. The need for a robust and comprehensive approach to PE emanates from the multifaceted health challenges prevalent in the twenty-first century. Thus, issues such as obesity, mental health disorders, and chronic diseases are on the rise, and the youth population is being significantly affected [11]. These health challenges, often rooted in lifestyle choices, underscore the exigency of instilling healthy habits early in life.

In this context, PE serves as a nexus and a catalytic platform through which young people not only learn about physical or theoretical components of health and well-being but also immerse themselves in practical experiences that develop ideas, habits, and attitudes toward health and PA [12]. The connection between PE and lifelong health is symbiotic. PE, in particular, serves as the foundational stage in which individuals are prepared with the skills, knowledge, and attitudes required for a future active lifestyle. The habits, preferences, and choices ingrained during these early stages have a domino effect, influencing subsequent life stages [13]. Youths who are exposed to a robust PE curriculum are more likely to transition into adulthood with a predilection for PA, a profound understanding of health, and resilience against lifestyle-related health challenges [14].

Collectively, the empirical evidence highlights the importance of PE and PA in the holistic development and lifetime health of youth. As the gateway to lifelong health, PE and PA embody an educational experience that encapsulates physical fitness, cognitive development, emotional intelligence, and social skills [15]. During today's health challenges, PE and PA stand out as beacons of hope, as they are forces capable of recalibrating society's health trajectory by instilling healthy habits from an early age [16].

7.2 Physical Activity and Physical Education: Definitions and Guidelines

PA refers to a wide range of body movements caused by skeletal muscle contractions that result in an increase in energy expenditure above basal values. This activity covers a wide range of forms and intensities. It includes structured activities such as exercise and sports, as well as less formal pursuits such as leisure activities, household chores, and tasks performed in professional or environmental settings [17]. The World Health Organization (WHO) has highlighted PA as a key component for maintaining a healthy lifestyle, reducing the risk of chronic diseases, and promoting mental health during childhood and adolescence [18].

The WHO recommends that children and adolescents aged 5–17 accumulate at least 60 min of moderate-to-vigorous intensity PA (MVPA) daily [19]. Despite our extensive knowledge, youth remain largely physically inactive and do not meet recommended activity levels. For instance, Tapia-Serrano et al.'s [20] meta-analysis involving 387,437 participants across 23 countries revealed that most young people, particularly adolescents and girls, fail to adhere to the three 24-hour movement guidelines. Furthermore, the authors found that 1 in 5 young people did not meet any of these recommendations. Similarly, *the Global Matrix 4.0 Physical Activity Report Card Grades* of 57 countries demonstrated that levels of PA and sedentary behavior among youth are of concern and may indicate a global crisis in these age groups [21].

PE, on the other hand, is an instructional process and a systematic and organized effort facilitated within the educational curriculum to instill knowledge, skills, and competencies related to PA and health [22]. Another related concept is the quality of PE (QPE). According to UNESCO, QPE is the planned, progressive, inclusive learning experience that forms part of the curriculum in the early years of primary and secondary education [23]. The QPE aims to develop students' physical competence, health-related physical fitness, self-responsibility, and enjoyment of PA so that they can be physically active for a lifetime. It integrates theoretical and practical learning experiences, fostering a comprehensive understanding and application of PA within and beyond the educational setting. In this respect, the WHO has made important conclusions: (1) PE should be valued within the school and not replaced by other subjects, courses or activities; (2) all schools should provide QPE as a core part of formal curricula; and (3) students' performance should be evaluated in terms of personal improvement and effort rather than by comparison to others [24].

The establishment of the *Global Observatory for Physical Activity* (GoPA!) in 2012 marked a significant milestone in the field of PA and public health. The GoPA! (http://www.globalphysicalactivityobservatory.com/) was established in 2012 and is unique in leading evidence- and expert-based systems for monitoring PA surveillance, research, and policy worldwide [25]. Until now, the GoPA! did not include specific indicators of PE or PA within the school setting. Hence, in alignment with the mission of the GoPA! and with the goal of monitoring and evaluating QPE and health-enhancing PA in schools, the Global Observatory for Physical Education (GoPE!) was launched in 2023. This initiative represents a significant advancement in the field, as it aims to comprehensively oversee school-based PA programs through surveillance, policy development, and research on a global scale. GoPE! underscores a commitment to enhancing PE and promoting active lifestyles among students worldwide, reflecting a coordinated effort to build healthier and more active generations [26].

7.3 Physical Activity Through Physical Education

Curricular PE is a school-based opportunity to influence movement habits by making PA a relevant component of a student's life [27]. PE lessons are a cornerstone in enhancing daily MVPA during school hours [28]. Research indicates that students who participate in PE are not only more physically active but also exhibit less sedentary behavior, contributing to overall better health outcomes [29]. This increase in PA during PE lessons is critical, especially in an era where sedentary lifestyles are becoming more prevalent among youth. Furthermore, there is a well-established, positive correlation between regular attendance in PE lessons and adherence to the WHO's PA guidelines. This correlation holds true across diverse demographics, transcending gender and age barriers [30]. In this context, the outstanding study by Uddin et al. [31], which analyzed a sample of 206,417 adolescents across 65 countries, showed that participation in PE classes correlates positively with increased PA levels, regardless of the participant's gender or age group. Moreover, the impact of PE extends beyond immediate physical health benefits. For instance, daily attendance in PE has been linked to the cultivation of healthy movement behaviors, a pattern that begins in adolescence and often continues into adulthood [32]. This long-term influence highlights the role of PE in inculcating lifelong habits of PA. By encouraging active participation in PE, schools play a pivotal role in shaping the future health and well-being of their students.

As stated previously, the WHO recommends that youth accumulate at least 60 min of MVPA daily; however, achieving this benchmark is contingent on multiple factors, including the quality and quantity of PE. A pivotal consideration in this discourse is the proportion of PE time allocated to achieve MVPA recommendations. Panels of researchers and relevant organizations advocate for students to engage in MVPA for at least 50% of the PE class duration. Some authors advocate for a more dynamic approach, recommending that students should engage in active movement for a substantial portion of their educational time in PE. Specifically, they suggest that 50–80% of the available learning time should be dedicated to physical activities, emphasizing the importance of integrating movement in most PE classes [33]. Despite this recommendation, the global picture of MVPA engagement during PE remains insufficient. Several systematic reviews have analyzed MVPA levels and correlates during PE lessons in children and adolescents [34–38]. Research has shown that the proportions of children and adolescents engaging in PE in MVPA are 44.8% and 40.5%, respectively [36, 37]. A recent study of data from eight systematic reviews that included 224 studies and involved more than 80,000 students revealed that students fail to meet the 50% recommendation of MVPA lesson time, irrespective of country, school stage, or gender [35]. Regardless, the evidence shows that PE contributes to total PA levels and predominantly at higher intensities [39]. Additionally, studies comparing days with and without PE classes have shown that less sitting time is present on PE class days [40, 41]. To date, only two systematic reviews have analyzed the effect of interventions in PE aimed at increasing PA [42, 43]. These studies concluded that, compared with control interventions, PE-based interventions increased students' MVPA during PE education lessons (range 14.3–24%).

The level of PA during PE classes can vary widely due to numerous influencing factors. A systematic review by Wang et al. [37] revealed that sex (boys), PE activities (team games), PE context (fitness activities, gameplay, and skill practice), class location (outdoors) and perceived competence were positively associated with MVPA and body mass index (BMI), larger class size, and PE activities (movement activities) were consistently and negatively related to MVPA. However, the elements that determine PA levels during a PE can be broadly classified as individual characteristics, environmental influences, and institutional components. For instance, at an individual level, the motivation and attitudes of students toward PA play a significant role. Self-determination theory (SDT) suggests that intrinsic motivation is crucial for engaging in PA [44, 45]. This finding is supported by research showing that intrinsically motivated students are more likely to participate actively in PE classes. In addition to motivation, perceived physical competence significantly impacts PE participation. Thus, students who feel competent in their physical abilities are generally more active during PE. Additionally, the actual physical fitness and health status of the students also influence their participation levels, with those with higher fitness levels often being more active. The social environment, including peer relationships and family and community support for PA, also plays a role [46]. On an institutional level, the design and content of the PE curriculum are significant determinants of student engagement. A curriculum that offers a variety of activities and accommodates different skill levels can increase participation. The qualifications and teaching styles of PE teachers are equally important. Teachers who adopt student-centered approaches and provide positive feedback can significantly enhance student motivation and, consequently, PA levels during PE classes [47]. At the institutional level, recent research has suggested the necessity of tailored intervention strategies based on specific country or regional requirements. In this context, a noteworthy study explored the association between attendance in PE classes and overall PA among adolescents in 50 low- and middle-income countries [48]. Using data from the *Global School-based Student Survey*, which included variables such as frequency of PE classes, PA levels, and sedentary behavior, the research analyzed responses from 187,386 adolescents aged 13–17 years. The findings revealed that only 14.9% of the adolescents met the PA guidelines, with 16.5% attending PE classes five or more days per week. The results showed that an increased frequency of PE class attendance was correlated with a greater likelihood of meeting PA guidelines, which was also observed for both male and female students. Specifically, the odds ratio of meeting PA guidelines increased with the number of days attending PE classes, reaching the highest likelihood for those attending five or more days per week.

Collectively, the levels of PA in PE classes are influenced by a complex interplay of individual, environmental, and institutional factors. Understanding these elements is vital for developing effective PE programs that engage students and promote lifelong PA habits through this subject. Future research and policy initiatives should aim at creating comprehensive PE programs that address these various influences to maximize the benefits of PA and PE for all students across the globe.

7.4 Health Benefits of Physical Education

7.4.1 Enhancing Physical Fitness

PE has emerged as a critical intervention for enhancing physical health in youth, addressing major global health challenges. The relevance of PE extends beyond immediate physical health benefits, playing a significant role in shaping long-term health. In this sense, PE has been recognized for its ability to improve physical fitness, which is an important health marker throughout the lifespan [49–51]. Extensive scientific research, including systematic reviews and meta-analytic investigations, has established the importance of PE for physical fitness. The most recent evidence suggests that well-designed PE programs can help improve young people's physical fitness and, in turn, physical health [52, 53]. Furthermore, recent evidence emphasizes the importance of customizing PE programs to enhance their effectiveness in improving physical fitness. Specifically, individualized approaches considering factors such as age, sex, and physical capabilities are imperative for maximizing the effectiveness of PE interventions targeting physical fitness components. In this sense, the systematic review of Lander et al. [53] focused on teacher training characteristics in school-based PE interventions aimed at improving fundamental movement skills and PA. Specifically, the study examined various interventions within the school-based PE context to enhance students' PA levels. Teacher training was found to play a crucial role in the success of these interventions. The article emphasizes the importance of equipping teachers with the tools and strategies necessary to promote physical fitness. Furthermore, teacher training should be ongoing and adaptable to changing student needs and trends in PE.

The meta-analyses of García-Hermoso et al. [52] investigated the impact of PE interventions on the physical fitness and motor skills of children and adolescents. A total of 56 articles were analyzed, and a total of 48,185 participants were included. The interventions were categorized as quality-based PE or quantity-based PE. Quality-based PE was associated with reductions in BMI, waist circumference, and body fat as well as increases in lean body mass, cardiorespiratory fitness, muscular strength, and fundamental movement skills. Quantity-based PE interventions were associated with increases in cardiorespiratory fitness, muscular strength, and speed agility. Subgroup analysis of quality-based PE revealed that physical fitness infusion interventions were linked to greater benefits in terms of BMI, body fat, lean body mass, CRF, and muscular strength. However, increasing PE exposure was not consistently associated with greater changes in health-related physical fitness outcomes, except for fundamental movement skills. The findings indicate that both quality-based and quantity-based PE can have positive effects on physical fitness and motor skills in children and adolescents, with fitness infusion interventions showing slightly greater benefits. In line with these results, other systematic reviews have investigated the effects of PE on cardiorespiratory fitness in youth [53]. This systematic review identified age and weight as significant factors influencing the efficacy of PE in promoting this physical fitness component. Specifically, the findings emphasize the need to prioritize overweight and obese students in PE programs targeting cardiorespiratory fitness. This is based on the observation that these students often face greater challenges in improving their cardiorespiratory fitness than their normal-weight counterparts. Additionally, the review highlights the differential impact of PE on younger versus older students. Studies focusing on younger students have consistently reported more significant improvements in cardiorespiratory fitness. In contrast, findings from research on older students suggest a potential vulnerability to declining levels of PA, which may impede improvements in cardiorespiratory fitness.

While our understanding of how to improve cardiorespiratory fitness through PE is growing, we can speculate about potential determinants. Several key determinants have been identified as essential for the effective improvement of cardiorespiratory fitness in educational settings. First, there is evidence that higher-intensity activities within PE classes are pivotal for enhancing cardiorespiratory fitness. In this sense, it has been demonstrated that high-intensity exercise, when integrated regularly or over sustained periods, has a significant impact on increasing cardiorespiratory endurance in young individuals [55–58]. Second, the diversity of exercise types within PE programs is crucial. A balanced mix of aerobic, strength, and flexibility exercises not only improves overall physical fitness but also caters to the varied interests and abilities of students, encouraging greater participation and engagement [59]. Additionally, tailoring PE programs to individual needs and developmental stages is fundamental. Personalized approaches that consider each student's unique physical capabilities and physical fitness levels can maximize the effectiveness of PE in improving cardiorespiratory fitness. Furthermore, the inclusion of educational components that teach students about the benefits of physical fitness and how to maintain it outside of school settings is vital. In summary, while additional research is needed to fully understand and optimize how PE can be used to improve cardiorespiratory fitness, the current evidence highlights the importance of intensity, diversity, personalization, and educational integration in PE programs.

Muscular fitness is an important aspect of general health, particularly in youth, where it builds the framework for active and healthy adulthood [60]. Children with low levels of muscular fitness often exhibit reduced motor skills, functional impairments, and negative health consequences [60]. Similarly, a recent manuscript by Faigenbaum et al. [61] focused on the foundational role of PE in developing muscular strength and fitness in youth. This study identified a decline in physical strength among today's children and adolescents, emphasizing the importance of early muscular strength for counteracting this trend. The authors argue that muscular fitness is crucial for motor skill development and overall physical capability. They advocate for integrating resistance training into PE curricula, highlighting its impact on long-term health and PA engagement. Aligned with this vision, Till et al. [62] advocated also for the integration of muscular fitness and conditioning into PE curricula and extracurricular activities, emphasizing the positive impact on students' PA levels, cognitive functions, mental health, and academic performance. This paper highlights the need for comprehensive strategies to incorporate muscular strength and conditioning in schools, recognizing the potential of these strategies to contribute significantly to a healthier society. The paper identifies several barriers to implementing this concept in schools. These include misconceptions about the safety and value of youth muscular fitness, a focus on sport-specific skills rather than overall fitness, and limited implementation of health and fitness activities in school curricula.

The role of PE in contributing to muscular fitness development has been identified in the scientific literature, with some systematic reviews and meta-analyses delineating the tangible impacts of well-curated PE programs [63, 64]. In the detailed systematic review and meta-analysis of Cox et al. [64], the focus was on assessing the impact of school-based PA interventions on muscular fitness in adolescent boys. The included interventions were specifically aimed at enhancing muscular fitness in adolescent boys and had a small-to-medium effect, with an overall effect size of $g = 0.32$. To further investigate the results, various forms of muscular fitness delivery were analyzed. Traditional resistance training methods, such as using weight machines and free weights, have shown significant effectiveness. Similarly, plyometric exercises, which involve explosive movements to improve power, demonstrated notable benefits. These results highlight the efficacy of well-structured PE programs in school settings, especially those incorporating traditional and plyometric resistance training. Furthermore, in the study of Villa-González et al. [63], which included a systematic review and meta-analysis aimed at evaluating the effectiveness of school-based exercise interventions in enhancing muscular fitness in children under 13 years of age, the potential of PE was also confirmed. The review included both randomized and nonrandomized controlled trials involving 1653 children (28% girls). The interventions, which mostly involved combined exercises targeting specific domains of muscular fitness, had significant moderate increases in local muscular endurance ($g = 0.65$, 95% CI 0.13 to 1.17, $p = 0.020$; I2 = 85.0%) and muscular strength and power ($g = 0.33$, 95% CI 0.16 to 0.51, $p = 0.001$; I2 = 59.3%). Notably, interventions with three or more sessions per week were associated with greater effectiveness. For local muscular endurance, interventions with ≥3 sessions per week showed greater increases in local muscular endurance than did those with <3 sessions per week, without significant differences in effect based on the length or duration of the interventions.

The multifaceted benefits of enhanced muscular fitness in youth are indisputable and range from improved physical performance and bone health to enhanced metabolic profiles and mental well-being [60]. The systematic incorporation of exercises targeting muscular fitness and endurance in PE programs has emerged as a cornerstone in extending these benefits [65, 66]. In summary, the landscape of scientific literature, enriched by systematic reviews and meta-analyses, highlights the compelling narrative of PE's instrumental role in elevating muscular fitness among youth. Tailoring PE curricula to incorporate a balanced, diverse array of exercises targeting muscular fitness development is not only an educational imperative but also a public health priority. The responsibility lies with educators, policymakers, and health professionals to assimilate scientific insights, continually refine PE interventions, and ensure their alignment with the dynamic needs of youth populations. As the scientific community further investigates the comprehensive impact of PE programs, it is evident that these interventions oriented toward improving muscular fitness are indispensable in achieving these goals.

7.4.2 Improving Academic Performance and Cognitive Health

Over the past two decades, a substantial body of research has consistently demonstrated the positive impact of school-based PA interventions on academic performance and cognition [67–71]. The current discourse has shifted from questioning the inclusion of PA during school hours as a means to enhance cognition and academic performance. Instead, the focus is now on optimizing these interventions within the educational framework. Critical considerations include determining the most effective methods, appropriate timing, and suitable conditions under which PA should be implemented in the school context. Additionally, identifying which moderating factors can be leveraged to amplify the benefits of PA on these critical development aspects is essential [72]. In this context, the intricate relationship between PE and academic performance and cognition during adolescence has garnered increased amounts of attention within the scientific community [73–76]. Thus, the importance of PE in the educational curriculum should be expanded beyond physical fitness and motor skill development, and PE should be positioned as a critical determinant of cognitive functioning and academic success. In this educational landscape, enhancing both the quantity and quality of PE appears to be a promising strategy for improving academic performance and cognition. Despite the limited literature on this topic, this section examines the most significant findings in the field. The aim is to elucidate the role of PE in bolstering academic and cognitive outcomes, thereby offering a clearer understanding of its potential benefits in the educational context.

In a systematic review conducted by Rasberry et al. [77], an analysis of 14 studies revealed that 11 studies demonstrated one or more positive correlations between PE and various aspects of cognitive skills, academic behavior, and academic performance. Notably, almost half (49.5%) of these correlations between PE and academic performance were positive, while the vast majority of the remaining correlations indicated no significant relationship. In 2020, Dudley et al. [78] posed a critical inquiry question: How does augmenting the portion of curriculum time dedicated to PE impact student learning? To address this, they conducted a systematic review coupled with a meta-analysis. The key finding from this study was that expanding the curriculum time for PE significantly enhances student learning outcomes. Specifically, the research revealed that increasing the time allocated to PE positively affects various aspects of student learning, although the extent of impact varies across different dimensions: cognitive ($d = 0.14$), affective ($d = 0.66$), and psychomotor ($d = 0.83$) skills. Overall, the effect across all three learning domains was moderate ($d = 0.41$). These findings are highly promising, especially when viewed in the context of John Hattie's influential 2008 work [79]. Compared to the effects of regular academic testing ($d = 0.34$), increasing the amount of time in the PE curriculum appears to have a more substantial impact on student learning. This finding suggests that enhancing PE in the school curriculum could be a more effective strategy for increasing performance in academic outcomes than traditional methods focused solely on academic performance assessments.

García-Hermoso et al. [80] aimed to evaluate the impact of interventions aimed at optimizing the quantity and quality of PE on cognition and academic performance through a systematic review and meta-analysis. By analyzing 19 trials with 8676 participants, it was found that interventions focused on improving the quality of PE notably enhanced cognitive performance ($g = 0.38$), especially in primary education, and improved academic performance, primarily in mathematics ($g = 0.15$). Consistent results were obtained for quality-based PE interventions using specific teaching strategies, but the results did not vary widely ($g = 0.12$). In contrast, interventions that simply increased the amount of PE time had a minimal and insignificant effect on academic performance ($g = 0.09$). Finally, the study concluded that there were no significant differences in academic performance between quantity-based, quality-based, or combined PE interventions. Furthermore, a meta-analysis by Cho et al. [81] revealed that school PE significantly boosts students' cognitive competencies, including intelligence and academic performance. The authors observed that aerobic exercise within PE had a more substantial effect than did model-based or traditional approaches. The study concludes that while PE positively affects students' cognitive outcomes, further research is needed to understand how different content and teaching methods uniquely affect cognitive abilities. Another recent meta-analysis scrutinized data from 135 studies involving more than 42,500 participants and assessed the influence of PE on cognitive, affective, social, and psychomotor domains. The study reports a small-to-medium positive effect of PE interventions on these learning outcomes, with the most notable impact observed in psychomotor learning. The findings underline the crucial role of PE in not only enhancing physical health but also contributing significantly to the cognitive, social, and emotional development of young individuals. The article emphasizes the need for high-quality, well-structured PE programs tailored to address the diverse and specific needs of youth to maximize their developmental benefits [54].

Collectively, the current research suggests that increasing the time dedicated to PE does not negatively affect academic performance or cognition, even if it results in less time for other academic subjects. This aligns with the findings of Zach's study [82], which indicates that there is a consensus among researchers that PE classes do not detract from youths' academic performance, even when PE takes precedence over other academic subjects. Trudeau's research [83] reinforces this claim, showing that integrating PA into the curriculum by reducing time for other subjects does not harm student academic performance. In contrast, allocating more time to other subjects at the expense of PE does not necessarily enhance grades and may adversely affect student health. A systematic review examining the connection between PE and academic performance in other curriculum learning areas, which analyzed 48 peer-reviewed articles out of 5599, yielded interesting results [84]. A key observation from this research is that increasing PA by adding more PE time had no detrimental effect on students' academic performance or grades in other academic subjects. The conclusion drawn is that while the effect of PE on academic performance and cognition in other learning areas varies, it certainly does not impair overall student performance.

Overall, the current literature has room for improvement, highlighting the need for further research to fully understand the relationships between PE and academic performance and cognitive function. Additionally, further investigation is necessary to determine the effects of different activities, teaching methods, and student subgroups. The existing research tentatively suggests that PE does not adversely impact students' performance in other academic subjects. In some cases, PE participation may even correlate with improved academic performance and cognitive development. This finding suggests a complex relationship between PE and academic performance and cognition, requiring detailed investigation to fully realize and leverage its potential benefits in this area.

7.4.3 Mitigating Obesity

The global prevalence of childhood obesity, a serious public health concern, has been alarming, with approximately 340 million children and adolescents affected worldwide as of 2016. This epidemic, fueled by obesogenic factors such as energy-dense diets and sedentary lifestyles, poses significant risks for noncommunicable diseases (NCDs), psychological issues, and a greater likelihood of obesity in adulthood [85]. As early as 2016, the WHO highlighted the importance of PE in its "Report of the Commission on Ending Childhood Obesity" [86]. The report specifically recommends the inclusion of QPE in school curricula, along with the provision of suitable and sufficient staff and facilities to support it. Similarly, in 2020, UNICEF also supported this approach, recommending mandatory QPE programs to combat youth obesity [87]. These findings reinforce the critical role of PE in confronting childhood obesity, demonstrating a unified commitment by organizations such as the WHO and UNICEF to fostering comprehensive health education in school settings.

School-based interventions have shown promising results in reducing excessive weight in young people [88–91]. In this context, the role of PE in schools is critically important for preventing and treating youth obesity [92]. While the potential of PE for combating obesity is evident, the specific mechanisms through which PE achieves this effect are not yet fully understood. Observational studies have shown the positive effects of enhancing the quality and quantity of PE on various adiposity measures. However, there is a lack of robust scientific evidence stemming from rigorous randomized trials that conclusively demonstrate these impacts. Regardless of these uncertainties, one thing is clear: PE must be equipped to address all youth conditions. This necessity aligns with the principle that 'every child of every size matters', emphasizing the inclusive beneficial nature of PE. This notion highlights the importance of adapting PE programs to be accessible and effective for children of diverse body types and abilities, ensuring that every child has the opportunity to benefit from PE [93]. Additionally, paying attention to enjoyment in PE sessions is pivotal for the success of these programs. This idea aligns with emerging evidence suggesting that fun and inclusive PE activities correlate with better body composition outcomes in youth [94, 95].

Specifically, one study has shown that increasing the PE duration from 90 to 270 min per week may not significantly reduce overweight or obesity, but it does help prevent children from becoming overweight or obese over a two-year follow-up period [96]. Interestingly, other research has indicated that transferring 18 children (i.e., NNT = 17.1, 95% CI = 11.0–226.1) from a typical PE class to an intensive PE program could prevent one case of overweight/obesity [97]. These findings highlight the nuanced impact of PE on obesity prevention, suggesting that both the quantity and quality of PE are important in addressing this public health challenge. Interestingly, Menschik et al. [98] reported that for each weekday that adolescents with a normal weight participated in PE, the odds of becoming overweight in adulthood decreased by 5% [98]. A meta-analysis by Dabravolskaj et al. [99] revealed that modifications to the PE curriculum can effectively improve obesity outcomes. The study revealed a significant decrease in BMI of −0.16 (95% CI: −0.3, −0.02), along with a reduced likelihood of being overweight or obese, with odds of 0.41 (95% CI: 0.23, 0.73). A recent randomized controlled trial assessed the impact of a large-scale, real-world, school-based PA intervention in Slovenia involving more than 34,000 participants aged 6–14 years across more than 200 schools. The intervention, which provided two to three additional PE sessions per week, was compared with a similar number of nonparticipants from the same schools. The findings revealed that BMI was consistently lower in the intervention group than in the control group, regardless of the duration of participation or initial weight. Notably, the impact on BMI was more pronounced after 3–4 years of participation, especially in children with obesity. The intervention began to effectively reverse obesity after 3 years, with the most significant changes observed after 5 years. This study demonstrated that school-based PA interventions can be effective at preventing and treating obesity, particularly by benefiting children with obesity the most. This study underscores the importance of implementing comprehensive and controlled PE initiatives in schools as a strategy to counteract the growing global prevalence of childhood obesity [100].

Interestingly, a recent study analyzed the cost-effectiveness of school-based obesity prevention interventions. The study utilized a microsimulation model incorporating intervention effects on multiple risk factors to estimate the cost-effectiveness and return on investment (ROI) for each program type. The findings of PE curriculum modification programs suggested that they were cost effective when the program costs were less than CA$416 per student in terms of the quality-adjusted life years (QALYs) gained. This program type remained cost-effective for up to CA$1987 per student when looking at the prevention of chronic disease per year. Additionally, if these interventions were implemented at a total discounted cost of CA$100 per student, the ROI, calculated through the avoidance of direct healthcare costs related to the treatment and management of chronic diseases, would be 484% [101]. The seminal work of Kahan and Mckenzie [102] clarified the potential and reality of PE in controlling overweight and obesity. The authors estimated energy expenditure (derived from PE frequency, duration, and intensity; mean student mass; and class size) from national recommendations and data from the 19 United States with PE duration guidelines under three scenarios: potential (quality PE, defined as 50% MVPA), reality (MVPA = 35%), and classroom instruction only. Students in schools following nationally recommended PE standards from grades 1 through 10 expended 35,000 to 90,000 more kilocalories than students who received classroom instruction. Either way, the results make it clear that even from conservative energy expenditure estimates, PE has great potential for helping to control child and adolescent overweight, especially when conducted at a dosage recommended by international standards.

7.5 Advancing Health Through Innovations in Physical Education

To this point, it is critical to think about and foresee the future trajectory of PE in the promotion of health. With each decade, our understanding of human health, educational methodologies, and societal needs has undergone significant shifts. These changes are not merely incremental; they are often revolutionary, challenging our long-held beliefs and practices in this field. As educators and researchers, it is our paramount duty to stay abreast of these changes, to adapt, and to innovate, ensuring that our practices are relevant, effective, and responsive to the needs of the times [103]. The field of PE and health, in particular, stands at a unique juncture. Historically, grounded in the development of physical skills and the promotion of health, it now faces an array of new challenges and opportunities. Societal changes, technological advancements, and a growing body of interdisciplinary research are all converging to expand the scope and depth of this field [104].

When imagining the future of PE in public health, the concept of physical literacy is crucial [105]. Physical literacy is a concept that is gaining increasing recognition in the field of PE and transcends the traditional boundaries of physical health, embodying a more holistic approach to well-being [106, 107]. Unlike the conventional focus on physical skills and physical fitness alone, physical literacy encompasses a wider spectrum of attributes, including emotional, cognitive, and social aspects. At its core, physical literacy is about developing a range of skills and attitudes that encourage individuals to embrace PA as a lifelong habit [6]. This concept is crucial in PE, as it shifts the focus from short-term goals, such as mastering a specific sport or improving physical fitness, to long-term engagement and well-being. It recognizes the role of PE in enhancing mental health, building social connections, and fostering a sense of competence and confidence that extends beyond the school context. In essence, physical literacy in PE means equipping individuals with the knowledge, skills, and attitudes necessary to value and engage in PA throughout their lives. Overall, the future of PE will push us to abandon a narrow view of PE rooted in fixed methods closely linked to traditional sports education or physical fitness aspects and will assist us in recognizing the accountability and educational value of PE in overall health beyond its contribution to physical health per se [108].

In recent years, the application of artificial intelligence has had a profound impact on all areas of human society, including PE [109]. Artificial intelligence algorithms can analyze vast amounts of data from various sources, including wearable technology and interactive physical fitness equipment, to provide personalized exercise recommendations and health monitoring. This customization can ensure that PE programs meet the specific needs of each individual, optimizing health outcomes. Moreover, artificial intelligence can facilitate the tracking of student progress, allowing for adjustments. The integration of artificial intelligence into PE also offers innovative ways to engage students, such as through gamified physical fitness challenges or virtual reality experiences, which can make PA more appealing and enjoyable. Artificial intelligence-driven analytics can assist educators in identifying trends and patterns in student engagement and sports performance, leading to more effective and responsive curriculum development. For instance, Zhang et al. [110] proposed virtual simulation technology using artificial intelligence in a virtual sports simulation teaching mode in PE.

Another key aspect of future developments in health promotion through PE will be the scalability of interventions. Scale-up is the process by which health interventions are shown to be efficacious on a small scale and/or under controlled conditions are expanded under real-world conditions into broader policy or practice [111]. To date, only three whole-of-school scalable programs in the PA field have been recognized [112]. In a recent Delphi study utilizing 46 experts in the field, the implementation of scalable school-based interventions to improve and promote physical fitness was ranked fourth in international priorities for the future of physical fitness research [113]. A good example of scalability is the Physically Active Children in Education (PACE) program, aimed at increasing PA minutes scheduled by classroom teachers each week; this program was evaluated for its scalability across multiple regions in New South Wales, Australia [114]. With 100 schools involved in an uncontrolled before-and-after study, the program ran for approximately 12 months. The outcomes assessed were the delivery of the evidence-based intervention in terms of scheduled PA minutes, implementation strategies (reach, dose, adherence, sustainability), and determinants such as acceptability and cost. The results indicated that the PACE was effective, with teachers increasing their average minutes of scheduled PA by 26.8 min per week. High adherence to implementation strategies was observed, with 90% of schools receiving all components and more than 50% adhering to most strategies. The program was well accepted, with over 50% agreement for all strategies.

In recent years, the role of health in PE has increasingly come under the spotlight, garnering significant public and political attention. Recognized for its vital contribution to the health and well-being of children and adolescents, PE is at the center of a growing discourse. Critical PE scholars challenge the dominant biomedical perspective on health, which they argue is too narrow in its focus on PA and disease prevention. They advocate for alternative, more holistic approaches to health, such as critical and salutogenic perspectives, which encompass a broader understanding of health. Wiklander's research [115] reveals that while PE teachers may initially possess a limited view of health, they show openness to these alternative perspectives. The study highlights that with adequate support and opportunities for professional development, PE teachers are capable of engaging in critical reflections and adapting their views, indicating a potential shift in the way health is approached within the context of PE [115]. As a cornerstone of holistic health promotion, modern PE will extend beyond traditional sports and physical fitness activities to encompass a broader spectrum of health-related issues. As such, the evolution of PE is crucial not only for physical fitness but also as a vital instrument in shaping healthier, more informed, and resilient students. In conclusion, the scope of health promotion via PE extends far beyond the realms discussed in this chapter. Continuous vigilance and adaptability are needed from both researchers and educators to respond effectively to ever-evolving social challenges. As societal needs and health paradigms shift, professionals in this field must remain at the forefront of innovation and change.

7.6 Recommendations

PE represents the primary mode of promoting PA within the school environment. In numerous countries, there are legal mandates that ensure that PE is a part of the curriculum for a significant portion of the mandatory schooling years. The research presented in this chapter highlights the significant role of PE in enhancing the physical and brain health of youth, potentially exceeding the benefits provided by other subjects in the school curriculum. Evidence-based studies have revealed that PE classes play a crucial role in optimizing youth health. This is particularly evident in the enhancement of physical fitness, recognized as an important marker of health, and the improvement of cognitive abilities and academic performance. The fundamental mission of PE is to educate people through movement by inducing the advantages of regular PA. The insights garnered from this chapter position PE as a vital element of the educational curriculum, indispensable and not to be overshadowed by other subjects. The recommendation emerging from this chapter is clear: PE should be a consistent, almost daily presence in educational programs worldwide.

The National Association for Sport and Physical Education (NASPE) recommends that elementary and secondary schools provide at least 150 min of PE every week. However, qualitative aspects of PE should not be underestimated. The QPE is deemed the optimal pedagogical approach for implementing PE to enhance various aspects of health [116]. From a youth's perspective, engaging in movement through play, games, exploration, and learning is naturally enjoyable. Youth inherently desire inclusion, recognition, and the opportunity to explore exciting ways to feel positive about their movements and themselves. Inclusive education, therefore, necessitates access to QPE, appropriate equipment and facilities, and opportunities for skill development with maximal participation. This approach encompasses age-appropriate content and experiences and relies on teachers who are not only knowledgeable but also invested in each child's progress and movement. A teacher's interest in each child's development and overall enjoyment are crucial components of this educational framework [117].

To maximize health benefits through PAs and PEs, implementing a comprehensive school curriculum program is essential. A prime example of this is the *Whole School, Whole Community, Whole Child* (WSCC) model, which is an evidence-based program that focuses on integrating health into the school environment [118]. Central to the WSCC model is the concept of a student-centered approach, underlining the crucial role of community support for schools, the interconnection between health and academic success, and the importance of implementing evidence-based policies and practices within educational settings. A key aspect of this framework is the *Comprehensive School Physical Activity Program* (CSPAP). This

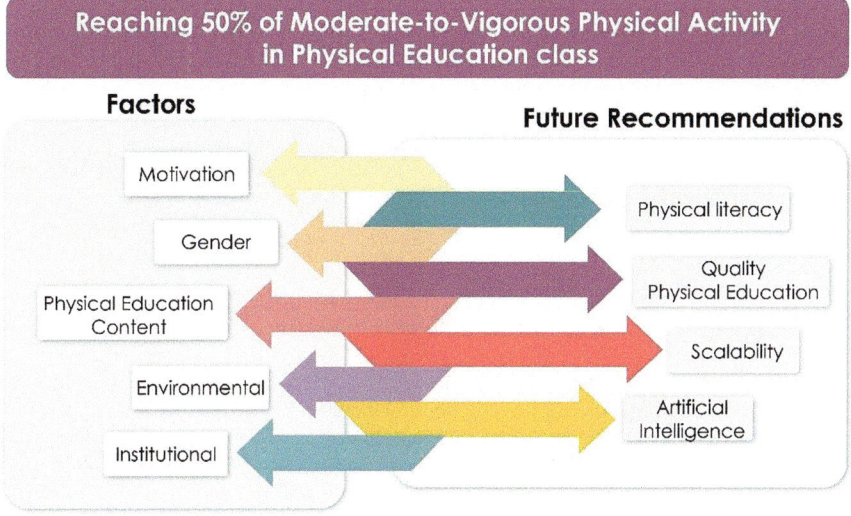

Fig. 7.1 Factors and future recommendations associated with achieving 50% compliance in physical education classes regarding moderate-to-vigorous intensity physical activity

multicomponent approach enables schools to provide multiple opportunities for students to be physically active. The aim is to ensure that students meet the recommended 60 min of PA daily and cultivate the knowledge, skills, and confidence necessary for lifelong PA. Such multifaceted approaches have proven more effective at enhancing daily PA levels and academic performance among students, thereby improving their overall health [119, 120]. Thus, adopting models such as the CSPAP is instrumental in actualizing a whole-school approach, transforming it into practical and actionable strategies that foster healthier youths.

Figure 7.1 summarizes the factors associated with achieving 50% compliance in PE classes regarding MVPA, along with future recommendations to accomplish this.

7.7 Conclusions

Research on the public health benefits of PE is being conducted, particularly regarding its comprehensive role in health beyond physical fitness, academic performance, cognition, and obesity-related factors. While PE classes are known to provide a significant amount of PA to students, the specifics of this provision, including its quantity and quality aspects, require additional inquiry. To date, evidence has shown that PE participation positively influences PA levels, physical fitness, and academic and cognitive performance. However, there is a need for more extensive research into how PE might contribute to preventing unhealthy behaviors and reducing the risk of diseases associated with physical inactivity or sedentary lifestyles. Given the potential implications of PE for public health, there is an urgent need for comprehensive research exploring both the immediate and long-term effects of PE on other health markers. Policymakers frequently recognize the importance of PE in health interventions, but the limited evidence supporting their health benefits may hinder their prioritization as a key public health strategy. Thus, it is crucial to expand the research scope to better understand the diverse impacts of PE on public health, thereby reinforcing its role in educational and health policies.

References

1. Quennerstedt M. Healthying physical education—on the possibility of learning health. Phys Educ Sport Pedagog. 2019;24(1):1–15. https://doi.org/10.1080/17408989.2018.1539705.
2. Fernandez-Rio J. Health-based physical education: a model for educators. J Phys Educ Recreat Danc. 2016;87(8):5–7. https://www.tandfonline.com/doi/full/10.1080/07303084.2016.1217123
3. Ladwig MA, Vazou S, Ekkekakis P. "My Best memory is when I was done with it": PE memories are associated with adult sedentary behavior. Transl J Am Coll Sport Med. 2018;3(16):119–29. https://journals.lww.com/01933607-201808150-00001
4. Rhodes RE, Kates A. Can the affective response to exercise predict future motives and physical activity behavior? A systematic review of published evidence. Ann Behav Med. 2015;49(5):715–31. https://academic.oup.com/abm/article/49/5/715/4562772
5. Quennerstedt M. Exploring the relation between physical activity and health—a salutogenic approach to physical education. Sport Educ Soc. 2008;13(3):267–83.
6. Cairney J, Dudley D, Kwan M, Bulten R, Kriellaars D. Physical literacy, physical activity and health: toward an evidence-informed conceptual model. Sport Med. 2019;49(3):371–83. http://link.springer.com/10.1007/s40279-019-01063-3
7. Sallis JF, McKenzie TL. Physical education's role in public health. Res Q Exerc Sport. 1991;62(2):124–37. http://www.tandfonline.com/doi/abs/10.1080/02701367.1991.10608701
8. Hills AP, Dengel DR, Lubans DR. Supporting public health priorities: recommendations for physical education and physical activity promotion in schools. Prog Cardiovasc Dis. 2015;57(4):368–74. https://linkinghub.elsevier.com/retrieve/pii/S003306201400142X
9. Sallis JF, McKenzie TL, Beets MW, Beighle A, Erwin H, Lee S. Physical education's role in public health. Res Q Exerc Sport. 2012;83(2):125–35. http://www.tandfonline.com/doi/abs/10.1080/02701367.2012.10599842
10. Martins J, Marques A, Gouveia ÉR, Carvalho F, Sarmento H, Valeiro MG. Participation in physical education classes and health-related behaviours among adolescents from 67 countries. Int J Environ Res Public Health. 2022;19(2):955. https://www.mdpi.com/1660-4601/19/2/955
11. Lister NB, Baur LA, Felix JF, Hill AJ, Marcus C, Reinehr T, et al. Child and adolescent obesity. Nat Rev Dis Prim. 2023;9(1):24. https://www.nature.com/articles/s41572-023-00435-4
12. Corbin CB. Conceptual physical education: a course for the future. J Sport Heal Sci. 2021;10(3):308–22. https://linkinghub.elsevier.com/retrieve/pii/S2095254620301435
13. Kingston Ú, Adamakis M, Lester D, Costa J. A scoping review on quality physical education programmes and their outcomes on primary-level pupils. Int J Environ Res Public Health. 2023;20(4):3575. https://www.mdpi.com/1660-4601/20/4/3575
14. Ekblom-Bak E, Ekblom Ö, Andersson G, Wallin P, Ekblom B. Physical education and leisure-time physical activity in youth are both important for adulthood activity, physical

performance, and health. J Phys Act Health. 2018;15(9):661–70. https://journals.humankinetics.com/view/journals/jpah/15/9/article-p661.xml
15. Bandeira A da S, Ravagnani FC de P, Barbosa Filho VC, de Oliveira VJM, de Camargo EM, Tenório MCM, et al. Mapping recommended strategies to promote active and healthy lifestyles through physical education classes: a scoping review. Int J Behav Nutr Phys Act. 2022;19(1):36. https://ijbnpa.biomedcentral.com/articles/10.1186/s12966-022-01278-0
16. Ramires VV, dos Santos PC, Barbosa Filho VC, Bandeira A da S, Marinho Tenório MC, de Camargo EM, et al. Physical education for health among school-aged children and adolescents: a scoping review of reviews. J Phys Act Heal. 2023;20(7):586–99. https://journals.humankinetics.com/view/journals/jpah/20/7/article-p586.xml
17. Caspersen CJ, Powell KE, Christenson GM. Physical activity, exercise, and physical fitness: definitions and distinctions for health-related research. Public Health Rep. 1985;100(2):126–31.
18. World Health Organization. WHO guidelines on physical activity and sedentary behaviour. World health. Organization. 2020:104.
19. Chaput JP, Willumsen J, Bull F, Chou R, Ekelund U, Firth J, et al. 2020 WHO guidelines on physical activity and sedentary behaviour for children and adolescents aged 5–17 years: summary of the evidence. Int J Behav Nutr Phys Act. 2020;17(1):141. https://ijbnpa.biomedcentral.com/articles/10.1186/s12966-020-01037-z
20. Tapia-Serrano MA, Sevil-Serrano J, Sánchez-Miguel PA, López-Gil JF, Tremblay MS, García-Hermoso A. Prevalence of meeting 24-hour movement guidelines from pre-school to adolescence: a systematic review and meta-analysis including 387,437 participants and 23 countries. J Sport Heal Sci. 2022;11(4):427–37. https://linkinghub.elsevier.com/retrieve/pii/S2095254622000205
21. Aubert S, Barnes JD, Demchenko I, Hawthorne M, Abdeta C, Abi Nader P, et al. Global matrix 4.0 physical activity report card grades for children and adolescents: results and analyses from 57 countries. J Phys Act Health. 2022;19(11):700–28. https://journals.humankinetics.com/view/journals/jpah/19/11/article-p700.xml
22. McKenzie TL, Lounsbery MAF. The pill not taken: revisiting physical education teacher effectiveness in a public health context. Res Q Exerc Sport. 2014;85(3):287–92. http://www.tandfonline.com/doi/abs/10.1080/02701367.2014.931203
23. United Nations Educational S and CO. Quality Physical Education (QPE): Guidelines for policy makers. 2015. 4–82 p. http://creativecommons.org/licenses/by-sa/3.0/igo/
24. World Health Organization. Promoting physical activity through schools: a toolkit. Geneva; 2021.
25. Ramirez Varela A, Salvo D, Pratt M, Milton K, Siefken K, Bauman A, et al. Worldwide use of the first set of physical activity country cards: the global Observatory for Physical Activity—GoPA! Int J Behav Nutr Phys Act. 2018;15(1):29. https://ijbnpa.biomedcentral.com/articles/10.1186/s12966-018-0663-7
26. Martins J, Onofre M, Hallal PC. Launch of the Global Observatory for Physical Education (GoPE!). J Phys Act Health. 2023;20(7):573–4. https://journals.humankinetics.com/view/journals/jpah/20/7/article-p573.xml
27. Cale L. Physical education's journey on the road to health. Sport Educ Soc. 2021;26(5):486–99. https://www.tandfonline.com/doi/full/10.1080/13573322.2020.1740979
28. Meyer U, Roth R, Zahner L, Gerber M, Puder JJ, Hebestreit H, et al. Contribution of physical education to overall physical activity. Scand J Med Sci Sports. 2013;23(5):600–6. https://onlinelibrary.wiley.com/doi/10.1111/j.1600-0838.2011.01425.x
29. da Silva DJ, Barbosa AO, Barbosa Filho VC, de Farias Júnior JC. Is participation in physical education classes related to physical activity and sedentary behavior? A systematic review. J Phys Act Health. 2022;19(11):786–808. https://journals.humankinetics.com/view/journals/jpah/19/11/article-p786.xml
30. de Jesus GM, de Oliveira Araujo RH, Dias LA, Barros AKC, dos Santos Araujo LDM, de Assis MAA. Attendance in physical education classes, sedentary behavior, and different

forms of physical activity among schoolchildren: a cross-sectional study. BMC Public Health. 2022;22(1):1461. https://bmcpublichealth.biomedcentral.com/articles/10.1186/s12889-022-13864-9
31. Uddin R, Salmon J, Islam SMS, Khan A. Physical education class participation is associated with physical activity among adolescents in 65 countries. Sci Rep. 2020;10(1):22128. https://www.nature.com/articles/s41598-020-79100-9
32. García-Hermoso A, Ezzatvar Y, López-Gil JF. Association between daily physical education attendance and meeting 24-hour movement guidelines in adolescence and adulthood. J Adolesc Health. 2023;73(5):896–902. https://linkinghub.elsevier.com/retrieve/pii/S1054139X23003245
33. Hobbs M, Daly-Smith A, McKenna J, Quarmby T, Morley D. Reconsidering current objectives for physical activity within physical education. Br J Sports Med. 2018;52(19):1229–30. https://bjsm.bmj.com/lookup/doi/10.1136/bjsports-2016-097328
34. Arenas D, Vidal-Conti J, Muntaner-Mas A. Gender differences in students' moderate to vigorous physical activity levels during primary school physical education lessons: a systematic review and meta-analysis. J Teach Phys Educ. 2024. https://doi.org/10.1123/jtpe.2024-0027
35. Iglesias D, Fernandez-Rio J, Rodríguez-González P. Moderate-to-vigorous physical activity in physical education: a review of reviews. J Teach Phys Educ. 2023;42(4):640–6. https://journals.humankinetics.com/view/journals/jtpe/42/4/article-p640.xml
36. Hollis JL, Williams AJ, Sutherland R, Campbell E, Nathan N, Wolfenden L, et al. A systematic review and meta-analysis of moderate-to-vigorous physical activity levels in elementary school physical education lessons. Prev Med (Baltim). 2016;86:34–54. http://linkinghub.elsevier.com/retrieve/pii/S009174351500345X
37. Wang L, Zhou Y. A systematic review of correlates of the moderate-to-vigorous physical activity of students in elementary school physical education. J Teach Phys Educ. 2021:1–16. https://journals.humankinetics.com/view/journals/jtpe/aop/article-10.1123-jtpe.2020-0197/article-10.1123-jtpe.2020-0197.xml
38. Hollis JL, Sutherland R, Williams AJ, Campbell E, Nathan N, Wolfenden L, et al. A systematic review and meta-analysis of moderate-to-vigorous physical activity levels in secondary school physical education lessons. Int J Behav Nutr Phys Act. 2017;14(1):52. http://ijbnpa.biomedcentral.com/articles/10.1186/s12966-017-0504-0
39. Kerr C, Smith L, Charman S, Harvey S, Savory L, Fairclough S, et al. Physical education contributes to total physical activity levels and predominantly in higher intensity physical activity categories. Eur Phys Educ Rev. 2018;24(2):152–64. http://journals.sagepub.com/doi/10.1177/1356336X16672127
40. Alderman BL, Benham-Deal T, Beighle A, Erwin HE, Olson RL. Physical education's contribution to daily physical activity among middle school youth. Pediatr Exerc Sci. 2012;24(4):634–48. https://journals.humankinetics.com/view/journals/pes/24/4/article-p634.xml
41. Mayorga-Vega D, Martínez-Baena A, Viciana J. Does school physical education really contribute to accelerometer-measured daily physical activity and non sedentary behaviour in high school students? J Sports Sci. 2018;36(17):1913–22. https://www.tandfonline.com/doi/full/10.1080/02640414.2018.1425967
42. Lonsdale C, Rosenkranz RR, Peralta LR, Bennie A, Fahey P, Lubans DR. A systematic review and meta-analysis of interventions designed to increase moderate-to-vigorous physical activity in school physical education lessons. Prev Med (Baltim). 2013;56(2):152–61. https://linkinghub.elsevier.com/retrieve/pii/S0091743512006068
43. Wong LS, Gibson AM, Farooq A, Reilly JJ. Interventions to increase moderate-to-vigorous physical activity in elementary school physical education lessons: systematic review. J Sch Health. 2021;91(10):836–45.
44. White RL, Bennie A, Vasconcellos D, Cinelli R, Hilland T, Owen KB, et al. Self-determination theory in physical education: a systematic review of qualitative studies. Teach Teach Educ. 2021;99:103247. https://linkinghub.elsevier.com/retrieve/pii/S0742051X20314384

45. Ryan RM, Deci EL. Self-determination theory and the facilitation of intrinsic motivation, social development, and well-being. Am Psychol. 2000;55(1):68–78. http://doi.apa.org/getdoi.cfm?doi=10.1037/0003-066X.55.1.68
46. Prochaska JJ, Rodgers MW, Sallis JF. Association of parent and peer support with adolescent physical activity. Res Q Exerc Sport. 2002;73(2):206–10. http://www.tandfonline.com/doi/abs/10.1080/02701367.2002.10609010
47. Sun H, Li W, Shen B. Learning in physical education: a self-determination theory perspective. J Teach Phys Educ. 2017;36(3):277–91. https://journals.humankinetics.com/view/journals/jtpe/36/3/article-p277.xml
48. Zhan X, Clark CCT, Bao R, Duncan M, Hong JT, Chen ST. Association between physical education classes and physical activity among 187,386 adolescents aged 13–17 years from 50 low- and middle-income countries. J Pediatr. 2021;97(5):571–8. https://linkinghub.elsevier.com/retrieve/pii/S0021755721000231
49. Raghuveer G, Hartz J, Lubans DR, Takken T, Wiltz JL, Mietus-Snyder M, et al. Cardiorespiratory fitness in youth: an important marker of health: a scientific statement from the American Heart Association. Circulation. 2020;142(7) https://www.ahajournals.org/doi/10.1161/CIR.0000000000000866
50. Ortega FB, Ruiz JR, Castillo MJ, Sjöström M. Physical fitness in childhood and adolescence: a powerful marker of health. Int J Obes. 2008;32(1):1–11.
51. Ortega FB, Cadenas-Sanchez C, Lee D, Chul, Ruiz J, Blair S, Sui X. Fitness and fatness as health markers through the lifespan: an overview of current knowledge. Prog prev med. 2018;3(2):e0013. http://ovidsp.ovid.com/ovidweb.cgi?T=JS&PAGE=reference&D=ovftt&NEWS=N&AN=01960908-201804000-00001
52. García-Hermoso A, Alonso-Martínez AM, Ramírez-Vélez R, Pérez-Sousa MÁ, Ramírez-Campillo R, Izquierdo M. Association of physical education with improvement of health-related physical fitness outcomes and fundamental motor skills among youths. JAMA Pediatr. 2020;174(6):e200223. https://jamanetwork.com/journals/jamapediatrics/fullarticle/2763829
53. Peralta M, Henriques-Neto D, Gouveia ÉR, Sardinha LB, Marques A. Promoting health-related cardiorespiratory fitness in physical education: a systematic review. Clemente FM, editor. PLoS One. 2020;15(8):e0237019. https://dx.plos.org/10.1371/journal.pone.0237019
54. Lander N, Eather N, Morgan PJ, Salmon J, Barnett LM. Characteristics of teacher training in school-based physical education interventions to improve fundamental movement skills and/or physical activity: a systematic review. Sport Med. 2017;47(1):135–61. http://link.springer.com/10.1007/s40279-016-0561-6
55. Costigan SA Eather N, Plotnikoff RC, Taaffe DR, Lubans DR. High-intensity interval training for improving health-related fitness in adolescents: a systematic review and meta-analysis. Br J Sports Med. 2015; 2014(April):1–9. http://bjsm.bmj.com/content/early/2015/06/18/bjsports-2014-094490.full%5Cn; http://bjsm.bmj.com/cgi/doi/10.1136/bjsports-2014-094490
56. Jurić P, Dudley DA, Petocz P. Does incorporating high intensity interval training in physical education classes improve fitness outcomes of students? A cluster randomized controlled trial. Prev Med Reports. 2023:102127. https://linkinghub.elsevier.com/retrieve/pii/S2211335523000189
57. Duncombe SL, Barker AR, Bond B, Earle R, Varley-Campbell J, Vlachopoulos D, et al. School-based high-intensity interval training programs in children and adolescents: a systematic review and meta-analysis. Harnish C, editor. PLoS One. 2022;17(5):e0266427. https://dx.plos.org/10.1371/journal.pone.0266427
58. Bauer N, Sperlich B, Holmberg HC, Engel FA. Effects of high-intensity interval training in school on the physical performance and health of children and adolescents: a systematic review with meta-analysis. Sport Med—Open. 2022;8(1):50. https://sportsmedicine-open.springeropen.com/articles/10.1186/s40798-022-00437-8
59. Lloyd RS, Oliver JL. The youth physical development model. Strength Cond J. 2012;34(3):61–72. https://journals.lww.com/00126548-201206000-00008

60. García-Hermoso A, Ramírez-Campillo R, Izquierdo M. Is muscular fitness associated with future health benefits in children and adolescents? A systematic review and meta-analysis of longitudinal studies. Sport Med. 2019;49(7):1079–94. http://link.springer.com/10.1007/s40279-019-01098-6
61. Faigenbaum AD, Ratamess NA, Kang J, Bush JA, Rebullido TR. May the force be with youth: Foundational strength for lifelong development. 2023;22(12):414–22.
62. Till K, Bruce A, Green T, Morris SJ, Boret S, Bishop CJ. Strength and conditioning in schools: a strategy to optimise health, fitness and physical activity in youths. Br J Sports Med. 2022;56(9):479–80. https://bjsm.bmj.com/lookup/doi/10.1136/bjsports-2021-104509
63. Villa-González E, Barranco-Ruiz Y, García-Hermoso A, Faigenbaum AD. Efficacy of school-based interventions for improving muscular fitness outcomes in children: a systematic review and meta-analysis. Eur J Sport Sci. 2022:1–16. https://www.tandfonline.com/doi/full/10.1080/17461391.2022.2029578
64. Cox A, Fairclough SJ, Kosteli MC, Noonan RJ. Efficacy of school-based interventions for improving muscular fitness outcomes in adolescent boys: a systematic review and meta-analysis. Sport Med. 2020;50(3):543–60. http://link.springer.com/10.1007/s40279-019-01215-5
65. Stricker PR, Faigenbaum AD, McCambridge TM, LaBella CR, Brooks MA, Canty G, et al. Resistance training for children and adolescents. Pediatrics. 2020;145(6) https://publications.aap.org/pediatrics/article/145/6/e20201011/76942/Resistance-Training-for-Children-and-Adolescents
66. Smith JJ, Eather N, Morgan PJ, Plotnikoff RC, Faigenbaum AD, Lubans DR. The health benefits of muscular fitness for children and adolescents: a systematic review and meta-analysis. Sport Med. 2014;44(9):1209–23. http://link.springer.com/10.1007/s40279-014-0196-4
67. Martin-Martinez C, Valenzuela PL, Martinez-Zamora M, Martinez-de-Quel Ó. School-based physical activity interventions and language skills: a systematic review and meta-analysis of randomized controlled trials. J Sci Med Sport. 2023;26(2):140–8. https://linkinghub.elsevier.com/retrieve/pii/S1440244022005047
68. Masini A, Marini S, Gori D, Leoni E, Rochira A, Dallolio L. Evaluation of school-based interventions of active breaks in primary schools: a systematic review and meta-analysis. J Sci Med Sport. 2020;23(4):377–84. https://linkinghub.elsevier.com/retrieve/pii/S144024401930800X
69. Sneck S, Viholainen H, Syväoja H, Kankaapää A, Hakonen H, Poikkeus AM, et al. Effects of school-based physical activity on mathematics performance in children: a systematic review. Int J Behav Nutr Phys Act. 2019;16(1):109. https://ijbnpa.biomedcentral.com/articles/10.1186/s12966-019-0866-6
70. Watson A, Timperio A, Brown H, Best K, Hesketh KD. Effect of classroom-based physical activity interventions on academic and physical activity outcomes: a systematic review and meta-analysis. Int J Behav Nutr Phys Act. 2017;14(1):114. http://ijbnpa.biomedcentral.com/articles/10.1186/s12966-017-0569-9
71. Norris E, van Steen T, Direito A, Stamatakis E. Physically active lessons in schools and their impact on physical activity, educational, health and cognition outcomes: a systematic review and meta-analysis. Br J Sports Med. 2020;54(14):826–38. https://bjsm.bmj.com/lookup/doi/10.1136/bjsports-2018-100502
72. Visier-Alfonso ME, Sánchez-López M, Álvarez-Bueno C, Ruiz-Hermosa A, Nieto-López M, Martínez-Vizcaíno V. Mediators between physical activity and academic achievement: a systematic review. Scand J Med Sci Sports. 2021; https://onlinelibrary.wiley.com/doi/10.1111/sms.14107
73. Donnelly JE, Hillman CH, Castelli D, Etnier JL, Lee S, Tomporowski P, et al. Physical activity, fitness, cognitive function, and academic achievement in children. Med Sci Sport Exerc. 2016;48(6):1197–222. http://content.wkhealth.com/linkback/openurl?sid=WKPTLP:landingpage&an=00005768-201606000-00027
74. Erickson KI, Hillman C, Stillman CM, Ballard RM, Bloodgood B, Conroy DE, et al. Physical activity, cognition, and brain outcomes: a review of the 2018 physical activity guidelines. Med Sci Sport Exerc. 2019;51(6):1242–51.

75. Singh AS, Saliasi E, van den Berg V, Uijtdewilligen L, de Groot RHM, Jolles J, et al. Effects of physical activity interventions on cognitive and academic performance in children and adolescents: a novel combination of a systematic review and recommendations from an expert panel. Br J Sports Med. 2019;53(10):640–7. http://bjsm.bmj.com/lookup/doi/10.1136/bjsports-2017-098136
76. Marqu es A, Santos DA, Hillman CH, Sardinha LB. How does academic achievement relate to cardiorespiratory fitness, self-reported physical activity and objectively reported physical activity: a systematic review in children and adolescents aged 6–18 years. Br J Sports Med. 2018;52(16):1039–9. http://bjsm.bmj.com/lookup/doi/10.1136/bjsports-2016-097361
77. Rasberry CN, Lee SM, Robin L, Laris BA, Russell LA, Coyle KK, et al. The association between school-based physical activity, including physical education, and academic performance: a systematic review of the literature. Prev Med (Baltim). 2011;52:S10–20. https://linkinghub.elsevier.com/retrieve/pii/S0091743511000557
78. Dudley D, Burden R. What effect on learning does increasing the proportion of curriculum time allocated to physical education have? A systematic review and meta-analysis. Eur Phys Educ Rev. 2020;26(1):85–100. http://journals.sagepub.com/doi/10.1177/1356336X19830113
79. Hattie J. Visible learning. Routledge; 2008.
80. García-Hermoso A, Ramírez-Vélez R, Lubans DR, Izquierdo M. Effects of physical education interventions on cognition and academic performance outcomes in children and adolescents: a systematic review and meta-analysis. Br J Sports Med. 2021;55(21):1224–32. https://bjsm.bmj.com/lookup/doi/10.1136/bjsports-2021-104112
81. Cho O, Choi W, Shin Y. The effectiveness of school physical education on students' cognitive competence: a systematic review and meta-analysis. J Sports Med Phys Fitness. 2022;62(4) https://www.minervamedica.it/index2.php?show=R40Y2022N04A0575
82. Zach S, Shoval E, Lidor R. Physical education and academic achievement—literature review 1997–2015. J Curric Stud. 2017;49(5):703–21. https://www.tandfonline.com/doi/full/10.1080/00220272.2016.1234649
83. Trudeau F, Shephard RJ. Physical education, school physical activity, school sports and academic performance. Int J Behav Nutr Phys Act. 2008;5(1):10. http://ijbnpa.biomedcentral.com/articles/10.1186/1479-5868-5-10
84. Lambert K, Ford A, Jeanes R. The association between physical education and academic achievement in other curriculum learning areas: a review of literature. Phys Educ Sport Pedagog. 2024;29(1):51–81. https://www.tandfonline.com/doi/full/10.1080/17408989.2022.2029385
85. García-Hermoso A, Ramírez-Vélez R, Saavedra JM. Exercise, health outcomes, and pædiatric obesity: a systematic review of meta-analyses. J Sci Med Sport. 2019;22(1):76–84. https://doi.org/10.1016/j.jsams.2018.07.006.
86. World Health Organization. Report of the commission on ending childhood obesity. World Health Organization; 2016. https://iris.who.int/handle/10665/204176
87. UNICEF. UNICEF advocacy strategy guidance for the prevention of overweight and obesity in children and adolescents. New York: UNICEF; 2020.
88. Doak CM, Visscher TLS, Renders CM, Seidell JC. The prevention of overweight and obesity in children and adolescents: a review of interventions and programmes. Obes Rev. 2006;7(1):111–36. https://onlinelibrary.wiley.com/doi/10.1111/j.1467-789X.2006.00234.x
89. Katz DL, O'Connell M, Njike VY, Yeh MC, Nawaz H. Strategies for the prevention and control of obesity in the school setting: systematic review and meta-analysis. Int J Obes. 2008;32(12):1780–9. https://www.nature.com/articles/ijo2008158
90. Khambalia AZ, Dickinson S, Hardy LL, Gill T, Baur LA. A synthesis of existing systematic reviews and meta-analyses of school-based behavioural interventions for controlling and preventing obesity. Obes Rev. 2012;13(3):214–33. https://onlinelibrary.wiley.com/doi/10.1111/j.1467-789X.2011.00947.x
91. Hodder RK, O'Brien KM, Lorien S, Wolfenden L, Moore THM, Hall A, et al. Interventions to prevent obesity in school-aged children 6-18 years: an update of a Cochrane systematic review and meta-analysis including studies from 2015–2021. eClinicalMedicine. 2022;54:101635. https://linkinghub.elsevier.com/retrieve/pii/S2589537022003650

92. Kirk D. The 'obesity crisis' and school physical education. Sport Educ Soc. 2006;11(2):121–33. http://www.tandfonline.com/doi/full/10.1080/13573320600640660
93. Cale L, Harris J. 'Every child (of every size) matters' in physical education! Physical education's role in childhood obesity. Sport Educ Soc. 2013;18(4):433–52. http://www.tandfonline.com/doi/abs/10.1080/13573322.2011.601734
94. Jacob CM, Hardy-Johnson PL, Inskip HM, Morris T, Parsons CM, Barrett M, et al. A systematic review and meta-analysis of school-based interventions with health education to reduce body mass index in adolescents aged 10 to 19 years. Int J Behav Nutr Phys Act. 2021;18(1):1–22.
95. Liu Z, Xu HM, Wen LM, Peng YZ, Lin LZ, Zhou S, et al. A systematic review and meta-analysis of the overall effects of school-based obesity prevention interventions and effect differences by intervention components. Int J Behav Nutr Phys Act. 2019;16(1):1–12.
96. Klakk H, Chinapaw M, Heidemann M, Andersen LB, Wedderkopp N. Effect of four additional physical education lessons on body composition in children aged 8–13 years—a prospective study during two school years. BMC Pediatr. 2013;13(1):170. http://bmcpediatr.biomedcentral.com/articles/10.1186/1471-2431-13-170
97. Learmonth YC, Hebert JJ, Fairchild TJ, Møller NC, Klakk H, Wedderkopp N. Physical education and leisure-time sport reduce overweight and obesity: a number needed to treat analysis. Int J Obes. 2019;43(10):2076–84. https://www.nature.com/articles/s41366-018-0300-1
98. Menschik D, Ahmed S, Alexander MH, Blum RW. Adolescent physical activities as predictors of young adult weight. Arch Pediatr Adolesc Med. 2008;162(1):29. http://archpedi.jamanetwork.com/article.aspx?doi=10.1001/archpediatrics.2007.14
99. Dabravolskaj J, Montemurro G, Ekwaru JP, Wu XY, Storey K, Campbell S, et al. Effectiveness of school-based health promotion interventions prioritized by stakeholders from health and education sectors: a systematic review and meta-analysis. Prev Med Reports. 2020;19:101138. https://linkinghub.elsevier.com/retrieve/pii/S221133552030098X
100. Jurić P, Jurak G, Morrison SA, Starc G, Sorić M. Effectiveness of a population-scaled, school-based physical activity intervention for the prevention of childhood obesity. Obesity. 2023;31(3):811–22. https://onlinelibrary.wiley.com/doi/10.1002/oby.23695
101. Ekwaru JP, Ohinmaa A, Dabravolskaj J, Maximova K, Veugelers PJ. Cost-effectiveness and return on investment of school-based health promotion programmes for chronic disease prevention. Eur J Pub Health. 2021;31(6):1183–9. https://academic.oup.com/eurpub/article/31/6/1183/6342860
102. Kahan D, McKenzie TL. The potential and reality of physical education in controlling overweight and obesity. Am J Public Health. 2015;105(4):653–9. https://ajph.aphapublications.org/doi/full/10.2105/AJPH.2014.302355
103. Clark H, Coll-Seck AM, Banerjee A, Peterson S, Dalglish SL, Ameratunga S, et al. A future for the world's children? A WHO–UNICEF–Lancet Commission. Lancet. 2020;395(10224):605–58. https://linkinghub.elsevier.com/retrieve/pii/S0140673619325401
104. Dudley D, Beighle A, Erwin H, Cairney J, Schaefer L, Murfay K. Physical education-based physical activity interventions. In: The Routledge handbook of youth physical activity. Routledge; 2020. p. 489–503. https://www.taylorfrancis.com/books/9781000050660/chapters/10.4324/9781003026426-30.
105. Corbin CB. Implications of physical literacy for research and practice: a commentary. Res Q Exerc Sport. 2016;87(1):14–27. http://www.tandfonline.com/doi/full/10.1080/02701367.2016.1124722
106. Bailey R. Defining physical literacy: making sense of a promiscuous concept. Sport Soc. 2022;25(1):163–80. https://www.tandfonline.com/doi/full/10.1080/17430437.2020.1777104
107. Edwards LC, Bryant AS, Keegan RJ, Morgan K, Jones AM. Definitions, foundations and associations of physical literacy: a systematic review. Sport Med. 2017;47(1):113–26. http://link.springer.com/10.1007/s40279-016-0560-7

108. Lundvall S. Physical literacy in the field of physical education—a challenge and a possibility. J Sport Heal Sci. 2015;4(2):113–8. https://linkinghub.elsevier.com/retrieve/pii/S2095254615000228
109. Luan H, Geczy P, Lai H, Gobert J, Yang SJH, Ogata H, et al. Challenges and future directions of big data and artificial intelligence in education. Front Psychol. 2020:11. https://www.frontiersin.org/articles/10.3389/fpsyg.2020.580820/full
110. Zhang B, Jin H, Duan X. Physical education movement and comprehensive health quality intervention under the background of artificial intelligence. Front Public Heal. 2022;10. https://www.frontiersin.org/articles/10.3389/fpubh.2022.947731/full
111. McKay H, Naylor PJ, Lau E, Gray SM, Wolfenden L, Milat A, et al. Implementation and scale-up of physical activity and behavioural nutrition interventions: an evaluation roadmap. Int J Behav Nutr Phys Act. 2019;16(1):102. https://ijbnpa.biomedcentral.com/articles/10.1186/s12966-019-0868-4
112. Reis RS, Salvo D, Ogilvie D, Lambert EV, Goenka S, Brownson RC. Scaling up physical activity interventions worldwide: stepping up to larger and smarter approaches to get people moving. Lancet. 2016;388(10051):1337–48. https://linkinghub.elsevier.com/retrieve/pii/S0140673616307280
113. Lang JJ, Zhang K, Agostinis-Sobrinho C, Andersen LB, Basterfield L, Berglind D, et al. Top 10 international priorities for physical fitness research and surveillance among children and adolescents: a twin-panel Delphi study. Sport Med. 2023;53(2):549–64. https://link.springer.com/10.1007/s40279-022-01752-6
114. Hall A, Lane C, Wolfenden L, Wiggers J, Sutherland R, McCarthy N, et al. Evaluating the scaling up of an effective implementation intervention (PACE) to increase the delivery of a mandatory physical activity policy in primary schools. Int J Behav Nutr Phys Act. 2023;20(1):106. https://ijbnpa.biomedcentral.com/articles/10.1186/s12966-023-01498-y
115. Wiklander P, Fröberg A, Lundvall S. Searching for the alternative: a scoping review of empirical studies with holistic perspectives on health and implications for teaching physical education. Eur Phys Educ Rev. 2023;29(3):351–68. http://journals.sagepub.com/doi/10.1177/1356336X221147813
116. N. M, J T. Quality physical education (QPE): guidelines for policy makers. Paris: UNESCO Publishing; 2015.
117. Solmon MA. Optimizing the role of physical education in promoting physical activity: a social-ecological approach. Res Q Exerc Sport. 2015;86(4):329–37. http://www.tandfonline.com/doi/full/10.1080/02701367.2015.1091712
118. Lewallen TC, Hunt H, Potts-Datema W, Zaza S, Giles W. The whole school, whole community, whole child model: a new approach for improving educational attainment and healthy development for students. J Sch Health. 2015;85(11):729–39. http://www.pubmedcentral.nih.gov/articlerender.fcgi?artid=4606766&tool=pmcentrez&rendertype=abstract
119. Burns RD, Brusseau TA, Fu Y, Myrer RS, Hannon JC. Comprehensive school physical activity programming and classroom behavior. Am J Health Behav. 2016;40(1):100–7. http://openurl.ingenta.com/content/xref?genre=article&issn=1087-3244&volume=40&issue=1&spage=100
120. Brusseau TA, Hannon J, Burns R. The effect of a comprehensive school physical activity program on physical activity and health-related fitness in children from low-income families. J Phys Act Health. 2016;13(8):888–94.

Chapter 8
Active Travel to and from School

Adilson Marques, Tiago Ribeiro, and Miguel Peralta

8.1 Introduction

Modes of commuting play an important role in shaping spatial and societal organization and influencing quality of life and overall well-being. Active modes of commuting are important in education, public health, and urban planning. Among young people, active travel to and from school emphasizes the use of human-powered modes of commuting, such as walking and cycling, over motorized vehicles like cars and buses.

In recent years, the trend of using passive travel modes, especially motorized vehicles, for school commutes has raised concerns. Sedentary lifestyles and the overreliance on cars contribute to rising rates of childhood obesity and related health issues. Moreover, increased traffic congestion and air pollution around schools affect students' well-being and raise environmental concerns. Given that a significant proportion of adolescents fail to meet recommended levels of physical activity (PA) [1], active commuting to school can substantially contribute to boosting their PA levels. This assertion is further strengthened by the fact that school-related activities occur daily, providing a consistent opportunity for regular PA [2]. Thus, active travel offers a promising solution to address these issues by promoting PA, reducing traffic, and lowering carbon emissions.

While active travel offers numerous benefits, it also faces various challenges. Safety concerns, including traffic accidents and crime, can deter parents from allowing their children to walk or cycle to school. Insufficient infrastructure, such as sidewalks, bike lanes, and safe crossing points, can hinder active travel initiatives. This chapter explores these challenges and highlights the need for strategies and policies that can mitigate them, promoting safer and more accessible routes for

---

A. Marques (✉) · T. Ribeiro · M. Peralta
CIPER, Faculty of Human Kinetics, University of Lisbon, Lisbon, Portugal
e-mail: amarques@fmh.ulisboa.pt

students. The chapter also considers the role of parents and educators in promoting active travel to and from school. Parental attitudes and perceptions can significantly influence a child's mode of transportation, so understanding and addressing their concerns is crucial. Teachers and schools can incorporate active travel into their curricula and extracurricular activities, further promoting its adoption among students.

This chapter explores the multifaceted dimensions of active travel behavior to and from school, its benefits, challenges, and potential to transform how we think about education and urban design.

8.2 Concepts and Determinants of Active Travel

Promoting active travel to school may be an important strategy to improve children's and adolescents' PA levels. However, to get to a point where promoting active travel is possible and meaningful, we need to understand what we mean by active travel, the prevalence of this behavior, and how internal and external factors impact opportunities for and engagement in active travel.

8.2.1 What Are Active, Passive, and Independent Mobility?

Active travel (also known as active commuting or active transportation) entails human-powered means of getting from one place to another, encompassing activities like walking, cycling, and even skating or skateboarding. It strongly emphasizes physical exertion as the primary method for covering to moderate distances, typically within urban or suburban settings. On the other hand, passive or non-active travel involves using modes of transportation that require low-activity engagement, such as sitting or standing for extended periods while transported. In contrast to passive travel options such as cars or public transit, active travel requires individuals to actively engage in physical effort to propel themselves to their destinations. Among young people, particularly children and adolescents, active travel opportunities occur in several contexts, including commuting to school or engaging in leisure activities.

Although active and passive travel behavior is separated here as different concepts, real-life behavior is more complex. For example, travel-to-school behavior is more fluid than fixed. It may encompass both active and passive travel in the same trip. Also, the availability of new fully or partly electric-powered devices, such as bicycles, skateboards, and scooters, blurs the line separating active and passive transportation modes as they allow them to be active but at a lower intensity level.

Another important concept associated with travel behavior in youth is independent mobility. Youth's independent mobility denotes the autonomy of children and adolescents to navigate their neighborhoods by themselves, i.e., without adult supervision [3]. Thus, it encompasses traveling independently, alone or with friends, around the neighborhood to a range of destinations, including schools, shops, parks, or playgrounds, using either an active (e.g., walking, cycling) or passive (e.g., public transport) mode of transportation. Despite incorporating both modes of transport, independent mobility is thought to be important in facilitating opportunities for active travel.

8.2.2 How Often Do Young People Engage in Active Travel?

Dutch children demonstrate notably high levels of active travel to and from school. A comprehensive study conducted across five major Dutch cities involving children aged 6–11 revealed that an impressive 67% of them opt for walking as their mode of commuting to school, while an additional 27% choose to cycle [4]. When combined, these percentages exceed 90% of children who actively engage in walking or cycling for their school journeys. Similarly, in Denmark, active travel accounted for a substantial 85.4% share of all school-related journeys (Christiansen et al., 2014 [12]). In this Danish study, while 15.9% of adolescents opted for walking, including roller-skating and skateboarding, the significant majority, accounting for almost 70%, chose cycling as their preferred mode of transport to and from school. The Netherlands and Denmark are well-known examples of European countries where most young people and adults engage in active travel, but do not represent the overall reality of active travel to and from school worldwide or even in Europe.

Another example of a European country with an important percentage of children and adolescents who actively commute is Germany, with an estimated prevalence of 78% [5]. Despite being a seemingly high figure, this prevalence has declined over the years, dropping from 84.8% in 2003 to 78.3% in 2017. With the decrease in active travel, there is naturally an increase in passive modes of transportation, which is more pronounced among younger children, those with lower socioeconomic status, and in smaller cities. A study comprising data from 28 other studies conducted in Spain found that the prevalence of active travel to and from school was around 60% [6]. This study also allowed for an analysis of temporal trends in active travel, showing no significant variation from 2010 to 2017. Other European countries, such as Portugal, present a lower prevalence of active travel behavior. A study using data from the World Health Organization's Health Behavior in School-Aged Children 2018 survey revealed that only 37% of adolescents reported active commute to and from school [7]. These studies highlight that active travel behavior can vary significantly between countries, even in the same continent, and point to a stagnation or decreasing trend in active travel behavior.

Most studies about active travel to school behavior have been conducted in European or North American countries with high economic development. However, some recent research has allowed us to observe and compare the prevalence of active travel among children and adolescents in countries with medium and low economic development. In the three most comprehensive studies [8–10], which encompass countries with different levels of economic development, it was evident that, on average, about 40% of children and adolescents use an active mode of transport for their school commutes. Among the countries studied, Japan and Nepal stand out with a prevalence of 86%, followed by Zimbabwe (80%) and Denmark (70%). On the other hand, Canada (36.8%), the United States (38%), and Chile (15%) have lower rates of active transportation usage for school commutes. It was also clear that most countries displayed a stable or decreasing trend in active travel behavior [8]. These investigations contribute to the idea that there is a significant variance in active travel behavior among children and adolescents. In this regard, understanding the determining factors that can explain these differences is important.

8.2.3 What Influences Young People's Active Travel Behavior?

Analyzing the determinants of active commuting is not always easy because it is a complex behavior with explanatory variables related to the physical (i.e., built and natural) environment, individual and psychological factors, and, since we are dealing with young people, the role of parents and family. Thus, engagement in active travel sits on multilevel interactions between individuals and their social and cultural environments with physical environments and policies [11].

Environmental factors are one of the greatest determinants of active travel behavior. Researchers have explored various facets of the constructed surroundings concerning active commuting to school, yielding diverse findings. Children and adolescents residing in urban areas seem to exhibit a higher inclination for active commuting to school [11], as do those residing in neighborhoods with greater walkability and the availability of local recreational facilities [12]. In some regions, low residential density and mixed land use have also shown a connection with active school travel [13]. However, their significance was not observed in other locations [14].

Conversely, challenges to active travel to and from school may arise when traffic signals or pedestrian crossings are lacking. Students must navigate freeways, highways, or major arterial roads to reach their schools [14]. Also, in areas with substantial traffic volume, children and adolescents were less likely to walk when connectivity was high but more inclined to walk when traffic levels were low [15].

Research on school transportation choices has consistently indicated that a short distance to school is the most influential factor in predicting active school travel. A comprehensive review explored the factors linked to active school travel [16]. The school's proximity to home had the strongest correlation with active travel to school. Although this review was performed some years ago, the results remain up to date. Data from students attending schools in the UK [17], Canada [13], and Spain [18] unequivocally demonstrate that the distance between home and school stands out as the most significant individual-level factor associated with active commuting to school.

Psychological and social factors also have a role in determining young people's active travel behavior. Parents' perceptions and availability linked to an increased likelihood of actively commuting to school encompass perceptions of neighborhood safety, parent-perceived importance of social interaction and fathers' work flexibility [12, 15, 19, 20]. On the other hand, parental perceptions of convenience concerns about traffic safety and fears of stranger danger are associated with discouraging active travel behavior [15, 20]. Additionally, socioeconomic status has been associated with the decision regarding school transportation modes. Most research has linked children from higher-income households to a reduced likelihood of actively commuting to school and a higher likelihood of being driven to school [11].

Lastly, individual non-modifiable factors that may influence active travel behavior include sex and age. Boys tend to commute actively to and from school more frequently than girls across all age groups [15, 19]. However, this difference may diminish somewhat as children grow older. Boys, in particular, are more inclined to use bicycles for their school commute, with reported bicycling rates approximately three times higher for boys than girls [21]. This gender disparity in active school travel aligns with boys' overall higher prevalence of PA [21], and it can be partly attributed to varying levels of independent mobility. Also, cultural factors may lead some parents to be more protective of girls and impose greater restrictions on their ability to travel independently. Research findings regarding the impact of age on school transportation choices exhibit greater variability. Several studies have suggested that younger students, spanning various age groups, are more inclined to engage in active commuting than their older counterparts [11, 22]. However, contrary findings have emerged in other studies, indicating the opposite relationship [23]. As one might anticipate, with new travel options, such as driving, the rates of walking and biking tend to decrease as children reach the age at which they can drive [23]. Nevertheless, it is important to note that the effects of age do not appear to follow a consistent pattern. Older students typically cover greater distances on foot when traveling to school than their younger peers, often resulting in longer average travel distances. This shift can be attributed to the fact that elementary school students typically attend nearby neighborhood schools, while commute distances increase as they transition to more distant middle and secondary schools.

8.3 Movement Behaviors and Active Travel to and from School

Promoting active travel behavior to and from school can promote healthier lifestyles among young people around the globe [24]. Movement behaviors, including PA, sedentary behavior, and sleep, are important to a healthier lifestyle.

8.3.1 Physical Activity and Active Travel Behavior

Physical activity is associated with several health benefits among youth, including cardiovascular, metabolic, bone, and mental health [25]. Numerous strategies can potentially improve children's and adolescents' PA levels. Active travel to and from school is a low-cost and sustainable behavior suggested to be an effective strategy to increase overall PA [26].

A systematic review comprising 68 studies revealed that students who actively commuted to school were more active than their passive-traveling peers [27]. In that study, active travel interventions also led to increased PA. This was corroborated by a recent meta-analysis (analyzing only device-measured PA) showing that active travel to and from school contributed to 48% of the World Health Organization's recommendations for 60 min of daily moderate-to-vigorous PA [28]. These two reviews clearly show that active travel behavior improves PA levels among young people. However, most included studies were conducted in high-income countries from Europe and North America.

To fill this knowledge gap, two studies have examined the association between active travel behavior and PA in middle- and low-income countries [9, 24]. In one of them, including 80 countries ranging from high- to low-income, adolescents actively commuting to school for at least three days a week had double the odds of meeting the PA recommendations [24]. Furthermore, these odds were greater for students from low-income countries than those from high-income countries. The other study, with data from 63 middle- and low-income countries, showed that boys and girls who actively traveled to and from school were 42% and 66% more likely to achieve the PA recommendations [9].

Young people's active travel behavior may impact present and future PA levels. A Finnish cohort study from 1962 to 2020 revealed that although active traveling to school during childhood was not associated with increased active travel behavior in adulthood, it was related to greater leisure-time PA engagement during early and middle adulthood [29]. Also, a link between childhood active travel behavior and increased step counts in adulthood was found. Therefore, active travel to and from school during childhood may contribute to future PA and should be encouraged and promoted from an early age.

The link between active travel behavior and PA is well-documented in the literature for both boys and girls and different countries and regions, making this one of the most promising global strategies to promote PA.

8.3.2 Sedentary Behavior, Sleep, and Active Travel Behavior

Sedentary behavior (e.g., sitting and screen time) and sleep are important health behaviors. However, unlike PA, the link between active travel behavior and the other moment behaviors, i.e., sedentary behavior and sleep, is studied less.

A systematic review conducted in 2013 showed that only five studies examined the association between active travel to and from school and sedentary behavior [30]. In that review, three of the five studies presented no significant correlation. The other two reported a reduction in sedentary time among active commuters. More recent research, published after that systematic review, has provided similar findings. On the one hand, a comprehensive study with 80 high- to low-income countries revealed that adolescents actively commuting to school for at least three weekdays had 17% lower odds of having high sedentary behavior levels [24]. On the other hand, some studies have indicated that active travel behavior was positively associated with PA but not with sedentary time [30, 31]. Furthermore, prospective studies investigating the relationship between change in school travel mode and sedentary behavior have also demonstrated conflicting results, ranging from a significant inverse association with after-school sedentary time [32] to no effect [33]. The link between active travel and sedentary behaviors is inconsistent and may be moderated by external factors. Thus, more research on this topic is warranted.

Research on the association between sleep and active travel behavior is scarce. It has mostly been focused on the effect of sleep on active commuting to and from school and not the other way around. Cross-sectional research from Equator and Spain has demonstrated that young people meeting the sleep duration recommendations or have better sleep quality are more likely to actively commute to school than their peers not meeting the recommendations or with poorer sleep [34, 35]. Inversely, in a study conducted in Brazil, adolescents who actively traveled to and from school had lower sleep duration than those who passively commuted to school [36]. Sleep duration and quality are associated with young people's health, quality of life, and PA levels. However, very little is known of its association with active travel behaviors. To ascertain the possible role of active traveling to and from school in promoting sleep, and vice versa, should be a future research priority.

8.4 Benefits of Active Travel to and from School

Active travel to and from school, including walking, cycling, and others, such as skateboards or scooters, have direct benefits for those who do it, but also for the general economy, health, and sustainability [27, 37–39]. Figure 8.1 presents a conceptual summary of those benefits.

8.4.1 How Can Active Travel Impact Health?

Several investigations have shown that active travel is associated with positive health outcomes. The health benefits of active travel behavior are probably due, in large part, to the extent it improves PA levels. Among adults, active commuting reduces the risk of all-cause mortality, cardiovascular disease incidence, and type 2

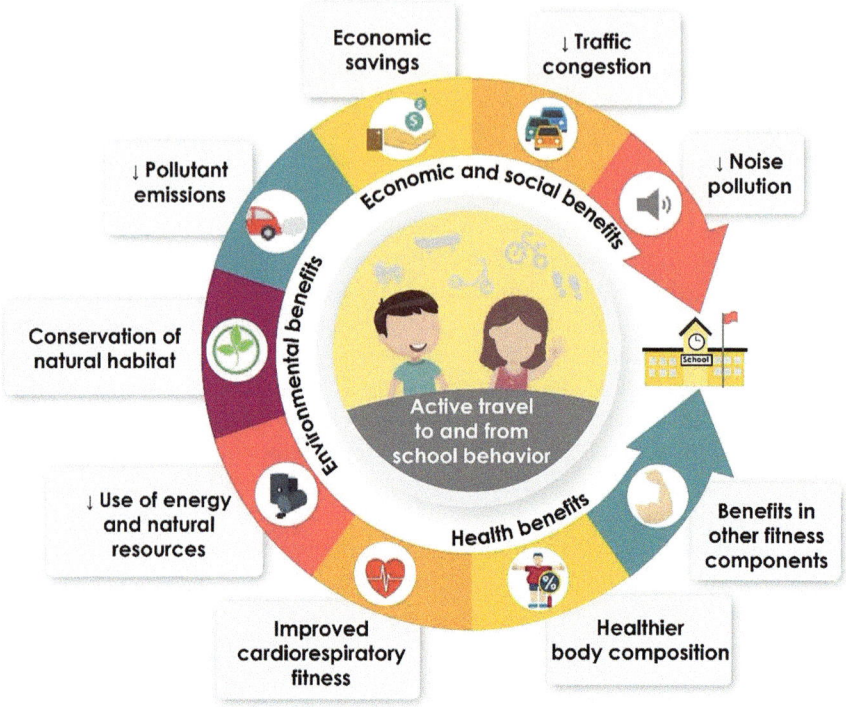

Fig. 8.1 Overview examples of the benefits of active travel behavior to and from school

diabetes [39]. For children and adolescents, active travel to and from school has been associated with healthier body composition and cardiorespiratory fitness [40, 41]. However, the evidence is less consistent.

Childhood overweight and obesity prevalence is considerably high [42], being recognized as a worldwide epidemic with important consequences [43]. Increasing PA levels effectively hinders this problem, as it increases daily energy expenditure. Active travel to and from school as an approach to promote PA can positively impact young people's overweight and obesity. A first systematic review, published in 2011, showed that in only 11 out of 23 studies (48%), active travel behavior was related to healthier body composition (more beneficial weight status or lower body fat) [40]. Notwithstanding, sensitivity analysis showed that when lower-quality studies were excluded, this percentage increased to 56% (5 out of 9 studies). Similarly, a systematic review of longitudinal studies concluded that robust evidence of the effectiveness of active commuting for reducing obesity is lacking [41].

More recent research has continued to investigate the role of active travel in reducing obesity. For example, in an investigation from eight Latin American countries, adolescents who cycled to and from school were less likely to be overweight and obese [44]. Conversely, in the same adolescents, walking was not associated with any obesity indicator. Another example is from a longitudinal study performed in the UK, where switching to physically active forms of travel to school had a beneficial impact on obesity indicators, making this association more apparent for children with lower socioeconomic status [45]. These findings suggest that intensity may play a part and that promoting active travel may be more effective for those who need the most. Nonetheless, more evidence is needed to consistently affirm that active travel behavior benefits weight status in young people.

Cardiorespiratory fitness is an important health marker in youth, PA being the primary means of improving it. Several systematic reviews have connected active travel behavior to and from school to an increase in or better cardiorespiratory fitness [27, 40, 41, 46]. Most of the included studies indicated that cycling, over walking, is associated with increased fitness. Thus, investigations focused on cycling present better results than those focused on walking. Also, active travel behavior change is related to cardiorespiratory fitness improvements. A 6-year longitudinal study demonstrated that change in commuting to school mode, from non-cycling to cycling, predicted better cardiorespiratory fitness at follow-up [47].

Other components of health-related fitness, such as muscle strength, endurance, and power and flexibility, have been studied to a lesser extent and have been inconsistently associated with active travel behavior [40, 46]. Findings suggest a positive to non-significant association between active travel to and from school.

8.4.2 Other Benefits of Active Travel

Beyond the impact on children and adolescents' PA and health, active travel to and from school can have environmental, economic, and social benefits, as it aligns with policies to decrease the use of motorized transport, reduce greenhouse gas emissions, and promote lifelong sustainable development [48].

Active travel behavior is closely linked to independent mobility, and both are associated with greater PA and autonomy. Young people who can travel with friends and play outdoors accumulate more PA [27, 30]. Furthermore, children who actively travel to school and are unaccompanied by an adult have greater self-efficacy, autonomy, and perceptions of safety [49, 50].

Globally, any active commuting behavior, whether to school, work, or anywhere else, promotes health and the environment. Reduced pollutant emissions, decreased usage of energy and natural resources, and conservation of natural habitat are benefits of active travel, which can improve health [51]. For example, the motorized transport sector accounts for nearly a third of end-stage energy use, contributing directly to greenhouse gas emissions. Changing transportation mode to active traveling could reduce this burden.

Additional benefits include decreased traffic congestion, economic savings, and reduced noise pollution [52]. Active travel emerges as a pragmatic and sustainable avenue for increasing PA, yielding benefits beyond human health enhancements. As the Institute of Medicine underscores, active transportation offers an excellent opportunity for individuals to engage in PA while fostering family and community involvement, thereby contributing to sustainability [53].

8.5 Promoting Active Travel Among Young People

The benefits of active commuting are multiple, encompassing health, autonomy, and sustainability. However, in the past few decades, a decline in active travel behavior has been observed among children and adolescents. This scenario reinforces the need to develop and implement strategies to promote active travel behavior to and from school, as this is the most frequent opportunity for young people.

Active travel behavior is influenced by several determinants, including environmental, psychological, social, and individual factors. Strategies for promoting active commuting must take all these into account. Thus, decision-makers and schools must provide proper conditions and implement strategies to promote active travel among young people and encourage and empower them and their parents to travel actively.

8.5.1 How Can We Promote Active Travel to and from School?

Several strategies can be implemented to promote active travel behavior among young people. These strategies can mainly be implemented by decision-makers responsible for the built environment outside and inside schools and housing policies or directed to parents and young people by working on individual and psychological determinants.

Proximity to school is a key determinant of young people's active travel behavior. In broad terms, those who live closer to school tend to actively travel to school rather than using a car or other modes of transport based on inactive behaviors. Therefore, the first approach to promote active travel behavior is to allocate young people to schools close to their homes [54]. However, research shows that this alone is not enough. The built environment surrounding the school must also allow for a safe and efficient trip. Thus, two groups of young people can be distinguished for active travel promotion: those who live closer to the school and those who live more distant [55].

For those who live closer, who are more likely to travel to school actively [54–56], a strategy for decision-makers is to promote increased safety around the school, especially at peak times (morning, lunchtime, and afternoon) so that parents and children feel safe and confident to actively travel to school [57]. Moreover, restricting traffic and limiting the area around the school for young people to walk or cycle is an important strategy for increasing safety, reducing traffic, and ensuring that a part of the travel is active [55, 58].

For those who live further away, cycling can be a quicker and more active way to travel to and from school [59, 60]. Therefore, cycling, apart from being a more sustainable mode of transport and associated with greater PA benefits, is an important aspect of active travel to and from school. Strategies to promote cycling to school include improvements to the built environment, e.g., creating cycle paths and attractive green spaces around it [61], but also social or financial support. Taking into account social inequalities, policies must be implemented for the purchase of bicycles and related equipment (e.g., helmet, lights, lock), or a public bicycle sharing system should be offered for the use of bicycles and minimum related equipment so that young people can cycle to school [62]. Good examples of how this strategy can be used have already been implemented [62, 63].

Sometimes, especially for young people who live further away from school, using an active mode of travel to and from school during the whole trip is not a feasible option. In these cases, providing a public transport service and network that allows young people to travel to school autonomously and that interconnects with routes specifically designed for active travel can improve the number of active travelers, as at least part of the trip can be performed actively [64]. Also, other means of active travel, such as skateboards, scooters, or skates, which particularly attract young people, should not be neglected despite being less common [65]. Building skateparks and attractive environments in the local communities may increase the number of practitioners in leisure activities, which may lead to actively adopting these means to travel to school [65].

Different strategies may be implemented at the school level to promote active travel behavior among young people, some more focused on infrastructures and others more focused on behavior change [62, 66]. Alongside these strategies, the role modeling of teachers and school staff may be important to encourage parents and children to adopt active travel behavior [56].

Schools should support students' active travel behavior and provide them with resources that enable them to be active when traveling to and from school. It is important to establish a safe place for young people to keep their bicycles and other means of transport [57]. Therefore, bicycles should preferably be stored inside the school. Furthermore, providing individual lockers for students is crucial. The lockers allow storing equipment related to the mode of transport and schoolbooks and other school materials, aiming at reducing the weight of backpacks [67, 68]. Carrying heavy backpacks is not only harmful to young people's health, with marked postural consequences, but along with that, it is a known barrier to actively traveling to and from school [57, 69].

Another way schools can support students' active travel behavior is through teaching. Schools especially impact young people's learning and abilities, capacitating them with skills and competencies that support their academic knowledge and daily life activities. In this sense, physical education classes can indeed contribute to promoting active travel by promoting physical literacy and by teaching cycling skills so that children have the motivation, confidence, and skill to know how to ride [62, 70]. For that purpose, physical education curricula should incorporate skating and cycling programs, and schools must have the necessary materials (e.g., skates and bicycles) to develop such classes. Ideally, skating and cycling skills should be developed from the youngest ages, as they represent a critical period for consolidating habits that could remain longer [71, 72].

Digital technologies can also help improve adolescents' active travel behavior within the school setting. In physical education or any other classes, teachers can fix weekly or monthly step targets or even organize competitions that can be easily recorded by students' smartphones [73, 74]. Such strategies encourage children and adolescents to walk to and from school more often. Digital technologies, especially smartphone apps, help young people become more engaged in adopting active behaviors [73, 74].

At the inter- and intra-individual levels, encouraging, educating, capacitating, and empowering parents and young people are key strategies to promote active travel [57, 75]. This includes knowledge about the benefits of active commuting to and from school and its barriers and facilitators [75]. Also, fostering social support from parents and friends can increase the likelihood of engaging in active travel to and from school, as these are known predictors of active commuting [76]. Besides attitudinal perceptions, environmental perceptions are also associated with children and adolescents' active travel behavior. Thus, improving the perception of safety and providing more supportive environments may help promote active commuting to and from school.

Overall, strategies that promote active travel to and from school should be incorporated into wider policies to improve PA, neighborhood walkability, and public transport networks. Notwithstanding, specific PA interventions can effectively increase active travel among young people.

8.5.2 Interventions Promoting Active Travel to and from School

PA-based interventions aimed at increasing young people's active travel are largely based on behavioral change techniques, including behavioral, environmental, informational, or multi-component approaches [62]. Although several interventions are reported in the literature, many are ineffective [26]. Effective interventions to promote active travel tend to have a holistic and multi-component approach, including informing, empowering, and creating opportunities for young people to actively travel to and from school [62]. The Active Living by Design community action is a useful model for community change interventions, which includes the 5P's: preparation, promotion, program, policy, and physical projects [75, 77, 78]. This model covers the five phases that should underpin an intervention to promote active travel to and from school since it is a community-orientated model [78].

Various interventions have already been implemented to promote active travel to and from school, leading to improvements in overall PA and active travel behavior.

Four examples of PA-based interventions with different characteristics are briefly presented:

(1) *Implementing walking buses at schools.* Walking school buses are a group of people who go to school together, usually organized by the parents of the children at each school. Moreover, walking school buses can include both young people walking and cycling. This initiative, which has been running since the 2000s in different places, has improved the number of people actively travelling to school and their PA levels [79].
(2) *The RIDE2SCHOOL project.* An intervention-based project developed in Australia aimed at promoting active travel to school, especially by cycling. It is a project with various initiatives related to active travel and has shown very positive results. A notable example is the bike education program of RIDE2SCHOOL, aimed to increase young people's cycling skills and competencies, which has led to an increase in the active travel of young people in several schools [80].
(3) *The Promoting Active Travel to School in Europe project.* This project is based on improving young people's technical cycling skills and includes parents in awareness-raising and participation. It is an initiative aimed at increasing active travel to school, especially cycling among young people, in five European countries. This initiative involved students in learning sessions and physical education classes and participating in active travel to and from school [81].
(4) *Beat the street project.* A 12-month community-wide project aimed at increasing active travel through a game system that awards points for passing through different locations in the city. This project, unlike previous ones, is not directly related to the school, but it is an initiative with promising results. This way of promoting active travel was first implemented in England. It could be an ally to transport to school, promoting active travel and increasing PA levels. It is an innovative community initiative with high potential that has increased PA levels [82].

Several systematic reviews have analyzed interventions aimed at promoting active travel to and from school [62, 66, 75, 77, 83]. Although many interventions are unsuccessful, some effectively increase PA or active travel behavior. These investigations have shown that interventions specifically focused on active transportation to school may be more effective than those with a broader focus. Furthermore, most interventions are implemented in schools and directed at young people and their parents. At this level, the most effective intervention is the walking/cycling bus [62]. In its classical form, the walking/cycling school bus allows young people, especially the youngest, to travel to school accompanied by an adult actively, thus promoting safety, compliance with the school timetables and sociability with their peers [79, 84]. On the other hand, interventions based on physical education and training children in active travel modes, such as cycling or skating, are less frequent and effective [62, 66, 75].

8.6 Conclusions

Most young people are not active enough to benefit their health [1]. Active travel behavior, particularly when active traveling to and from school, can help mitigate this important public health problem. Active commuting, encompassing activities like walking and cycling, offers an excellent means of incorporating PA into the daily routines of students [9]. By choosing active transportation modes to get to school, children and adolescents can engage regularly in PA that might otherwise be missing from their lives. Unlike planned exercise sessions, active commuting is seamlessly integrated into daily schedules, ensuring that young people engage in PA consistently.

The benefits of increasing PA through active commuting extend beyond health. One of the foremost and most consistent advantages is the enhancement of cardiorespiratory fitness [27, 40, 41, 46]. The regularity of daily walking and especially cycling to school leads to improved cardiovascular fitness and health. Moreover, active travel behavior contributes to greater energy expenditure, essential in managing body weight and composition [40, 41]. By promoting active transportation, we also contribute to reducing the use of motorized transport, alleviating greenhouse gas emissions, and fostering lifelong sustainable development [48].

Rates of active travel behavior in youth seem to be decreasing in most countries, highlighting the need for policies and strategies that increase the number of active commuters. Active travel behavior is influenced by environmental, psychological, social, and individual factors; thus, such strategies can mainly be implemented by decision-makers responsible for the built environment outside and inside schools' and housing policies or directed to parents and young people. Effective interventions to promote active travel to and from school tend to have a comprehensive, multi-component approach involving information dissemination, empowerment, and creating opportunities for young people to engage in active commuting [62].

References

1. Guthold R, Stevens GA, Riley LM, Bull FC. Global trends in insufficient physical activity among adolescents: a pooled analysis of 298 population-based surveys with 1.6 million participants. Lancet Child Adolesc Health. 2020;4(1):23–35. https://doi.org/10.1016/S2352-4642(19)30323-2.
2. Marques A, Henriques-Neto D, Peralta M, Martins J, Demetriou Y, Schonbach DMI, et al. Prevalence of physical activity among adolescents from 105 low, middle, and high-income countries. Int J Environ Res Public Health. 2020;17(9) https://doi.org/10.3390/ijerph17093145.
3. Riazi N, Faulkner G. Children's independent mobility. In: Larouche R, editor. Children's active transportation. Elsevier; 2018. p. 77–91.
4. Helbich M. Children's school commuting in The Netherlands: does it matter how urban form is incorporated in mode choice models? Int J Sustain Transp. 2017;11(7):507–17. https://doi.org/10.1080/15568318.2016.1275892.

5. Reimers AK, Marzi I, Schmidt SCE, Niessner C, Oriwol D, Worth A, et al. Trends in active commuting to school from 2003 to 2017 among children and adolescents from Germany: the MoMo study. Eur J Pub Health. 2020;31(2):373–8. https://doi.org/10.1093/eurpub/ckaa141.
6. Gálvez-Fernández P, Herrador-Colmenero M, Esteban-Cornejo I, Castro-Piñero J, Molina-García J, Queralt A, et al. Active commuting to school among 36,781 Spanish children and adolescents: a temporal trend study. Scand J Med Sci Sports. 2021;31(4):914–24. https://doi.org/10.1111/sms.13917.
7. Loureiro N, Loureiro V, Grao-Cruces A, Martins J, Gaspar de Matos M. Correlates of active commuting to school among Portuguese adolescents: an ecological model approach. Int J Environ Res Public Health. 2022;19(5) https://doi.org/10.3390/ijerph19052733.
8. Felez-Nobrega M, Werneck AO, Bauman A, Haro JM, Koyanagi A. Active school commuting in adolescents from 28 countries across Africa, the Americas, and Asia: a temporal trends study. Int J Behav Nutr Phys Act. 2023;20(1):1. https://doi.org/10.1186/s12966-022-01404-y.
9. Peralta M, Henriques-Neto D, Bordado J, Loureiro N, Diz S, Marques A. Active commuting to school and physical activity levels among 11 to 16 year-old adolescents from 63 low- and middle-income countries. Int J Environ Res Public Health. 2020;17(4) https://doi.org/10.3390/ijerph17041276.
10. Gonzalez SA, Aubert S, Barnes JD, Larouche R, Tremblay MS. Profiles of active transportation among children and adolescents in the global matrix 3.0 initiative: a 49-country comparison. Int J Environ Res Public Health. 2020;17(16) https://doi.org/10.3390/ijerph17165997.
11. Babey SH, Hastert TA, Huang W, Brown ER. Sociodemographic, family, and environmental factors associated with active commuting to school among US adolescents. J Public Health Policy. 2009;30(1):S203–S20. https://doi.org/10.1057/jphp.2008.61.
12. Christiansen LB, Toftager M, Schipperijn J, Ersbøll AK, Giles-Corti B, Troelsen J. School site walkability and active school transport—association, mediation and moderation. J Transp Geogr. 2014;34:7–15. https://doi.org/10.1016/j.jtrangeo.2013.10.012.
13. Mammen G, Stone MR, Buliung R, Faulkner G. School travel planning in Canada: identifying child, family, and school-level characteristics associated with travel mode shift from driving to active school travel. J Transp Health. 2014;1(4):288–94. https://doi.org/10.1016/j.jth.2014.09.004.
14. Timperio A, Ball K, Salmon J, Roberts R, Giles-Corti B, Simmons D, et al. Personal, family, social, and environmental correlates of active commuting to school. Am J Prev Med. 2006;30(1):45–51. https://doi.org/10.1016/j.amepre.2005.08.047.
15. Sener IN, Lee RJ, Sidharthan R. An examination of children's school travel: a focus on active travel and parental effects. Transp Res A Policy Pract. 2019;123:24–34. https://doi.org/10.1016/j.tra.2018.05.023.
16. Stewart O. Findings from research on active transportation to school and implications for safe routes to school programs. J Plan Lit. 2010;26(2):127–50. https://doi.org/10.1177/0885412210385911.
17. Easton S, Ferrari E. Children's travel to school—the interaction of individual, neighbourhood and school factors. Transp Policy. 2015;44:9–18. https://doi.org/10.1016/j.tranpol.2015.05.023.
18. Rodríguez-López C, Salas-Fariña ZM, Villa-González E, Borges-Cosic M, Herrador-Colmenero M, Medina-Casaubón J, et al. The threshold distance associated with waking from home to school. Health Education and Behavior. 2017;44(6):857–66. https://doi.org/10.1177/1090198116688429.
19. Leslie E, Kremer P, Toumbourou JW, Williams JW. Gender differences in personal, social and environmental influences on active travel to and from school for Australian adolescents. J Sci Med Sport. 2010;13(6):597–601. https://doi.org/10.1016/j.jsams.2010.04.004.
20. Ikeda E, Hinckson E, Witten K, Smith M. Assessment of direct and indirect associations between children active school travel and environmental, household and child factors using structural equation modelling. Int J Behav Nutr Phys Act. 2019;16(1):32. https://doi.org/10.1186/s12966-019-0794-5.

21. van Sluijs EMF, Fearne VA, Mattocks C, Riddoch C, Griffin SJ, Ness A. The contribution of active travel to children's physical activity levels: cross-sectional results from the ALSPAC study. Prev Med. 2009;48(6):519–24. https://doi.org/10.1016/j.ypmed.2009.03.002.
22. Wong BYM, Faulkner G, Buliung R, Irving H. Mode shifting in school travel mode: examining the prevalence and correlates of active school transport in Ontario, Canada. BMC Public Health. 2011:11. https://doi.org/10.1186/1471-2458-11-618.
23. Deka D. An explanation of the relationship between adults' work trip mode and children's school trip mode through the Heckman approach. J Transp Geogr. 2013;31:54–63. https://doi.org/10.1016/j.jtrangeo.2013.05.005.
24. Khan A, Mandic S, Uddin R. Association of active school commuting with physical activity and sedentary behaviour among adolescents: a global perspective from 80 countries. J Sci Med Sport. 2021;24(6):567–72. https://doi.org/10.1016/j.jsams.2020.12.002.
25. Chaput JP, Willumsen J, Bull F, Chou R, Ekelund U, Firth J, et al. 2020 WHO guidelines on physical activity and sedentary behaviour for children and adolescents aged 5–17 years: summary of the evidence. Int J Behav Nutr Phys Act. 2020;17(1):141. https://doi.org/10.1186/s12966-020-01037-z.
26. Larouche R, Mammen G, Rowe DA, Faulkner G. Effectiveness of active school transport interventions: a systematic review and update. BMC Public Health. 2018;18(1):206. https://doi.org/10.1186/s12889-017-5005-1.
27. Larouche R, Saunders TJ, John Faulkner GE, Colley R, Tremblay M. Associations between active school transport and physical activity, body composition, and cardiovascular fitness: a systematic review of 68 studies. J Phys Act Health. 2014;11(1):206–27. https://doi.org/10.1123/jpah.2011-0345.
28. Campos-Garzon P, Sevil-Serrano J, Garcia-Hermoso A, Chillon P, Barranco-Ruiz Y. Contribution of active commuting to and from school to device-measured physical activity levels in young people: a systematic review and meta-analysis. Scand J Med Sci Sports. 2023;33(11):2110–24. https://doi.org/10.1111/sms.14450.
29. Kaseva K, Lounassalo I, Yang X, Kukko T, Hakonen H, Kulmala J, et al. Associations of active commuting to school in childhood and physical activity in adulthood. Sci Rep. 2023;13(1):7642. https://doi.org/10.1038/s41598-023-33518-z.
30. Schoeppe S, Duncan MJ, Badland H, Oliver M, Curtis C. Associations of children's independent mobility and active travel with physical activity, sedentary behaviour and weight status: a systematic review. J Sci Med Sport. 2013;16(4):312–9. https://doi.org/10.1016/j.jsams.2012.11.001.
31. Huang C, Memon AR, Yan J, Lin Y, Chen ST. The associations of active travel to school with physical activity and screen time among adolescents: do individual and parental characteristics matter? Front Public Health. 2021;9:719742. https://doi.org/10.3389/fpubh.2021.719742.
32. Atkin AJ, Foley L, Corder K, Ekelund U, van Sluijs EM. Determinants of three-year change in children's objectively measured sedentary time. PLoS One. 2016;11(12):e0167826. https://doi.org/10.1371/journal.pone.0167826.
33. Werneck AO, Jago R, Kriemler S, Andersen LB, Wedderkopp N, Northstone K, et al. Association of change in the school travel mode with changes in different physical activity intensities and sedentary time: a international Children's Accelerometry database study. Prev Med. 2021;153:106862. https://doi.org/10.1016/j.ypmed.2021.106862.
34. Villa-Gonzalez E, Huertas-Delgado FJ, Chillon P, Ramirez-Velez R, Barranco-Ruiz Y. Associations between active commuting to school, sleep duration, and breakfast consumption in Ecuadorian young people. BMC Public Health. 2019;19(1):85. https://doi.org/10.1186/s12889-019-6434-9.
35. Martinez-Gomez D, Veiga OL, Gomez-Martinez S, Zapatera B, Calle ME, Marcos A, et al. Behavioural correlates of active commuting to school in Spanish adolescents: the AFINOS (physical activity as a preventive measure against overweight, obesity, infections, allergies, and cardiovascular disease risk factors in adolescents) study. Public Health Nutr. 2011;14(10):1779–86. https://doi.org/10.1017/S1368980010003253.

36. Pereira EF, Moreno C, Louzada FM. Increased commuting to school time reduces sleep duration in adolescents. Chronobiol Int. 2014;31(1):87–94. https://doi.org/10.3109/07420528.2013.826238.
37. Baker G, Pillinger R, Kelly P, Whyte B. Quantifying the health and economic benefits of active commuting in Scotland. J Transp Health. 2021;22:101111. https://doi.org/10.1016/j.jth.2021.101111.
38. Lin Y, Yang X, Liang F, Huang K, Liu F, Li J, et al. Benefits of active commuting on cardiovascular health modified by ambient fine particulate matter in China: a prospective cohort study. Ecotoxicol Environ Saf. 2021;224:112641. https://doi.org/10.1016/j.ecoenv.2021.112641.
39. Dinu M, Pagliai G, Macchi C, Sofi F. Active commuting and multiple health outcomes: a systematic review and meta-analysis. Sports Med. 2019;49(3):437–52. https://doi.org/10.1007/s40279-018-1023-0.
40. Lubans DR, Boreham CA, Kelly P, Foster CE. The relationship between active travel to school and health-related fitness in children and adolescents: a systematic review. Int J Behav Nutr Phys Act. 2011;8:5. https://doi.org/10.1186/1479-5868-8-5.
41. Saunders LE, Green JM, Petticrew MP, Steinbach R, Roberts H. What are the health benefits of active travel? A systematic review of trials and cohort studies. PLoS One. 2013;8(8):e69912. https://doi.org/10.1371/journal.pone.0069912.
42. Garrido-Miguel M, Cavero-Redondo I, Alvarez-Bueno C, Rodriguez-Artalejo F, Moreno LA, Ruiz JR, et al. Prevalence and trends of overweight and obesity in European children from 1999 to 2016: a systematic review and meta-analysis. JAMA Pediatr. 2019;173(10):e192430. https://doi.org/10.1001/jamapediatrics.2019.2430.
43. Di Cesare M, Soric M, Bovet P, Miranda JJ, Bhutta Z, Stevens GA, et al. The epidemiological burden of obesity in childhood: a worldwide epidemic requiring urgent action. BMC Med. 2019;17(1):212. https://doi.org/10.1186/s12916-019-1449-8.
44. Ferrari G, Drenowatz C, Kovalskys I, Gomez G, Rigotti A, Cortes LY, et al. Walking and cycling, as active transportation, and obesity factors in adolescents from eight countries. BMC Pediatr. 2022;22(1):510. https://doi.org/10.1186/s12887-022-03577-8.
45. Laverty AA, Hone T, Goodman A, Kelly Y, Millett C. Associations of active travel with adiposity among children and socioeconomic differentials: a longitudinal study. BMJ Open. 2021;11(1):e036041. https://doi.org/10.1136/bmjopen-2019-036041.
46. Henriques-Neto D, Peralta M, Garradas S, Pelegrini A, Pinto AA, Sanchez-Miguel PA, et al. Active commuting and physical fitness: a systematic review. Int J Environ Res Public Health. 2020;17(8) https://doi.org/10.3390/ijerph17082721.
47. Cooper AR, Wedderkopp N, Jago R, Kristensen PL, Moller NC, Froberg K, et al. Longitudinal associations of cycling to school with adolescent fitness. Prev Med. 2008;47(3):324–8. https://doi.org/10.1016/j.ypmed.2008.06.009.
48. Bearman N, Singleton AD. Modelling the potential impact on CO emissions of an increased uptake of active travel for the home to school commute using individual level data. J Transp Health. 2014;1(4):295–304. https://doi.org/10.1016/j.jth.2014.09.009.
49. Lu W, McKyer EL, Lee C, Ory MG, Goodson P, Wang S. Children's active commuting to school: an interplay of self-efficacy, social economic disadvantage, and environmental characteristics. Int J Behav Nutr Phys Act. 2015;12:29. https://doi.org/10.1186/s12966-015-0190-8.
50. Herrador-Colmenero M, Villa-Gonzalez E, Chillon P. Children who commute to school unaccompanied have greater autonomy and perceptions of safety. Acta Paediatr. 2017;106(12):2042–7. https://doi.org/10.1111/apa.14047.
51. Jochem C, Leitzmann M. A call for integrating active transportation into physical activity and sedentary behaviour guidelines. Lancet Planet Health. 2023;7(2):e112–e3. https://doi.org/10.1016/S2542-5196(23)00001-3.
52. Garrard J. Active transport: children and young people. An overview of recent evidence. VicHealth. 2009;
53. IoM. Educating the student body: taking physical activity and physical education to school. Washington DC: The National Academies Press; 2013.

54. Nelson NM, Foley E, O'Gorman DJ, Moyna NM, Woods CB. Active commuting to school: how far is too far? Int J Behav Nutr Phys Act. 2008;5(1):1. https://doi.org/10.1186/1479-5868-5-1.
55. Ikeda E, Stewart T, Garrett N, Egli V, Mandic S, Hosking J, et al. Built environment associates of active school travel in New Zealand children and youth: a systematic meta-analysis using individual participant data. J Transp Health. 2018;9:117–31. https://doi.org/10.1016/j.jth.2018.04.007.
56. Buttazzoni A, Nelson Ferguson K, Gilliland J. Barriers to and facilitators of active travel from the youth perspective: a qualitative meta-synthesis. SSM Popul Health. 2023;22:101369. https://doi.org/10.1016/j.ssmph.2023.101369.
57. Aranda-Balboa MJ, Chillón P, Saucedo-Araujo RG, Molina-García J, Huertas-Delgado FJ. Children and parental barriers to active commuting to school: a comparison study. Int J Environ Res Public Health. 2021;18(5) https://doi.org/10.3390/ijerph18052504.
58. Iiritano G, Petrungaro G, Trecozzi MR. Limited traffic zone for walk safety around the schools. Transportation Research Procedia. 2022;60:204–11. https://doi.org/10.1016/j.trpro.2021.12.027.
59. Goodman A, Rojas IF, Woodcock J, Aldred R, Berkoff N, Morgan M, et al. Scenarios of cycling to school in England, and associated health and carbon impacts: application of the 'propensity to cycle tool'. J Transp Health. 2019;12:263–78. https://doi.org/10.1016/j.jth.2019.01.008.
60. Loh V, Sahlqvist S, Veitch J, Thornton L, Salmon J, Cerin E, et al. From motorised to active travel: using GPS data to explore potential physical activity gains among adolescents. BMC Public Health. 2022;22(1):1512. https://doi.org/10.1186/s12889-022-13947-7.
61. Ferrari G, Oliveira Werneck A, Rodrigues da Silva D, Kovalskys I, Gómez G, Rigotti A, et al. Association between perceived neighborhood built environment and walking and cycling for transport among inhabitants from Latin America: the ELANS study. Int J Environ Res Public Health. 2020;17(18):6858.
62. Schönbach DMI, Altenburg TM, Marques A, Chinapaw MJM, Demetriou Y. Strategies and effects of school-based interventions to promote active school transportation by bicycle among children and adolescents: a systematic review. Int J Behav Nutr Phys Act. 2020;17(1):138. https://doi.org/10.1186/s12966-020-01035-1.
63. Estevan I, Queralt A, Molina-García J. Biking to school: the role of bicycle-sharing programs in adolescents. J Sch Health. 2018;88(12):871–6. https://doi.org/10.1111/josh.12697.
64. Durand CP, Pettee Gabriel KK, Hoelscher DM, Kohl HW 3rd. Transit use by children and adolescents: an overlooked source of and opportunity for physical activity? J Phys Act Health. 2016;13(8):861–6. https://doi.org/10.1123/jpah.2015-0444.
65. Cook S, Stevenson L, Aldred R, Kendall M, Cohen T. More than walking and cycling: what is 'active travel'? Transp Policy. 2022;126:151–61. https://doi.org/10.1016/j.tranpol.2022.07.015.
66. Jones RA, Blackburn NE, Woods C, Byrne M, van Nassau F, Tully MA. Interventions promoting active transport to school in children: a systematic review and meta-analysis. Prev Med. 2019;123:232–41. https://doi.org/10.1016/j.ypmed.2019.03.030.
67. Winters M, Buehler R, Götschi T. Policies to promote active travel: evidence from reviews of the literature. Curr Environ Health Reports. 2017;4(3):278–85. https://doi.org/10.1007/s40572-017-0148-x.
68. NeJhaddadgar N, Tavafian SS, Ziapour A, Mehedi N, Jamshidi AR, Gahvareh R. Effects of school-based educational program on backpack carrying behavior in teenage students. J Prim Care Community Health. 2022;13:21501319221086251. https://doi.org/10.1177/21501319221086251.
69. Janakiraman B, Ravichandran H, Demeke S, Fasika S. Reported influences of backpack loads on postural deviation among school children: a systematic review. J Educ Health Promot. 2017;6:41. https://doi.org/10.4103/jehp.jehp_26_15.
70. van Hoef T, Kerr S, Roth R, Brenni C, Endes K. Effects of a cycling intervention on adolescents cycling skills. J Transp Health. 2022;25:101345. https://doi.org/10.1016/j.jth.2022.101345.

71. Mercê C, Branco M, Catela D, Lopes F, Rodrigues LP, Cordovil R. Learning to cycle: are physical activity and birth order related to the age of learning how to ride a bicycle? Children (Basel). 2021;8(6) https://doi.org/10.3390/children8060487.
72. Strömmer S, Barrett M, Woods-Townsend K, Baird J, Farrell D, Lord J, et al. Engaging adolescents in changing behaviour (EACH-B): a study protocol for a cluster randomised controlled trial to improve dietary quality and physical activity. Trials. 2020;21(1):859. https://doi.org/10.1186/s13063-020-04761-w.
73. Yu H, Kulinna PH, Lorenz KA. An integration of Mobile applications into physical education programs. Strategies. 2018;31(3):13–9. https://doi.org/10.1080/08924562.2018.1442275.
74. Gil-Espinosa FJ, Nielsen-Rodríguez A, Romance R, Burgueño R. Smartphone applications for physical activity promotion from physical education. Educ Inf Technol (Dordr). 2022;27(8):11759–79. https://doi.org/10.1007/s10639-022-11108-2.
75. Pang B, Kubacki K, Rundle-Thiele S. Promoting active travel to school: a systematic review (2010–2016). BMC Public Health. 2017;17(1):638. https://doi.org/10.1186/s12889-017-4648-2.
76. Panter JR, Jones AP, van Sluijs EM, Griffin SJ. Attitudes, social support and environmental perceptions as predictors of active commuting behaviour in school children. J Epidemiol Community Health. 2010;64(1):41–8. https://doi.org/10.1136/jech.2009.086918.
77. Chillón P, Evenson KR, Vaughn A, Ward DS. A systematic review of interventions for promoting active transportation to school. Int J Behav Nutr Phys Act. 2011;8:10. https://doi.org/10.1186/1479-5868-8-10.
78. Bors P, Dessauer M, Bell R, Wilkerson R, Lee J, Strunk SL. The active living by design National Program: community initiatives and lessons learned. Am J Prev Med. 2009;37(6, Supplement 2):S313–S21. https://doi.org/10.1016/j.amepre.2009.09.027.
79. Smith L, Norgate SH, Cherrett T, Davies N, Winstanley C, Harding M. Walking school buses as a form of active transportation for children—a review of the evidence. J Sch Health. 2015;85(3):197–210. https://doi.org/10.1111/josh.12239.
80. Crawford S, Garrard J. A combined impact-process evaluation of a program promoting active transport to school: understanding the factors that shaped program effectiveness. J Environ Public Health. 2013;2013:816961. https://doi.org/10.1155/2013/816961.
81. Schönbach DMI, Chillón P, Marques A, Peralta M, Demetriou Y. Study protocol of a school-based randomized controlled trial to promote cycling to school among students in Germany using intervention mapping: the ACTS project. Front Public Health. 2021;9. https://doi.org/10.3389/fpubh.2021.661119.
82. Harris MA. Beat the street: a pilot evaluation of a community-wide gamification-based physical activity intervention. Games Health J. 2018;7(3):208–12. https://doi.org/10.1089/g4h.2017.0179.
83. Villa-Gonzalez E, Barranco-Ruiz Y, Evenson KR, Chillon P. Systematic review of interventions for promoting active school transport. Prev Med. 2018;111:115–34. https://doi.org/10.1016/j.ypmed.2018.02.010.
84. Koester M, Bejarano CM, Davis AM, Brownson RC, Kerner J, Sallis JF, et al. Implementation contextual factors related to community-based active travel to school interventions: a mixed methods interview study. Implement Sci Commun. 2021;2(1):94. https://doi.org/10.1186/s43058-021-00198-7.

Chapter 9
Physical Activity Opportunities During School Recess

Antonio García-Hermoso ⓘ

9.1 Introduction

Recess plays a significant role in a child's school day, providing a necessary break from the structured academic environment [1]. The US Centers for Disease Control and Prevention (CDC) define recess as "regularly scheduled periods within the elementary-school day for unstructured physical activity (PA) and play." Despite some controversy, various terms, such as "school recess," "break time," and "playtime," have also been utilized to characterize specific time intervals during the day or the combined duration of all recess periods in a day (e.g., morning, lunchtime, and afternoon).

During recess periods, students have the unique opportunity to engage in physical fitness activities, nurture social interactions, and enhance their overall well-being [2]. It is a time when they can stretch their legs, play, and simply be kids, offering a break from the demands of cognitive tasks [3]. These moments not only address the basic need for movement but also foster essential skills that extend beyond the playground, encompassing social development, emotional well-being, and physical health [4]. Additionally, recess plays a crucial role in helping young children develop social skills that they may not otherwise acquire in more formal and structured classroom environments [5].

To fully maximize the benefits of recess, it is imperative to take into account several key factors that shape this essential experience. Teachers and staff play pivotal roles not only in supervising but also in actively participating in recess periods [6]. They act as facilitators, encouraging and guiding students in their activities. Their involvement goes beyond mere observation; it includes promoting fair play,

---

A. García-Hermoso (✉)
Navarrabiomed, Hospital Universitario de Navarra, Universidad Pública de Navarra (UPNA), IdiSNA, Pamplona, Navarra, Spain
e-mail: antonio.garciah@unavarra.es

resolving conflicts, and ensuring that all students have the opportunity to participate and enjoy this valuable break from the academic routine [2]. Moreover, perceived and constructed school environments, encompassing aspects such as the playground layout, availability of equipment, and overall atmosphere, exert a profound influence on the type and level of PA that occurs during these breaks [7–12]. A well-designed, stimulating, and safe playground with a variety of equipment can encourage diverse physical activities, from team sports to imaginative play. The overall atmosphere, whether welcoming and inclusive or more restrictive, can significantly impact how students engage during recess [13].

By carefully examining and thoughtfully addressing these factors, schools can greatly enhance recess experience. This, in turn, contributes to the development of healthier, happier, and more engaged students. Moreover, it fosters a positive and supportive school environment that prioritizes the holistic well-being of students, recognizing that recess is not just a break from learning but an integral part of their overall education [14].

9.2 Benefits of Recess for the Whole Child

Like physical education (PE) and physical and mental health [15–17], recess offers distinct advantages [14]. Although additional studies are needed for confirmation, recess seems to have positive effects on various aspects of children's well-being [18]. Below, each of these possible benefits is outlined, along with several relevant studies.

9.2.1 Physical Activity Benefits

Unstructured play, which takes the form of recess in school settings, is characterized by self-directed activities driven by the enjoyment it brings rather than by a specific goal [19]. Research indicates that children are active approximately 40% of the time during unstructured play, whereas in structured activities such as soccer, their activity levels drop to less than 25% [20]. Several studies have assessed the influence of recess on PA levels among youth and overall PA accumulation. In 2005, Ridgers and Stratton [21] recommended that children participate in moderate to vigorous PA (MVPA) for a minimum of 40% of the recess duration. This recommendation is supported by a systematic review, which suggested that recess can contribute to achieving 40% of MVPA daily [22]. When provided with a 20-min recess period during the school day, they typically participate in approximately 10–15 min of MVPA, surpassing the activity levels reported in other school-based PA interventions [22]. Supporting this, one study indicated that a minimum of 30 min of daily recess is linked to twice the likelihood of meeting recommended PA levels, a finding reported by parents/guardians and confirmed by accelerometer data [23]. This was also observed by another study that used data from 6- to 11-year-old participants ($n = 499$) in the 2012 National Youth Fitness Survey and suggested that providing 30 min of recess 4–5 days a week is associated with a twofold increase in the likelihood of children meeting recommended PA levels [24].

In contrast, a nationally representative sample of 10- to 11-year-olds from Scotland showed that the majority of children dedicated minimal time—averaging only 20% of the recess duration—to participating in MVPA during the morning recess [25], as measured by accelerometers. However, it is important to remember that various factors, such as sex [26], climate [27], duration of recess [28], and/or space per child [29, 30], can influence the amount of MVPA performed during recesses in children, potentially explaining the differences observed in various studies.

9.2.2 Cognition and Academic Achievement Benefits

According to the "cognitive immaturity" hypothesis, breaking must be incorporated to optimize student learning [3]. Research indicates that recess positively influences both academic achievement and cognitive competence in students [3]. Moreover, brain-based learning theory advocates not only taking breaks but also engaging in PA to enhance cognitive benefits. Additionally, evidence suggests that PA before academic instruction is linked to improved academic progress in elementary students [31]. In a study by Dagli [32], the impact of recess of different durations on students' reading achievement was investigated. The results indicated that recess neither enhances nor hinders academic performance. Nevertheless, students who experienced an additional 16 to 30 min of recess demonstrated improved performance on reading tests. This study also suggested that the impact of recess on academic achievement depends on the interplay of recess frequency, duration, and classroom learning times [32]. By analyzing various schedules for 391 students, researchers found no single optimal combination for recess. Instead, they emphasized considering recess within the broader school schedule context. Students who experienced 1 day of recess per week tended to have higher reading scores. On the other hand, students with ≤15 min of daily recess had the lowest mean reading scores. Moreover, educational institutions that have increased the daily recess duration by twofold (offering multiple recess opportunities) have demonstrated an enhancement in math performance [33]. Esteban-Cornejo et al. [34] assessed PA during recess using accelerometers and examined academic outcomes in mathematics and language based on school-provided records for a sample of 1780 individuals aged 6–18 years. The study revealed that recess PA had no discernible impact on academic indicators in either a positive or negative direction for participants spanning elementary through high school levels.

Attention to classroom tasks has also been studied as a means of measuring children's motivation for and engagement with schoolwork; recess is one way to help maintain the attention needed for various learning experiences [3]. Break time plays a vital role in maintaining focus because students, especially boys and those with attention deficit hyperactivity disorder, exhibit increased attentiveness, productivity, and efficiency after recess in contrast to before recess [35]. This effect is particularly pronounced when individuals engage in a sustained period of outdoor free play. Additionally, as the duration of uninterrupted work periods increases, students, particularly younger children, show a decline in attentiveness, productivity, and efficiency [35]. Brez and Sheets [36] studied 99 elementary students and found that sustained attention significantly increased after recess, but creativity measures did not significantly change. Moreover, when breaks for recess are strategically scheduled to align with academic lessons, children exhibit increased focus and engagement during those lessons [37].

9.2.3 Behavioral and Socioemotional Benefits

As recess commonly represents one of the limited opportunities on school days for play and social interaction [4], recess can play a role in fostering positive social and emotional development and promoting social-emotional learning. Various approaches have been employed to explore this subject. For instance, research indicates that when recess is characterized by unstructured activities and encourages free play, it can contribute to social development and problem-solving skills and improve a child's overall school experience [38]. In other words, recess offered chances for social well-being and a sense of school belonging. Following this, the consistent provision of at least one recess lasting 15 min or more during the school day has been shown to enhance students' preparedness for learning, as indicated by Stapp and Karr [39], and to elicit positive evaluations of student behavior by teachers [40]. Finally, it has been recently observed that positive recess experiences among students can result in increased involvement in healthier lifestyle behaviors and the development of more favorable social-emotional profiles [41].

9.2.4 Physical Benefits

Although most related studies have focused on recessing time and its contribution to daily PA, as well as cognitive and socioemotional aspects, various cross-sectional works have also examined physical aspects such as anthropometric and cardiometabolic parameters and physical fitness, revealing contradictory and inconclusive results. For example, Fernandes and Sturm [42] examined data from the Early Childhood Longitudinal Study—the Kindergarten Cohort for 8246 students from 1998–2004—focusing on recess and body mass index (BMI). The findings revealed that a duration of daily recess within 20 min had a significant negative association with BMI, resulting in a 0.74-unit decrease. Moreover, each additional hour of recess per week correlated with a 0.30-unit decrease in BMI percentiles, indicating a negative relationship between recess and BMI. Ansari et al. [43] substantiated this hypothesis by finding that a daily 60-min outdoor playtime was the threshold at which BMIs consistently started to decrease in preschool children. Additionally, a systematic review conducted by Gray et al. [44] revealed that for each additional hour of recess provided weekly, the BMI percentile decreases by an additional 0.30, indicating that more than 30 min of additional recess time is necessary to observe more substantial differences. These findings confirm that PA during elementary school recesses has the potential to significantly contribute to daily energy expenditure [45].

In contrast, two additional studies do not corroborate these results. More precisely, a previously mentioned study that utilized information from the 2012 National Youth Fitness Survey proposed that providing 30 min of recess 4–5 days a week is connected to increased PA levels but is not correlated with weight status, adiposity, or fitness [24]. Similar findings were also observed in an analysis using data from the National Health and Nutrition Examination Survey (NHANES; 2013–2016) [23], which extended to cardiometabolic outcomes.

9.3 Considerations for Recess

Recess design and layout play pivotal roles in promoting PA among children during recess [9, 46]. A well-planned layout, including play areas, green spaces, and climbing structures, can inspire movement and exploration [29]. Along with diverse activities such as team games and running areas, open and secure spaces contribute to increased PA [30, 47]. Supervision and staff participation are crucial for ensuring safe engagement in games and activities [1, 2]. School staff can organize games, mediate disputes, and set an example for active play [1, 2, 48]. Additionally, the availability of resources and equipment, such as sports gear and play structures [49, 50], influences the quantity and variety of PAs children can enjoy during recess [29, 46, 50]. Among adolescents, promoting the availability of equipment and relaxing limitations in bringing sports gear to school might boost PA during school recess [51].

Another factor to consider in the development and implementation of recess interventions is whether the PA levels of children and adolescents vary across seasons. While some studies report no significant differences between seasons [21, 27], others suggest that children may be more active in spring [52] or in cooler conditions [53]. Meteorological conditions, including temperature and rainfall, can impact the PA of children. Research suggests that children tend to be more active at colder temperatures [27, 28], while rain may act as a barrier [13], leading to lower activity levels. Additionally, high ambient temperatures can also affect activity levels [54]. However, ensuring that students have suitable clothing and making indoor recess an occasional alternative, rather than the standard, can help sustain PA levels during adverse weather conditions [55]. Finally, taking into account clothing, it seems that school uniforms could also influence the levels of PA among students [56].

9.4 Interventions to Enhance Physical Activity During Recess

Several systematic reviews and meta-analyses have investigated the effectiveness of intervention strategies, but the majority of them are narrative and demonstrate mixed outcomes [7–12]. Generally, interventions during recess can be classified as unstructured [57], structured, or a combination of both, known as multicomponent programs. The following sections discuss some common intervention strategies, acknowledging that the list is not exhaustive. Figure 9.1 summarizes these interventions and their classifications.

9.4.1 Unstructured Recess

In unstructured recess, children have the freedom to choose the games they want to participate in without being obligated to perform specific activities. This autonomy allows them to freely select games and activities, including both active and inactive options. Various unstructured strategies, such as playground modifications, colorful markings (e.g., hopscotch, targets, mazes), and/or physical structures (e.g., soccer goals, fencing), and the addition of game equipment, such as ropes, balls, and hoops,

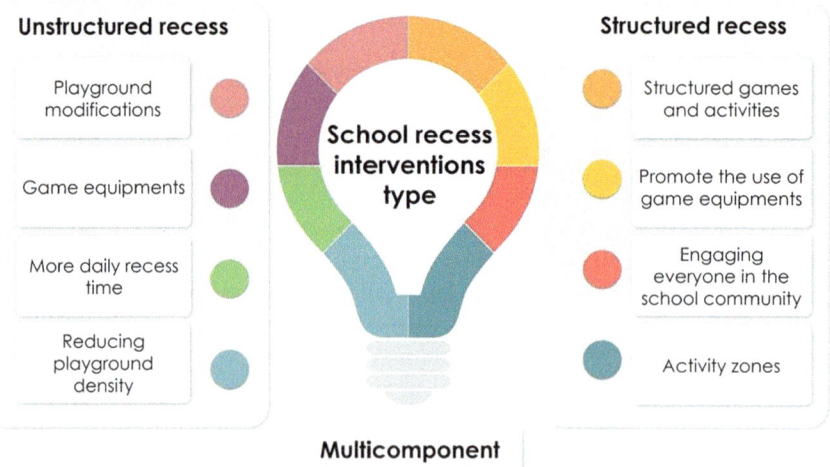

Fig. 9.1 Interventions type to enhance physical activity during recess

are part of these unstructured approaches. In other studies, interventions have been implemented that involve an increase in the daily time dedicated to recess or reducing playground density.

9.4.1.1 Playground Markings and/or Physical Structures

Multicolored playground markings are a cost-effective method for increasing children's daily PA levels, as observed in various studies of both preschoolers [58] and schoolchildren [59–62]. However, the results are inconclusive, with some preschool studies indicating an insufficient impact on MVPA and vigorous PA. A potential "novelty effect" in response to these markings might contribute to short-term improvements in activity levels [60]. Additionally, repainting playgrounds could reignite enthusiasm for PA engagement, potentially influenced by the intervention duration [58–61]. Two of these studies revealed that interventions are effective for both sexes [58, 59].

Interventions involving playground markings and physical structures have also been explored. Ridgers et al. investigated the impact of combining playground markings with physical structures on recess PA across the short term (6 weeks) [63], medium term (24 weeks) [12], and long term (52 weeks) [64]. Initially, the intervention effectively increased MVPA and vigorous PA, with these improvements persisting into the medium term. However, in the long term, the intervention seemed to lose its effectiveness, as there was no noticeable increase in PA compared to that in the control group.

Finally, several studies have investigated the impact of significant school playground renovations on children's activity levels. These renovations involved diverse changes, such as introducing age-appropriate play equipment, shaded areas [65–67], outdoor gyms [68], and green spaces and natural elements (e.g., hills, trees, boulders, and logs) [69, 70]. However, existing research presents mixed findings, with some studies indicating no significant differences in recess activity levels post renovation [66, 68], while others suggest increased activity in redesigned school playgrounds compared to control schools [65, 67, 69, 70]. For example, Raney et al. [69] and van Dijk-Wesselius et al. [70] enhanced playgrounds by incorporating additional green spaces and natural elements. These interventions resulted in a 5–19% increase in MVPA among 1st–5th grade students during postintervention assessments, as well as at the 4-month and 1-year follow-ups, in comparison to control students utilizing traditional playground equipment.

9.4.1.2 Game Equipment

Several studies have been conducted in preschoolers and children who have analyzed the inclusion of play equipment in recess, yielding equally contradictory results. In a short-term study of preschoolers, the inclusion of game equipment in the playground intervention did not result in changes in recess PA [58]. These findings suggest that additional equipment, guidance, and teacher support may be necessary for promoting PA in preschoolers. For schoolchildren, the effectiveness of play equipment during recess has varied [71, 72], with some even using recycled materials (e.g., car tires, milk crates, buckets) [73–75]. Verstraete et al. reported a decrease in vigor and MVPA in the morning after the equipment was introduced but an increase during lunchtime [72]. The rotation of loose equipment in intervention schools did not necessarily counter novelty effects. In contrast, Lopes et al. reported that game equipment increased vigorous PA during recess but led to decreases in moderate-intensity activity [71]. The results suggest that recycled materials can increase activity levels in the short term [73–75], but further research is needed to establish the longer-term effects of these materials. Overall, the availability of gaming equipment alone did not consistently predict PA levels, and its impact differed by sex [72] and weight status [76]. Most of these studies also show reductions in children's sedentary time [73, 74, 77].

Finally, although evidence among adolescents is limited, existing research suggests that loose equipment can increase PA [78]; however, preferences for activity types may vary by sex [79].

9.4.1.3 Increase in Recess Time

Another strategy employed to boost PA in the school environment involves increasing the time allocated to recess. Several studies have explored the impact of increasing recess time on PA levels in school settings. For instance, Brusseau and Kulinna [80] investigated how the duration of MVPA varied when children were given either a single 20-min outdoor recess or multiple 15-min recess sessions throughout the day. On average, students showed an increase of approximately 4 min in MVPA when provided with multiple outdoor recess opportunities without a structured format, and in some instances, their activity time even doubled. In a similar vein, Razak et al. [81] explored the differences in MVPA among children aged 3–6 who experienced either a single 60-min recess or three 15-min unstructured outdoor play breaks during childcare. The findings revealed that children with multiple breaks engaged in an average of 6 additional minutes of MVPA during play and an extra 20 min of MVPA throughout the day. Consequently, shorter, more frequent play breaks are linked to more substantial increases in MVPA when compared to a single continuous session [81].

9.4.1.4 Reducing Playground Density During Recess

A reduction in playground density during recess has been associated with increased PA and decreased sedentary time in children. This is attributed to the fact that lower playground density affords more space and opportunities for children to participate in physical activities such as running and playing. Consequently, a decrease in sedentary time is observed. Two distinct pilot studies conducted in Belgium have examined the feasibility and efficacy of decreasing playground density to promote PA and mitigate sedentary behavior in preschoolers [82] and children [83]. In one study involving 9- to 12-year-old children, the intervention led to expanded play space, diminished sedentary time, and increased MVPA during recess [83]. The second study, conducted with preschoolers [82], exhibited parallel enhancements, affirming the viability of the intervention and its potential benefits, particularly in environments with heightened playground density. Both studies garnered positive feedback from school administrators, who expressed openness to considering this strategy in future interventions.

9.4.2 Structured Recess

Structured recess interventions seek to address the rising issue of childhood obesity by promoting enhanced PA [2]. Grounded in the belief that children benefit from guidance and support during recess, these interventions involve organized and supervised games and activities led by skilled adults such as teachers and staff [1]. Involving all stakeholders within the school community, including staff, students, parents, and other committed community members, is crucial for the success and longevity of recess.

Some strategies for engaging the school community include the following [84]:

- Establishing roles and responsibilities for supervising and facilitating recess [85].
- Mobilizing parents and other community members to provide ongoing support for recess in the school.
- Parents and community members were trained to assist recess supervisors or PA facilitators, and their time was encouraged to increase in support of recess activities.
- Engaging students in the planning and leadership of recess empowers them to play an active role in promoting PA during this period.

Some interventions prescribe specific activities for all children, while others provide a diverse array of organized choices for children to select from. Notably, a comprehensive review of interventions in preschools and primary schools underscores the effectiveness of involving teachers as advocates for PA in a semi structured recess setting. This approach offers children the valuable choice to participate in teacher-led activities, further enhancing the overall impact of the interventions [8]. Instances of these interventions encompass obstacle courses [86, 87] such as parkour [88], dance videos [89, 90], a designated weekly "recess activity" demonstration of active games [91–93], and orchestrated games within designated activity zones [76]. Other semi structured options, for instance, provide play materials and encourage children to use them during playtime [94].

Overall, structured recess interventions have proven effective at increasing the time devoted to MVPA [76, 87, 88, 93, 94] and generating greater energy expenditure during this period [92]. However, the results are heterogeneous, with some studies showing particularly pronounced benefits for boys [87], who typically exhibit higher activity levels during recess [50, 95]. Notably, Scruggs et al. [87] observed that girls liked structured recess less than boys did, and they liked "usual" recess periods less often. Furthermore, the structured recess intervention not only positively impacted PA but also received high praise from teachers in the participating classrooms, who highly rated it in terms of children's enjoyment [92]. These teachers observed positive social and teamwork skills among the children during game play, and this positive influence extended beyond recess [92]. Finally, among adolescents, organized activities during recess do not seem to be sufficient to increase PA levels [96].

9.4.3 Multicomponent Strategies

Multicomponent interventions in the context of school recess refer to strategies that combine various approaches across different levels of influence to enhance children's PA levels. These interventions typically address multiple factors that can impact PA during recess [50]. Examples include combining environmental changes such as modifying playgrounds with social support measures such as teacher encouragement or activity coaches [97–100]. Other combinations involve environmental changes coupled with policy adjustments, such as increasing access to playground areas, reducing rules, and providing staff training [101–104].

Several studies reported significantly increased PA in multicomponent intervention schools compared to controls [97–100, 102, 104]. The "Ready for Recess" study by Huberty et al. highlights this as an exemplary multicomponent intervention during school recess [102]. Over the course of an academic year, they implemented measures such as staff training, activity zone maps, playground equipment, and activity cards for third- to fifth-grade students in two primary schools. This intervention led to an increase in MVPA [102] and demonstrated cost-effectiveness in the first year of implementation in the two schools [105]. The PLAYgrounds program also proved effective at boosting PA levels in children during recess throughout 1 school year, with a more pronounced impact among girls and during the summer/autumn period [100]. Dose–response analyses further indicated more significant changes in schools that implemented more components, targeting higher activity intensities [97]. Nevertheless, it is essential to acknowledge that not all studies demonstrate noteworthy increases in PA through these multicomponent interventions [101, 103]. Among preschoolers, the study conducted by Tucker et al. [104] involved a combination of staff training, the provision of portable play equipment, and four instances of outdoor free play (four 30-min sessions). The results indicated that this intervention led to a 1.28-min increase in children's MVPA per hour compared to that of control services.

Although the evidence is limited, among adolescents, the introduction of organized activities, equipment provisions, sporting facilities, and student recess activators in recess interventions also yielded positive outcomes in terms of PA levels, particularly among boys [99].

9.5 Recess Interventions for Reducing Obesity

Limited research has investigated the impact of recess interventions on obesity rates. Normally, the focus has been on providing 30 min or less of recess daily over a 9- to 12-week period in a school year, using BMI as the measure of obesity [9, 92, 106]. Some interventions compare structured and unstructured play, while others emphasize the addition of loose parts and fewer rules during recess [92, 103, 106]. No significant differences were observed in these studies, which included 30 min or less of recess, regardless of the anthropometric parameters used (i.e., BMI, waist circumference, or skinfolds). In contrast, studies reporting significant outcomes typically involve at least 60 min of unstructured, outdoor play and extend beyond a 6-month duration [43, 107]. Therefore, the inconclusive findings in previous studies are attributed to factors such as the duration of implementation (less than 6 months), limited time allocated for play (less than 60 min), and infrequent opportunities for play (two or fewer times per day) based on the literature.

9.6 Policies to Promote the Quality and Quantity of Recess Time

With the aim of ensuring the quality and quantity of recess time, the CDC launched a series of recommendations in 2017 as part of its Healthy Schools Initiative [84]: (a) ensure that all students from Kindergarten to 12th grade receive a minimum of 20 min of daily recess; (b) schedule recess before lunch; (c) prohibit the exclusion of students from recess for disciplinary reasons or academic performance in the classroom; (d) prohibit the replacement of PE with recess or the use of recess to meet time requirements for PE policies; (e) provide schools and students with adequate spaces, facilities, equipment, and supplies for recess; (f) ensure that spaces and facilities for recess meet or exceed recommended safety standards; (g) prohibit the use of PA during recess as punishment; and (h) provide staff members who lead or supervise recess with ongoing professional development. These policies and guidelines are designed to guarantee that children have consistent access to daily recess and that such recess are not unjustly withheld, ultimately promoting the physical, social, and emotional well-being of students.

In this regard, a recent study indicated that while surveillance reveals commendable practices in ensuring playground safety and providing recess for younger children, there is insufficient information available for older youth. Additionally, a discrepancy exists between the current surveillance data and the recommendations outlined by the CDC [108].

Challenges in implementing school recess policies include inconsistent application, budget limitations, varying school needs, prioritization of academic goals over PA, and insufficient advocacy. The mere existence of policies does not ensure enforcement, and the one-size-fits-all approach may not address diverse school requirements. Budget constraints and the perception of academic priorities may hinder effective implementation of these tools [109]. Additionally, the lack of strong advocacy from key stakeholders may undervalue the importance of recess policies [109]. Consequently, tackling these challenges necessitates a comprehensive approach that takes into account the distinct needs and resources of each school.

9.7 Conclusions and Future Considerations

This chapter underscores the crucial importance of recess during a child's school day, emphasizing its role as a necessary break from the structured academic environment. Defined by the US CDC as scheduled periods for unstructured PA and play, recess contributes to the physical, social, and emotional development of students. Teachers can play key roles in facilitating recess, encouraging fair play, resolving conflicts, and encouraging inclusive participation. The benefits range from PA and improve academic performance to positive socioemotional development, underscoring the need for thoughtful considerations in designing and implementing interventions to optimize the recess experience and contribute to the overall well-being of students.

Due to all the benefits associated with school recess, it is necessary to preserve this period and ensure that future generations have the opportunity to be in school environments that promote PA. Nonetheless, there are several areas lacking in the existing body of literature, such as interventions during recess specifically aimed at adolescents and the influence of recess policies on PA. Moreover, the majority of studies were cross-sectional designs conducted in the United States, indicating a need for further exploration of recess in diverse global contexts. Considering that recess and its associated activities are likely influenced by culture, investigating the impact of cultural factors, including cross-cultural comparisons, holds promise for enhancing recess experiences for children [110].

Lastly, recess poses challenges such as aggressive behaviors, bullying, and social exclusion among children, which are often intensified by minimal supervision and lack of structure [111, 112]. This period can be a source of fear for many children, influencing their social interactions and overall well-being [113]. Addressing these challenges is crucial for creating a safe and positive recess environment for all students.

References

1. Ramstetter CL, Murray R, Garner AS. The crucial role of recess in schools. J Sch Health. 2010;80(11):517–26.
2. Murray R, Ramstetter C. The crucial role of recess in school. Pediatrics. 2012;131(1):183–8.
3. Pellegrini AD, Bohn CM. The role of recess in children's cognitive performance and school adjustment. Educ Res. 2005;34(1):13–9.
4. McNamara L, Colley P, Franklin N. School recess, social connectedness and health: a Canadian perspective. Health Promot Int. 2017;32(2):392–402.
5. Pellegrini AD, Kato K, Blatchford P, Baines E. A short-term longitudinal study of children's playground games across the first year of school: implications for social competence and adjustment to school. Am Educ Res J. 2002;39:991–1015.
6. Centers for Disease Control and Prevention and SHAPE America. Strategies for recess in schools. Centers for Disease Control and Prevention; 2017. Available at: https://www.cdc.gov/healthyschools/physicalactivity/pdf/2019_04_25_SchoolRecess_strategies_508tagged.pdf. Accessed 26 Aug 2022.
7. Bassett DR, Fitzhugh EC, Heath GW, Erwin PC, Frederick GM, Wolff DL, et al. Estimated energy expenditures for school-based policies and active living. Am J Prev Med. 2013;44(2):108–13.
8. Ickes MJ, Erwin H, Beighle A. Systematic review of recess interventions to increase physical activity. J Phys Act Health. 2012;10(6):910–26.
9. Parrish AM, Chong KH, Moriarty AL, Batterham M, Ridgers ND. Interventions to change school recess activity levels in children and adolescents: a systematic review and meta-analysis. Sports Med. 2020;50(12):2145–73.
10. Erwin H, Abel M, Beighle A, Noland MP, Worley B, Riggs R. The contribution of recess to children's school-day physical activity. J Phys Act Health. 2012;9(3):442–8.
11. Escalante Y, García-Hermoso A, Backx K, Saavedra JM. Playground designs to increase physical activity levels during school recess: a systematic review. Health Educ Behav. 2014;41(2):138–44.
12. Ridgers ND, Stratton G, Fairclough SJ, Twisk JW. Long-term effects of a playground markings and physical structures on children's recess physical activity levels. Prev Med. 2007;44(5):393–7.
13. Willenberg LJ, Ashbolt R, Holland D, Gibbs L, MacDougall C, Garrard J, et al. Increasing school playground physical activity: a mixed methods study combining environmental measures and children's perspectives. J Sci Med Sport. 2009;13(2):210–6.
14. Hodges VC, Centeio EE, Morgan CF. The benefits of school recess: a systematic review. J Sch Health. 2022;92(10):959–67.
15. García-Hermoso A, Alonso-Martínez AM, Ramírez-Vélez R, Pérez-Sousa MÁ, Ramírez-Campillo R, Izquierdo M. Association of physical education with improvement of health-related physical fitness outcomes and fundamental motor skills among youths: a systematic review and meta-analysis. JAMA Pediatr. 2020;174(6):e200223.
16. García-Hermoso A, Ramírez-Vélez R, Lubans DR, Izquierdo M. Effects of physical education interventions on cognition and academic performance outcomes in children and adolescents: a systematic review and meta-analysis. Br J Sports Med. 2021;55(21):1224–32.
17. Lonsdale C, Rosenkranz RR, Peralta LR, Bennie A, Fahey P, Lubans DR. A systematic review and meta-analysis of interventions designed to increase moderate-to-vigorous physical activity in school physical education lessons. Prev Med. 2013;56(2):152–61.
18. Bohn-Gettler CM, Pellegrini AD. Recess in primary school: the disjuncture between educational policy and scientific research. 2014 [citado 22 de noviembre de 2023]. Disponible en: https://psycnet.apa.org/record/2014-24562-012
19. Nijhof SL, Vinkers CH, van Geelen SM, Duijff SN, Achterberg EJM, van der Net J, et al. Healthy play, better coping: the importance of play for the development of children in health and disease. Neurosci Biobehav Rev. 2018;95:421–9.

20. Gray C, Gibbons R, Larouche R, Sandseter EBH, Bienenstock A, Brussoni M, et al. What is the relationship between outdoor time and physical activity, sedentary behaviour, and physical fitness in children? A systematic review. 2015 [citado 22 de noviembre de 2023]. Disponible en: https://open.library.ubc.ca/soa/cIRcle/collections/52383/52383/items/1.0378647
21. Ridgers ND, Stratton G. Physical activity during school recess: the liverpool sporting playgrounds project. Pediatr Exerc Sci [Internet]. 2005 [citado 22 de noviembre de 2023];17(3). Disponible en: https://search.ebscohost.com/login.aspx?direct=true&profile=ehost&scope=site&authtype=crawler&jrnl=08998493&asa=Y&AN=17799726&h=Bc769%2FSkpK42xKeNuE1UIa2cFjcsXf2SZCKYWNyIXTB7b9MU7BifBKFBVP3YhxS%2F5wQNtSCZ57ppLEOch3zBbQ%3D%3D&crl=c
22. Pulido Sanchez S, Iglesias GD. Evidence-based overview of accelerometer-measured physical activity during school recess: an updated systematic review. Int J Environ Res Public Health. 2021;18(2):578.
23. Clevenger KA, Belcher BR, Berrigan D. Associations between amount of recess, physical activity, and cardiometabolic traits in US children. Transl J Am Coll Sports Med. 2022;7(3):e000202.
24. Clevenger KA, McNarry MA, Mackintosh KA, Berrigan D. Association of recess provision with elementary school-aged children's physical activity, adiposity, and cardiorespiratory and muscular fitness. Pediatr Exerc Sci. 2022;35(2):99–106.
25. Wong LS, Reilly J, McCrorie P, Harrington D. Physical activity levels during school recess in a nationally representative sample of 10–11-year-olds. Pediatr Exerc Sci [Internet]. 2023 [citado 22 de noviembre de 2023]. Disponible en: https://strathprints.strath.ac.uk/85486/
26. Ridgers ND, Saint-Maurice PF, Welk GJ, Siahpush M, Huberty J. Differences in physical activity during school recess. J Sch Health. 2011;81(9):545–51.
27. Ridgers ND, Stratton G, Clark E, Fairclough SJ, Richardson DJ. Day-to-day and seasonal variability of physical activity during school recess. Prev Med. 2006;42(5):372–4.
28. Stanley RM, Ridley K, Dollman J. Correlates of children's time-specific physical activity: a review of the literature. Int J Behav Nutr Phys Act [Internet]. 2012 [citado 22 de noviembre de 2023];9(50). Disponible en: https://www.cabdirect.org/cabdirect/abstract/20123166553
29. Ridgers ND, Fairclough SJ, Stratton G. Variables associated with children's physical activity levels during recess: the A-CLASS project. Int J Behav Nutr Phys Act. 2010;7:74.
30. Escalante Y, Backx K, Saavedra JM, García-Hermoso A, Domínguez AM. Play area and physical activity in recess in primary schools. Kinesiology. 2012;44(2):123–9.
31. Pontifex MB, Saliba BJ, Raine LB, Picchietti DL, Hillman CH. Exercise improves behavioral, neurocognitive, and scholastic performance in children with attention-deficit/hyperactivity disorder. J Pediatr. 2013;162(3):543–51.
32. Yesil DU. Recess and reading achievement of early childhood students in public schools. Educ Policy Anal Arch. 2012;20(10):n10.
33. Erwin H, Fedewa A, Wilson J, Ahn S. The effect of doubling the amount of recess on elementary student disciplinary referrals and achievement over time. J Res Child Educ. 2019;33(4):592–609.
34. Esteban-Cornejo I, Martinez-Gomez D, Garcia-Cervantes L, Ortega FB, Delgado-Alfonso A, Castro-Piñero J, et al. Objectively measured physical activity during physical education and school recess and their associations with academic performance in youth: the UP&DOWN study. J Phys Act Health. 2017;14(4):275–82.
35. Holmes RM, Pellegrini AD, Schmidt SL. The effects of different recess timing regimens on preschoolers' classroom attention. Early Child Dev Care [Internet]. 2006 [citado 22 de noviembre de 2023]. Disponible en: https://psycnet.apa.org/record/2006-20004-005
36. Brez C, Sheets V. Classroom benefits of recess. Learn Environ Res [Internet]. 2017 [citado 22 de noviembre de 2023]. Disponible en: https://psycnet.apa.org/record/2017-23916-001
37. Fagerstrom T, Mahoney K. Give me a break! Can strategic recess scheduling increase on-task behaviour for first graders? Ont Action Res. 2006;9(2):1.

38. Haapala HL, Hirvensalo MH, Laine K, Laakso L, Hakonen H, Kankaanpää A, et al. Recess physical activity and school-related social factors in Finnish primary and lower secondary schools: cross-sectional associations. BMC Public Health [Internet]. 2014 [citado 22 de noviembre de 2023];14. Disponible en: https://search.ebscohost.com/login.aspx?direct=true&profile=ehost&scope=site&authtype=crawler&jrnl=14712458&AN=153133745&h=Q%2BLjv79ttLOYnoiTco6JxPolqTDZR%2FTxxr1w0BDaeCwkuO2MdPbvU%2FAMyq2XPTf%2F5RFJAtGDoNh08LhWrktMcg%3D%3D&crl=c
39. Stapp AC, Karr JK. Effect of recess on fifth grade students' time on-task in an elementary classroom. Int Electron J Elem Educ [Internet]. 2018 [citado 22 de noviembre de 2023];10(4). Disponible en: https://search.ebscohost.com/login.aspx?direct=true&profile=ehost&scope=site&authtype=crawler&jrnl=13079298&AN=128873187&h=xHQYaWbKiJTR7JSTqwWvh94O%2BTVGTY2HPKCDOQS5ZMrzXG2gLLUVTJ92qq1xO77tGz6%2Bf%2BBgcgh3bsXxx4wU4Q%3D%3D&crl=c
40. Barros RM, Silver EJ, Stein RE. School recess and group classroom behavior. Pediatrics [Internet]. 2009 [citado 22 de noviembre de 2023]. Disponible en: https://psycnet.apa.org/record/2010-00478-009
41. Massey WV, Szarabajko A, Thalken J, Perez D, Mullen SP. Memories of school recess predict physical activity enjoyment and social-emotional well-being in adults. Psychol Sport Exerc. 2021;55:101948.
42. Fernandes MM, Sturm R. The role of school physical activity programs in child body mass trajectory. J Phys Act Health. 2011;8(2):174–81.
43. Ansari A, Pettit K, Gershoff E. Combating obesity in head start: outdoor play and change in children's body mass index. J Dev Behav Pediatr. 2015;36(8):605–12.
44. Gray HL, Buro AW, Ikan JB, Wang W, Stern M. School-level factors associated with obesity: a systematic review of longitudinal studies. Obes Rev. 2019;20(7):1016–32.
45. Kahan D, Poulos A. Models of school recess for combatting overweight in the United States. Prev Med Rep. 2022;31:102081.
46. Ridgers ND, Parrish AM, Salmon J, Timperio A. School recess physical activity interventions. En: the Routledge handbook of youth physical activity [Internet]. Routledge; 2020 [citado 29 de noviembre de 2023]. p. 504–22. Disponible en: https://www.taylorfrancis.com/chapters/edit/10.4324/9781003026426-31/school-recess-physical-activity-interventions-nicola-ridgers-anne-maree-parrish-jo-salmon-anna-timperio
47. Clevenger KA, Sinha G, Howe CA. Comparison of methods for analyzing global positioning system and accelerometer data during school recess. Meas Phys Educ Exerc Sci. 2019;23(1):58–68.
48. Sumpner C, Blatchford P. What do we know about breaktime? Results from a national survey of breaktime and lunchtime in primary and secondary schools. Br Educ Res J. 1998;24(1):79–94.
49. Haug E, Torsheim T, Sallis JF, Samdal O. The characteristics of the outdoor school environment associated with physical activity. Health Educ Res [Internet]. 2010 [citado 30 de noviembre de 2023];25(2). Disponible en: https://search.ebscohost.com/login.aspx?direct=true&profile=ehost&scope=site&authtype=crawler&jrnl=02681153&asa=Y&AN=50640900&h=vE8RbkDFuAU0ykbRmfgGSd5L0WpRPGblBhVquzFQKMuHXzQgOcWGaubYdzPTRzLmCJ3llJlfImWkPFbn2og44A%3D%3D&crl=c
50. Ridgers ND, Salmon J, Parrish AM, Stanley RM, Okely AD. Physical activity during school recess: a systematic review. Am J Prev Med. 2012;43(3):320–8.
51. Ridgers ND, Timperio A, Crawford D, Salmon J. What factors are associated with adolescents' school break time physical activity and sedentary time? PLoS One. 2013;8(2):e56838.
52. Saint-Maurice PF, Welk GJ, Silva P, Siahpush M, Huberty J. Assessing children's physical activity behaviors at recess: a multi-method approach. Pediatr Exerc Sci [Internet]. 2011 [citado 19 de diciembre de 2023];23(4). Disponible en: https://search.ebscohost.com/login.aspx?direct=true&profile=ehost&scope=site&authtype=crawler&jrnl=08998493&AN=69

934989&h=Kw7ylWbR9cEJ6O849tY0qJkH60yI4YXHh3NLNcAzfmMg6jOv0xHIgWR erhONJDLiT7UfAI%2FSxNGPO5sfojqGKQ%3D%3D&crl=c
53. Ridgers ND, Salmon J, Timperio A. Seasonal changes in physical activity during school recess and lunchtime among Australian children. J Sports Sci. 2017;36(13):1508–14.
54. Lanza K, Alcazar M, Durand CP, Salvo D, Villa U, Kohl HW. Heat-resilient schoolyards: relations between temperature, shade, and physical activity of children during recess. J Phys Act Health. 2022;20(2):134–41.
55. Button BLG, Martin G. Exploring extreme weather and recess policies, practices, and procedures in the Canadian context. Int J Environ Res Public Health. 2023;20(1):814.
56. Ryan M, Ricardo LIC, Nathan N, Hofmann R, van Sluijs E. Are school uniforms associated with gender inequalities in physical activity? A pooled analysis of population-level data from 135 countries/regions. J Sport Health Sci [Internet]. 2024 [citado 14 de abril de 2024]. Disponible en: https://www.sciencedirect.com/science/article/pii/S2095254624000206
57. Hyndman B. Where to next for school playground interventions to encourage active play? An exploration of structured and unstructured school playground strategies. J Occup Ther Sch Early Interv. 2015;8(1):56–67.
58. Cardon G, Labarque V, Smits D, de Bourdeaudhuij I. Promoting physical activity at the pre-school playground: the effects of providing markings and play equipment. Prev Med. 2009;48(4):335–40.
59. Blaes A, Ridgers ND, Aucouturier J, Van Praagh E, Berthoin S, Baquet G. Effects of a playground marking intervention on school recess physical activity in French children. Prev Med. 2013;57(5):580–4.
60. Stratton G, Mullan E. The effect of multicolor playground markings on children's physical activity level during recess. Prev Med. 2005;41(5/6):828–33.
61. Stratton G. Promoting children's physical activity in primary school: an intervention study using playground markings. Ergonomics. 2000;43(10):1538–46.
62. Loucaides CA, Jago R, Charalambous I. Promoting physical activity during school break times: piloting a simple, low cost intervention. Prev Med. 2009;48(4):332–4.
63. Ridgers ND, Stratton G, Fairclough SJ, Twisk JW. Children's physical activity levels during school recess: a quasi-experimental intervention study. Int J Behav Nutr Phys Act [Internet]. 2007 [citado 30 de noviembre de 2023];4. Disponible en: https://search.ebscohost.com/login.aspx?direct=true&profile=ehost&scope=site&authtype=crawler&jrnl=14795868&AN=28774180&h=q8XqG2hM3QNG8ckp8WaBpxWoXQNrhl8hJ7RWL9Fv4%2B0CexJ2hNA75c9ZNwD4Agdk%2BcKKrNHHh6dz7n1P%2BYCmEg%3D%3D&crl=c
64. Ridgers ND, Fairclough SJ, Stratton G. Twelve-month effects of a playground intervention on children's morning and lunchtime recess physical activity levels. J Phys Act Health [Internet]. 2010 [citado 30 de noviembre de 2023];7(2). Disponible en: https://search.ebscohost.com/login.aspx?direct=true&profile=ehost&scope=site&authtype=crawler&jrnl=15433080&AN=49718376&h=5YZoGDeOs53NBRpBJALoLn%2F%2Fl4dIdotD1ZT6q2Ow7Mllx%2BdRtjUOOJaq%2FA8eLLBRbYRVIDSOwGmqgnOtdSPsLw%3D%3D&crl=c
65. Brink LA, Nigg CR, Lampe SM, Kingston BA, Mootz AL, van Vliet W. Influence of schoolyard renovations on children's physical activity: the Learning Landscapes Program. Am J Public Health. 2010;100(9):1672–8.
66. Anthamatten P, Brink L, Lampe S, Greenwood E, Kingston B, Nigg C. An assessment of schoolyard renovation strategies to encourage children's physical activity. Int J Behav Nutr Phys Act [Internet]. 2011 [citado 30 de noviembre de 2023];8. Disponible en: https://search.ebscohost.com/login.aspx?direct=true&profile=ehost&scope=site&authtype=crawler&jrnl=14795868&AN=61036248&h=1%2BJ%2BpPQtEJ41b%2FzH8bfT1VQX%2FJUvs4%2Ffdxe0mOuHdtC0%2BxTBmfCI64SYTbfBiF1pV5OA7iiRoxh%2FGKCtJJYWrw%3D%3D&crl=c
67. Barnas J, Wunder C, Ball S. In the zone: an investigation into physical activity during recess on traditional versus zoned playgrounds. Phys Educ [Internet]. 2018 [citado 30 de noviembre de 2023];75(1). Disponible en: https://www.cabdirect.org/cabdirect/abstract/20183078708

68. Hamer M, Aggio D, Knock G, Kipps C, Shankar A, Smith L. Effect of major school playground reconstruction on physical activity and sedentary behaviour: Camden active spaces. BMC Public Health [Internet]. 2017 [citado 30 de noviembre de 2023];17(552). Disponible en: https://www.cabdirect.org/cabdirect/abstract/20173269688
69. Raney MA, Hendry CF, Yee SA. Physical activity and social behaviors of urban children in green playgrounds. Am J Prev Med. 2019;56(4):522–9.
70. van Dijk-Wesselius JE, Maas J, Hovinga D, van Vugt M, van den Berg AE. The impact of greening schoolyards on the appreciation, and physical, cognitive and social-emotional well-being of schoolchildren: a prospective intervention study. Landsc Urban Plan. 2018;180:15–26.
71. Lopes L, Lopes V, Pereira B. Physical activity levels in normal weight and overweight Portuguese children: an intervention study during an elementary school recess. Int Electron J Health Educ. 2009;12:175–84.
72. Verstraete SJ, Cardon GM, De Clercq DL, De Bourdeaudhuij IM. Increasing children's physical activity levels during recess periods in elementary schools: the effects of providing game equipment. Eur J Public Health. 2006;16(4):415–9.
73. Bundy A, Engelen L, Wyver S, Tranter P, Ragen J, Bauman A, et al. Sydney playground project: a cluster-randomized trial to increase physical activity, play, and social skills. J Sch Health. 2017;87(10):751–9.
74. Engelen L, Bundy AC, Naughton G, Simpson JM, Bauman A, Ragen J, et al. Increasing physical activity in young primary school children-it's child's play: a cluster randomised controlled trial. Prev Med. 2013;56(5):319–25.
75. Hyndman BP, Benson AC, Ullah S, Telford A. Evaluating the effects of the Lunchtime Enjoyment Activity and Play (LEAP) school playground intervention on children's quality of life, enjoyment and participation in physical activity. BMC Public Health. 2014;14(1):164.
76. Huberty JL, Beets MW, Beighle A, Welk G. Environmental modifications to increase physical activity during recess: preliminary findings from ready for recess. J Phys Act Health. 2011;8:S249–56.
77. Hyndman BP, Lester L. The effect of an emerging school playground strategy to encourage children's physical activity: the accelerometer intensities from movable playground and lunchtime activities in youth (AIM-PLAY) study. Child Youth Environ. 2015;25(3):109.
78. Yu H, Kulinna PH, Mulhearn SC. The effectiveness of equipment provisions on rural middle school students' physical activity during lunch recess. J Phys Act Health [Internet]. 2021 [citado 5 de diciembre de 2023];18(3). Disponible en: https://search.ebscohost.com/login.aspx?direct=true&profile=ehost&scope=site&authtype=crawler&jrnl=15433080&AN=149084552&h=%2BP4wy0TcQVgGzlPrrOpcKAIkwlanF1OPzZV8LftjqFDlJziWaflLu4XB8qi9GKkddKqzHzFbyHVNxlip%2B7ciCw%3D%3D&crl=c
79. Klinker CD, Schipperijn J, Christian H, Kerr J, Ersbøll AK, Troelsen J. Using accelerometers and global positioning system devices to assess gender and age differences in children's school, transport, leisure and home based physical activity. Int J Behav Nutr Phys Act [Internet]. 2014 [citado 3 de diciembre de 2023];11. Disponible en: https://search.ebscohost.com/login.aspx?direct=true&profile=ehost&scope=site&authtype=crawler&jrnl=14795868&AN=94507658&h=t5f01zLBJbSbwfP6EHQiHFEm%2FaQanRpJ1cDqPl4Wt8NVVI8Vj7JBFJEoBoCt7PxLz0HPy1pFPFKPN7ZaGYKMpw%3D%3D&crl=c
80. Brusseau TA, Kulinna PH. An examination of four traditional school physical activity models on children's step counts and MVPA. Res Q Exerc Sport. 2015;86(1):88–93.
81. Razak LA, Yoong SL, Wiggers J, Morgan PJ, Jones J, Finch M, et al. Impact of scheduling multiple outdoor free-play periods in childcare on child moderate-to-vigorous physical activity: a cluster randomised trial. Int J Behav Nutr Phys Act. 2018;15(1):34.
82. Van Cauwenberghe E, De Bourdeaudhuij I, Maes L, Cardon G. Efficacy and feasibility of lowering playground density to promote physical activity and to discourage sedentary time during recess at preschool: a pilot study. Prev Med. 2012;55(4):319–21.

83. D'Haese S, Van Dyck D, De Bourdeaudhuij I, Cardon G. Effectiveness and feasibility of lowering playground density during recess to promote physical activity and decrease sedentary time at primary school. BMC Public Health. 2013;13:1154.
84. Control C for D, Prevention, Health SAS of, Educators P. Strategies for recess in schools. Centers for Disease Control and Prevention, US Department of Health and …; 2017.
85. Zavacky F, Michael SL. Keeping recess in schools. J Phys Educ Recreat Dance. 2017;88(5):46–53.
86. Stellino MB, Sinclair CD, Partridge JA, King KM. Differences in children's recess physical activity: recess activity of the week intervention. J Sch Health. 2010;80(9):436–44.
87. Scruggs PW, Beveridge SK, Watson DL. Increasing children's school time physical activity using structured fitness breaks. Pediatr Exerc Sci [Internet]. 2003 [citado 1 de diciembre de 2023];15(2). Disponible en: https://search.ebscohost.com/login.aspx?direct=true&profile=ehost&scope=site&authtype=crawler&jrnl=08998493&AN=9749361&h=wCKK23B9v%2FVE3HoylIOCGYcCyVE%2FGn8lZrE%2Fww3aJCGBYP2R8A74kcS2nKZXwRxa1d%2BC%2FBGkIrkd6Pq3YjjBQQ%3D%3D&crl=c
88. Vanluyten K, Cheng S, Roure C, Seghers J, Ward P, Iserbyt P. Participation and physical activity in organized recess tied to physical education in elementary schools: an interventional study. Prev Med Rep. 2023;35:102355.
89. Erwin H, Koufoudakis R, Beighle A. Children's physical activity levels during indoor recess dance videos. J Sch Health. 2013;83(5):322–7.
90. Duncan M, Staples V. The impact of a school-based active video game play intervention on children's physical activity during recess. Hum Mov. 2010;1(11):95–9.
91. Efrat MW. Exploring effective strategies for increasing the amount of moderate-to-vigorous physical activity children accumulate during recess: a quasi-experimental intervention study. J Sch Health. 2013;83(4):265–72.
92. Howe CA, Freedson PS, Alhassan S, Feldman HA, Osganian SK. A recess intervention to promote moderate-to-vigorous physical activity. Pediatr Obes. 2012;7(1):82–8.
93. Lassiter JW, Campbell AL. Effect of an elementary school walking program on physical activity and classroom behavior. Phys Educ. 2019;76(2):485–502.
94. Volmut T, Šimunic B. Effect of unstructured 15-minute active recess on children's daily physical activity. J Phys Educ Sport [Internet]. 2021 [citado 1 de diciembre de 2023];21(1). Disponible en: https://search.ebscohost.com/login.aspx?direct=true&profile=ehost&scope=site&authtype=crawler&jrnl=22478051&AN=148527910&h=uW3RXdjevp4DsKtYrEMKfvjHRNYJKuhQqNI9QtcA0ShSgEzdQ4PQq6TVH7qwH5MxrZlw2XQzqD7xOs0FKgXUKw%3D%3D&crl=c
95. Escalante Y, Backx K, Saavedra JM, García-Hermoso A, Domínguez AM. Relationship between daily physical activity, recess physical activity, age and sex in scholar of primary school, Spain. Rev Esp Salud Publica. 2011;85(5):481–9.
96. Sutherland R, Campbell E, Lubans DR, Morgan PJ, Okely AD, Nathan N, et al. 'Physical Activity 4 Everyone' school-based intervention to prevent decline in adolescent physical activity levels: 12 month (mid-intervention) report on a cluster randomised trial [Internet]. 2016 [citado 3 de diciembre de 2023]. Disponible en: https://pubmed.ncbi.nlm.nih.gov/26359346/
97. Van Kann DH, de Vries SI, Schipperijn J, de Vries NK, Jansen MW, Kremers SP. A multicomponent schoolyard intervention targeting children's recess physical activity and sedentary behavior: effects after 1 year. J Phys Act Health. 2017;14(11):866–75.
98. Farbo D, Maler LC, Rhea DJ. The preliminary effects of a multi-recess school intervention: using accelerometers to measure physical activity patterns in elementary children. Int J Environ Res Public Health. 2020;17(23):E8919.
99. Haapala HL, Hirvensalo MH, Laine K, Laakso L, Hakonen H, Lintunen T, et al. Adolescents' physical activity at recess and actions to promote a physically active school day in four Finnish schools. Health Educ Res. 2014;29(5):840–52.

100. Janssen M, Twisk JW, Toussaint HM, van Mechelen W, Verhagen EA. Effectiveness of the PLAYgrounds programme on PA levels during recess in 6-year-old to 12-year-old children. Br J Sports Med. 2015;49(4):259–64.
101. Parrish AM, Okely AD, Batterham M, Cliff D, Magee C. PACE: a group randomised controlled trial to increase children's break-time playground physical activity. J Sci Med Sport. 2016;19(5):413–8.
102. Huberty JL, Siahpush M, Beighle A, Fuhrmeister E, Silva P, Welk G. Ready for recess: a pilot study to increase physical activity in elementary school children. J Sch Health. 2011;81(5):251–7.
103. Farmer VL, Williams SM, Mann JI, Schofield G, McPhee JC, Taylor RW. The effect of increasing risk and challenge in the school playground on physical activity and weight in children: a cluster randomised controlled trial (PLAY). Int J Obes (Lond). 2017;41(5):793–801.
104. Tucker P, Vanderloo LM, Johnson AM, Burke SM, Irwin JD, Gaston A, et al. Impact of the Supporting Physical Activity in the Childcare Environment (SPACE) intervention on preschoolers' physical activity levels and sedentary time: a single-blind cluster randomized controlled trial. Int J Behav Nutr Phys Act. 2017;14(1):120.
105. Wang H, Li T, Siahpush M, Chen LW, Huberty J. Cost-effectiveness of ready for recess to promote physical activity in children. J Sch Health. 2017;87(4):278–85.
106. Casolo A, Sagelv EH, Bianco M, Casolo F, Galvani C. Effects of a structured recess intervention on physical activity levels, cardiorespiratory fitness, and anthropometric characteristics in primary school children. 2019 [citado 19 de diciembre de 2023]. Disponible en: https://munin.uit.no/handle/10037/16555
107. Nally S, Carlin A, Blackburn NE, Baird JS, Salmon J, Murphy MH, et al. The effectiveness of school-based interventions on obesity-related behaviours in primary school children: a systematic review and meta-analysis of randomised controlled trials. Children. 2021;8(6):489.
108. Clevenger KA, Dunton GF, Katzmarzyk PT, Pfeiffer KA, Berrigan D. Adherence to recess guidelines in the United States using nationally representative data: implications for future surveillance efforts. J Sch Health [Internet]. 2023 [citado 22 de noviembre de 2023]. Disponible en: https://europepmc.org/article/med/37317050
109. Ozenbaugh I, Thalken J, Logan S, Stellino MB, Massey WV. Parents' perceptions of school recess policies and practices. BMC Public Health. 2022;22:1575.
110. Bjornsen MA, Perryman KL, Cameron L, Thomas H, Howie EK. The impact of recess on students: a scoping review of developmental outcomes and methodological considerations. J Res Child Educ. 2024;0(0):1–16.
111. McNamara L, Vaantaja E, Dunseith A, Franklin N. Tales from the playground: transforming the context of recess through collaborative action research. Int J Play. 2015;4(1):49–68.
112. Vaillancourt T, Brittain H, Bennett L, Arnocky S, McDougall P, Hymel S, et al. Places to avoid: population-based study of student reports of unsafe and high bullying areas at school. Can J Sch Psychol [Internet]. 2010 [citado 18 de diciembre de 2023]. Disponible en: https://psycnet.apa.org/record/2010-04757-004
113. Bukowski WM, Laursen B, Hoza B. The snowball effect: friendship moderates escalations in depressed affect among avoidant and excluded children. Dev Psychopathol. 2010;22(4):749–57.

Chapter 10
Active Classrooms in School Curricula and Active Breaks

Abel Ruiz-Hermosa, David Sánchez-Oliva, and Mairena Sánchez-López

10.1 Why Reduce Sitting in the Classroom?

A worrying and persistent problem with significant implications for both health and academic performance is the high prevalence of sedentary behavior (SB) in children and adolescents. An SB is defined as "any waking behavior characterized by an energy expenditure ≤1.5 metabolic equivalents while in a sitting, reclining, or lying position" [1]. Regardless of physical activity (PA) level, SB has been associated with adverse effects on cardiometabolic health, symptoms of depression, decreased self-esteem, and reduced ability to focus and concentrate on classroom tasks in children and adolescents [2–4]. Furthermore, childhood SB tends to persist into adolescence [5] and adulthood [6]. It is important to note that the longest periods of uninterrupted sedentary time for children and adolescents typically occur during school hours. Studies show that European children and adolescents spend approximately 65–70% of their school time in a sedentary state [7]. Although there are no specific recommendations, various health institutions suggest that young people take breaks from prolonged sitting as often as possible [2]. Given the health, psychosocial, and cognitive risks associated with SB, the reported health benefits of different levels of PA, the knowledge that SB tends to persist into adulthood, and

A. Ruiz-Hermosa
Faculty of Sport Sciences, Universidad de Extremadura, Cáceres, Spain

School of Education, Universidad de Castilla-La Mancha, Ciudad Real, Spain

D. Sánchez-Oliva
Faculty of Sport Sciences, Universidad de Extremadura, Cáceres, Spain

M. Sánchez-López (✉)
School of Education, Universidad de Castilla-La Mancha, Ciudad Real, Spain
e-mail: Mairena.Sanchez@uclm.es

© The Author(s), under exclusive license to Springer Nature Switzerland AG 2024
A. García-Hermoso (ed.), *Promotion of Physical Activity and Health in the School Setting*, https://doi.org/10.1007/978-3-031-65595-1_10

interventions aimed at reducing these behaviors and increasing PA at different intensity levels in children and adolescents seem imperative.

10.2 The Link Between Physical Activity and Academic Performance at School

Recent studies have suggested that PA has beneficial effects on neurocognitive functioning [8, 9] and academic performance [10]. However, the associations between PA and cognitive and academic performance are complex and may be influenced by multiple mediators [11, 12]. Various mechanisms have been proposed to explain this relationship. For example, increases in cardiorespiratory fitness (CRF) lead to increased cerebral blood flow, which promotes cerebral angiogenesis and neurogenesis and improves oxygen saturation. This in turn triggers increased neurotransmitter levels and changes in neurotrophin regulation, particularly in brain regions associated with executive function [13, 14]. Another theory is based on cognitive stimulation. In this context, it is suggested that engaging in physical activities that involve high cognitive and motor demands—such as novel, complex, and varied tasks performed under changing situational conditions—may induce cognitive stimulation [15, 16]. In addition, participation in PA could have a positive impact on mental well-being, self-esteem, stress, social connectedness, and engagement, all of which can be derived from PA and may also lead to improved academic performance. In addition, involvement in PA could have a positive impact on other health-related behaviors, such as sleep and diet, which are also associated with improved academic performance [12].

According to a systematic review aimed at investigating the mediators between PA and academic performance in children and adolescents [17], most studies have identified CRF as the only variable with a statistically significant mediating role. Cognition and mental well-being may also be potential mediators of the relationship between PA and academic performance. The evidence for other mediators, such as adiposity or behavioral variables, was less clear.

10.3 Classroom-Based Physical Activity: Exploring the Concept

School has been recognized as the ideal place to promote PA in children and adolescents. Throughout the school day, pupils have multiple opportunities for PA (physical education-PE, recess, break time, or active commuting). However, it has been reported that even with all these activities, students achieve only 50% of the official PA recommendations [18]. Integrating PA into the classroom not only provides pupils with opportunities to increase PA time and break long periods of SB but can also be seen as a strategy in line with new learner-centered pedagogical approaches where pupils are actively engaged in their learning.

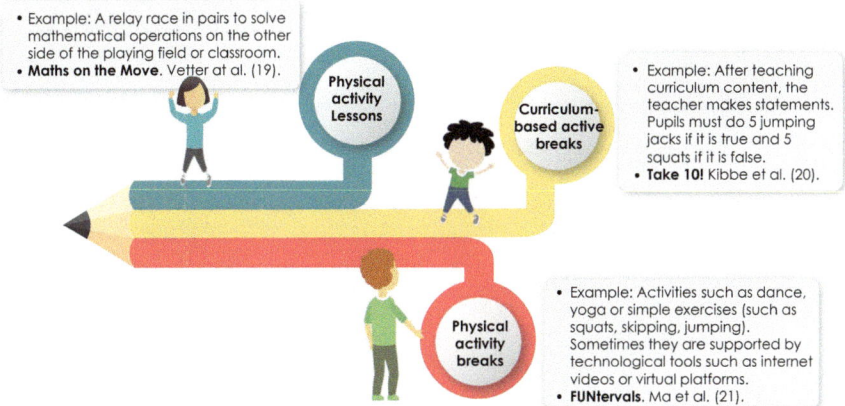

Fig. 10.1 Types of classroom-based physical activity [19–21]

In addition to classroom-based PAs, other terms such as "movement-based learning" or "active learning" have been used in the literature, especially when classroom-based PAs have a clear aim of promoting learning; these PA terms involve teachers incorporating PA into class time, either by integrating PA into lessons (PAL) or by adding short bursts of PA, either with curriculum content (curricular-based active breaks) or without (active breaks) (Fig. 10.1).

While the above classification is simple and useful for identifying the options available for integrating PAs in the classroom, it is generic and unspecific in relation to the integration of PAs in education to support cognition and learning. Thus, based on the theoretical framework of embodied cognition, which is based on the idea that the body and its interactions with the environment contribute to and are essential for cognition [22], a specific categorization of PA during academic time deserves to be mentioned [23].

This classification is based on a 2 × 2 matrix in which classroom PA proposals are grouped into one or another category according to their level of integration (low vs. high) and relevance to the learning content (low vs. high) (Fig. 10.2).

1. *High integration-high relevance:* PAs occur simultaneously and are meaningfully related to the learning task, while academic concepts are explained through movement.
2. *High integration-low relevance:* PAs occur simultaneously with the learning task but are not meaningfully related to the learning task.
3. *Low integration-high relevance:* PA (in this case, it would be more accurate to use the word "gestures," defined as subtle movements centered on the hands involving fine motor skills and requiring negligible energy expenditure) occurs before or after the learning task but is meaningfully related to the learning task.
4. *Low integration-low relevance:* PA preceding and not meaningfully related to the learning task (commonly referred to as "PA activity breaks").

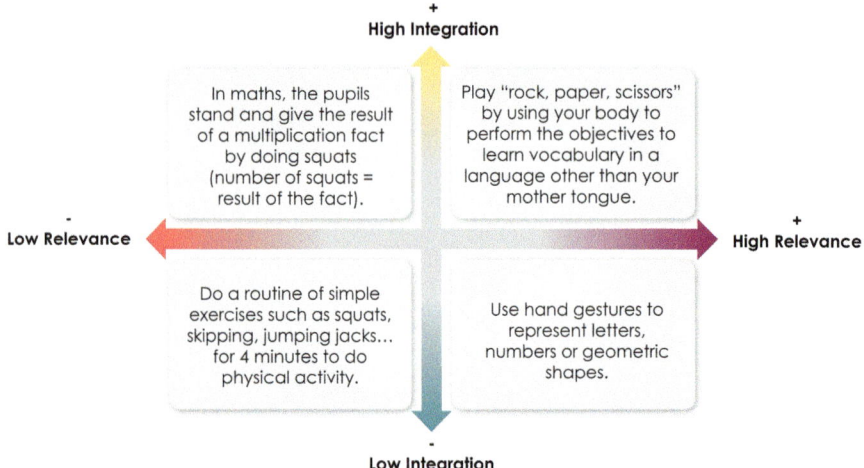

Fig. 10.2 Proposal for a 2 × 2 matrix based on the relevance of movements to cognitive/learning tasks and the integration of movements into cognitive/learning tasks to illustrate examples of activity types [24]. (Source: Adapted from Mavilidi et al. (2018). Fig. 1. Some modifications were made. https://doi.org/10.3389/fpsyg.2018.02079, licensed under the terms of the Creative Commons Attribution 4.0 International License (http://creativecommons.org/licenses/by/4.0/))

10.4 Classroom-Based Physical Activity: An Effective Strategy Beyond Breaking the Sedentary Time in the Classroom

Overall, according to the latest literature reviews, integrating PA into the classroom may offer a practical, low-cost, and effective approach to enhancing academic indicators, especially for acute positive effects on improving on-task and reducing off-task classroom behavior and selective attention [25–29]. It could also increase PA levels and reduce sedentary time during school days [25–27]. Although the effect of classroom-based PAs on students' well-being or enjoyment of school has been little studied, the results are promising [30–32]. To date, very few studies have analyzed the effect of integrated PA in the classroom on physical fitness and obesity, and the results are inconsistent [33–36].

Finally, beyond the benefits for students, integrated PA in the classroom can promote the health and well-being of teachers [37, 38] and may promote positive learning and a social climate in the school [39].

The integration of PA into the classroom offers numerous potential benefits, including increased moderate-vigorous PA (MVPA) and reduced sedentary time during the school day, improved on-task time and classroom behavior, enhanced well-being and enjoyment of school, decreased body fat, improved physical fitness, and better health and well-being for teachers. Additionally, it promotes a positive learning and social climate within the classroom. A more detailed description of the findings for each type of classroom-integrated PA strategy is given below.

10.5 Physically Active Lesson

10.5.1 An Approach to the Physical Active Lessons Concept

In recent years, there has been a growing debate about the need to increase the number of hours of physical education (PE) per week in schools. However, this is not a simple issue, as an increase in the number of hours of PE would mean a decrease in the number of hours of other subjects. As long as this is not a reality, it is necessary to resort to other types of methodologies that incorporate movement into the teaching-learning process.

A recent systematic review and meta-analysis of school-based PA interventions concluded that the most promising types of interventions involve extending opportunities by replacing time spent in SB with more physically active activities [40]. Physically active lessons (PALs) are academic lessons that include PA during teaching-learning activities involving subjects other than PE (e.g., math) without reducing the time devoted to the content of those subjects [26]. That is, PAL has the potential to reduce school sedentary time while maintaining educational value.

Therefore, what may be the reasons why teachers implement PAL? This methodology can be divided into two types: (1) health reasons and (2) motivational reasons. In terms of health, there is no doubt that the PAL methodology leads to moderate to vigorous physical activity, an element that can help students meet the WHO recommendations. Consequently, increasing PA can lead to an increase in fitness and may also be associated with the improvement of fundamental movement skills. As far as motivational benefits are concerned, there is no doubt that having an academic lesson outside the usual classroom context within four walls creates a certain motivation and good attitude toward the students. In addition, this method helps students socialize themselves, as many of the activities must be carried out in groups through cooperative tasks. Finally, PAL activities usually involve cognitive challenges, which increase students' motivation [41, 42].

10.5.2 Evidence for Physical Active Lessons Implementation

In recent years, there has been a significant increase in the implementation of PAL in schools and, as a result, an increase in the amount of research attempting to demonstrate the effects of this type of methodology. In this sense, a reference study was conducted by Norris et al. [43], who carried out a systematic review and meta-analysis to evaluate the effects of physically active learning on PA, health, education, and cognitive indicators. The review included 42 studies (39 in preschool or primary education and 3 in secondary education). The results showed that physically active lesson-based interventions led to a significant increase in PA time during class and a moderate increase in total PA. In addition, classroom-based PA interventions also led to significant improvements in educational outcomes in terms of classroom time and a moderate improvement in overall academic performance. In contrast, there were no effects on cognitive or health markers such as executive function or fitness/fatness.

10.5.3 Physical Active Lessons Taxonomy

PAL can be divided into several categories. One way is to divide indoor and outdoor areas. Indoor PALs are active lessons that take place in the same space as other academic lessons. This strategy involves moving classroom elements (e.g., chairs and tables) to leave an open space in which movement can be incorporated. This is not always possible because it depends on the space available and can create other barriers, such as noise, for neighboring classes. However, when PAL is implemented, the most common option is to develop the lesson outdoors. This strategy has the disadvantage of the time needed to move to the playground but offers many advantages, such as the large space to be used, the ability to take students out of the usual monotonous context, or the possibility of using elements of the space (e.g., natural elements to work on science).

Another way of classifying PALs is by type of activity. In this sense, Ottesen and von Seelen [44] propose the following classification:

- *Games*. Playful activities to which academic subject content is added. Example: The students are divided into teams of seven or eight members. Each team member has a card with a whole number, a fractional number or a decimal number. Each team must cooperate so that, without verbal communication, they arrange themselves in a row in such a way that the numbers are arranged in order from smallest to largest.
- *Structuring the teaching*. Include activities in which all the space in the classroom is organized to encourage movement. For example, pupils stand up, and the aim is to solve problems based on their own data. Before each problem, they perform a test that consists of performing the maximum number of repetitions of a given exercise (e.g., squats, lunges, jumping jacks, or burpees) for 1 min. Each student then records the number of repetitions and performs the problem. Example problems: (1) If you did X number of squats in 1 min, how many squats would you do in 9 min? (2) If you did X number of strides at 100% for 1 min, how many strides would you do at 30%. (3) Calculate 15% of the number of jumping jacks done. (4) Calculate 15% of the number of jumping jacks done.

- *Physical manifestations of the academic subject*. Activities in which the students enact the academic subject content. An example of an activity in this category is one in which students stand in a straight line separated from each other. The teacher indicates a type of angle (e.g., a straight angle), and the students must represent the angle indicated by the teacher with their arms.
- In situ *activities*. This category includes activities that are normally carried out in nature, outdoor activities, and the local environment, working with the specific content found in these spaces. An example of an activity could be one in which a color is initially associated with each type of angle (e.g., blue rectangle, green acute-angled, and orange obtuse-angled). Individual or paired pupils must find different types of angles in the classroom or playground for a given time by adhering to the color associated with each angle (e.g., rectangle, acute-angled, or obtuse-angled). When the time is up, the whole class goes around the different marked points and identifies whether they are correct or not.
- *Creative and esthetic learning activities*. This category includes physical activities that involve creative, esthetic, and productive activities, such as drama, music, and other expressive activities. An example of this category would be the performance of a drama about the content of a particular subject. Historically, for example, students could act out a historical war.

On the other hand, since the main objective of PAL is to learn through movement and since it is movement that generates learning experiences in students, we propose a classification of the activities according to the integration of movement into the academic content. We can therefore make this classification as follows:

- *Activities with forced inclusion of movement*. In this type of activity, movement is included to make the activity active, but the activity itself can develop without the inclusion of movement. This type of activity includes those where pupils must move from one side of the room to the other to develop the activity (see two examples https://www.youtube.com/watch?v=TIyElogqYig and https://www.youtube.com/watch?v=yq9Aoonvjyk).
- *Activities based on the result of movement*. In this type of activity, the movement is the first thing to be included, and the integration of the subsequent content is conditioned by the results obtained in practicing this physical challenge (see two examples https://www.youtube.com/watch?v=VhtprE_REv8&embeds_referring_euri=https%3A%2F%2Feumoveproject.eu%2F&source_ve_path=OTY3MTQ&feature=emb_imp_woyt and https://www.youtube.com/watch?v=kayJf3fyfOM).
- *Activities through movement*. In these activities, we use movement to reflect academic content; i.e., they have to use their own body in movement to complete the proposed challenge (see two examples https://www.youtube.com/watch?v=V29rK-_dl8U and https://www.youtube.com/watch?v=d_cAgmxsTJk&embeds_referring_euri=https%3A%2F%2Feumoveproject.eu%2F&source_ve_path=OTY3MTQ&feature=emb_imp_woyt).
- *Activities where the outcome requires movement*. A challenge containing the academic content is set, and the students must move to the place associated

with that outcome (see two examples https://www.youtube.com/watch?v=kyajt4dXgy4 and https://www.youtube.com/watch?time_continue=37&v=NvjzF4DP-ao&embeds_referring_euri=https%3A%2F%2Feumoveproject.eu%2F&source_ve_path=Mjg2NjIsMjg2NjIsMjg2NjY&feature=emb_logo).

10.5.4 Examples of Good Practices

In recent years, the body of related knowledge has increased. As a result, recently, several proposals have appeared, usually in the context of transnational research projects, which make practical suggestions for the implementation of PAL in the real world.

Undoubtedly, one of the most significant proposals is the one put forward by the ACTivate project (https://www.activateyourclass.eu/), an Erasmus+-funded project that aims to establish a cocreation working group of researchers, teachers, and other school stakeholders to develop an innovative Europe-wide open access education program, web portal, and community of practice for implementing PAL in practice [45].

Another proposal is made from the EUMOVE Project (https://eumoveproject.eu/), another Erasmus+-funded project aimed at creating a set of educational resources to enable the educational community to promote healthy lifestyles from schools [46]. One of the educational resources is the PAL Toolkit (https://eumove-project.eu/physicallyactive-lessons-toolkit/), a repository of videos with examples of activities (developed in a real context) within the PAL perspective. In addition, users can filter the list of activities by selecting from two categories: academic level (primary or secondary) and subject (mathematics, natural sciences, languages, or social sciences). Each activity also included the materials needed to carry out the activity in five different languages (English, Spanish, Portuguese, French, and Italian). Additionally, for Spanish speakers, derived from the EUMOVE project, Grao-Cruces et al. [47] published a book derived from the EUMOVE project describing a comprehensive set of activities to implement PAL in mathematics for secondary schoolteachers.

10.5.5 First Steps in the Implementation of Physically Active Lessons

When starting the PAL implementation process, it is important to keep in mind the motto "Think big and start small." Here are some recommendations for starting your PAL implementation:

– *Choose simple content for the first session.* The simpler the content is, the easier it is to devise a strategy for inclusion in PALs. We need to ensure that we can do what we have designed.

- *Activities that do not require too much complex structuring are used.* In the initial process of PAL implementation, it is advisable to start with activities that are easy for students to understand, that do not require a complex system of student organization and that require little material.
- *The materials used for activity were easy to prepare and use.* Preparing materials is an extra time commitment for teachers, so it is ideal not to spend too much time preparing materials so that they can be used regularly.
- *Design activities that involve small groups.* Distributing the organization of the class into small groups allows us to keep track of all the students and ensure that everyone is working. It also makes it easier for us to monitor all the processes that each student is using and to give more individual attention to their needs.
- *Prepare some rules that will be key and communicate them to your students.* Before starting this process, it would be very useful to draw up rules with the aim of facilitating the development of the class and to try to teach them to the students from the beginning, looking for the necessary fluency.
- *Create a space that you control.* Before designing an activity and/or a lesson, we should have identified the space we are going to use. Look for a space where you can hold the attention of all your pupils and where you can move quickly from one pupil to another to attend to them when they need you.

10.6 Active Breaks

10.6.1 An Approach to the Active Break Concept

Active breaks are short bouts of PA (usually between 5 and 10 min) implemented by teachers during or between curricular lessons so that schoolchildren can break with the periods of SB during the school day and, consequently, improve their health and promote learning. It is a simple methodology that can be implemented in daily class routines, has a short duration and has a low cost and does not require specific space or materials. Although active breaks are usually implemented in the classroom, it is also possible to carry out these PA periods in the hallway or even on the playground once the students have internalized the dynamics and organization time is minimized. In addition, active breaks are flexible in their implementation, as each teacher can choose the time of the school day that best suits them and their students.

10.6.2 Types of Active Breaks

Given that most interventions, when referring to the type of active breaks, define them as with/without cognitive engagement or with/without curricular content [48] and that there is no universal classification of the types of active breaks, we propose a classification based on the key mechanisms that explain the effect between PA and academic performance. It should be noted that this classification is only one way to help in the design of programrs [17]. Moreover, a type of activity should not be considered exclusive to one category, as in most cases, an activity falling into one block could fit, although to a minor degree, into the other two categories. Active breaks can therefore be divided into three blocks or types of active breaks according to their main purpose:

1. *Active breaks aimed at improving cardiorespiratory fitness:* To achieve this objective, the proposals must significantly increase the heart rate of students and focus on developing muscle strength and aerobic resistance (e.g., up and down stairs, dancing, or exercise routines based on high-intensity interval training [HIIT]).
2. *Active breaks to improve cognitive processes:* The objective is to influence the development of executive functions (attention/inhibition, working memory, and/or cognitive flexibility). For example, the teacher assigns an exercise to different geometric figures, and when he names an object with that geometric shape, the students will have to perform the corresponding action. For greater difficulty, you can exchange the exercises with other figures after a while.
3. *Active breaks to improve aspects of mental well-being*: The main goal is to improve the classroom climate and promote the well-being of students. These active breaks include mainly recreational and cooperative proposals where students enjoy the movement, reduce their stress, and improve their self-esteem. Some examples of this type of active break include asking students to dance freely around the classroom and, if the music stops, to hug another student or proposing that students cooperate to achieve an objective, for example, arranging themselves on chairs in small groups according to their height.

On the other hand, active breaks should be divided into three distinct steps to ensure their correct implementation: the introduction, the development of the active break, and the cool down (Fig. 10.3).

10.6.3 Evidence for Active Break Implementation

In recent years, active breaks have gained special attention in the educational context, and consequently, there has been a significant increase in research on the effects of these short bursts of PA. In this sense, recent systematic reviews and meta-analyses have shown that school-based active breaks interventions lead to significant improvements in terms of MVPA and the number of steps taken by students [25, 27, 49, 50]. Moreover, previous studies have indicated that active breaks can be easily introduced in school lessons, demonstrating the sustainability and feasibility of this strategy [27, 50].

On the other hand, the effects of active breaks on cognitive performance have mixed results and are therefore inconclusive [27, 51]. These conflicting results could be related to the duration, intensity, and type of active break intervention [27, 52]. In this sense, it is possible that active breaks focused on cognitively engaging PAs could have a greater effect on cognitive functions than aerobic PAs alone [27].

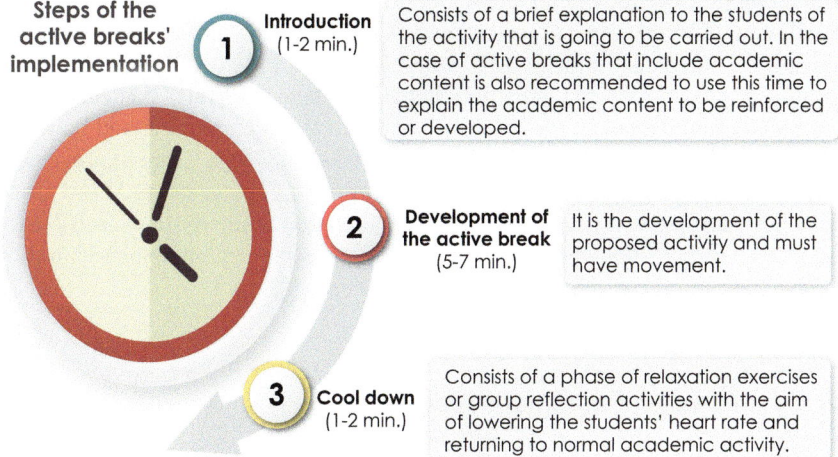

Fig. 10.3 Structure to ensure the correct implementation of the active breaks

In addition, a systematic review suggested that some attentional outcomes improved after active breaks of moderate/vigorous intensities [51]. However, additional research is needed to explore the potential role of active breaks in the cognitive performance of schoolchildren. However, studies have indicated that active breaks do not compromise students' attention or learning [50, 51, 53].

Similarly, there are no clear positive effects of active breaks on students' academic achievement scores (e.g., in specific subjects such as math or reading). Again, these results may be due to the different interventions or types of active breaks developed in the classroom. In this vein, it is possible that active breaks focused on the curricular content of a subject or that reinforce the content of previous lessons could have a greater effect on students' academic achievement scores [27]. On the other hand, most studies have shown positive effects of active breaks on the academic behavior of schoolchildren; thus, active breaks could be a way to improve students' learning and benefit teaching activities [27, 50, 51, 53]. In particular, several systematic reviews have noted that active breaks can improve the "time on task" and well-being of students [27, 50].

Regarding health-related physical fitness, very few studies have analyzed the impact of active breaks interventions on body composition and fitness levels. Therefore, there is insufficient evidence to draw a definitive conclusion, and additional research is needed. In this sense, Katz et al. [54] reported improvements in abdominal strength, upper-body strength, and trunk extensor strength following a 6-month active breaks intervention of 30 min per day. van den Berg et al. [55] observed no effect on schoolchildren's aerobic capacity after a 9-week active breaks intervention of 10 min per day. On the other hand, two studies found no improvements in the body mass index (BMI) of schoolchildren after intervention involving active breaks of 9 weeks [55] or 12 weeks [56], while other authors observed a decrease in BMI in the control group [54]. The *MOVI-da 10! One study* [48], after an intervention during a school year with two active breaks of 10 min per day, revealed no differences between the *MOVI-da10-enriched!* group (high-cognitive-demand PA integrated into the academic curriculum), the *MOVI-da10-Standard!* group (PA breaks with low cognitive demand, where curricular content was not reinforced), and the control group (BMI, abdominal circumference, and body fat). However, the *MOVI-da10-Enriched!* reported statistically significant improvements in all components of fitness (cardiorespiratory fitness, muscle strength, and speed-agility) compared with those of the control group. Similarly, the *MOVI-da10-Standard!* group exhibited improvements in muscle strength compared with those of the control group (results submitted for publication).

10.6.4 Examples of Good Practices

Below, we present some educational resources that could help teachers and stakeholders implement active breaks in the classroom:

10.6.4.1 Real-Time Active Breaks Platform of the EUMOVE Project

The EUMOVE project (https://eumoveproject.eu), described above, offers a free and easy-to-use digital tool to implement active breaks during academic lessons: The virtual platform for active breaks EUMOVE.

This platform involves a virtual cartoon avatar (called *EUMOVY*) that guides all active breaks and allows communication with users in five languages (Spanish, English, French, Italian, and Portuguese). In addition, this resource allows the customization of proposals to adapt them to the interests and objectives of teachers. Overall, this virtual platform allows the deployment of two types of active breaks:

- *The participants were actively broken with the academic content of different subjects while they were performing physical exercise.* Teachers can personalize and edit the content of different questions and up to four possible answers, each associated with an action or exercise (jumping jacks, squats, etc.) previously selected by the teacher. The question will be expressed by *EUMOVY* using a voice synthesis module (in the language chosen by the teacher), and the students must respond by carrying out the action/exercise associated with the answer they consider correct.
- *Active breaks aimed at performing physical exercise*: The avatar leads to an active break, and students must imitate the movements of the avatar. The teacher can choose from a list of movements or exercises, as well as methods (workouts or game models) and levels of difficulty, according to his/her preferences and the goals of the active break.

10.6.4.2 Active Breaks Programs of the MOVI Study

Other educational resources for implementing active breaks include the proposals of the *MOVI study*, led by a research group that has been conducting PA programs with schoolchildren for more than 15 years to prevent overweight/obesity; reduce cardiometabolic risk; and improve physical fitness, quality of life, and academic performance [57–60]. Overall, this research group has designed two different active breaks programs: the *MOVI-HIIT study* and the *MOVI-da 10! study*.

The *MOVI-HIIT* is a cluster-randomized controlled trial that included an active breaks intervention in the classroom for improving cognition, fitness, and body composition in children under 6 years of age (https://www.estudiomovi.com/movi-hiit-2). Specifically, the active breaks of this study were based on the HIIT protocol and included eight exercises of a functional movement for 20% at high intensity (80–90% of HR max) followed by 10% recovery (65–75% of HR max). Like the *EUMOVE project*, this study included a real-time active breaks platform to provide teachers with an easy way to implement active breaks during academic lessons (www.movihiit.es, free access web platform).

Similarly, the *MOVI-da 10! Study* [48] is a cluster-randomized controlled trial designed to evaluate the effectiveness of two types of active breaks programs (*MOVI-da10-enriched!* and *MOVI-da10-standard!*) for improving adiposity, physical fitness, and cognition in early childhood education students. The *MOVI-da10-enriched program* included active breaks with curricular contents of different subjects through coordination exercises (bilateral body coordination) and basic motor skills (balance, jumps, displacements, and handling of objects) of high cognitive demand. While the *MOVI-da10-standard!* included active breaks based on simple games or low-cognitive-demand activities without curricular content, such as dancing to the rhythm of a musical instrument, moving around the class, and following the teacher's instructions (running, touching the floor, jumping, getting on the chair). This document is a summary of all the activities that were part of the study here: https://ruidera.uclm.es/items/04d96534-fe68-4025-9ac1-000fc01a 033f [61].

10.7 Common Challenges for Teachers in Implementing Classroom-Based Physical Activity

There is no doubt that integrating PAs in the classroom is a major challenge for any teacher because it is a complete change in their methodology—a methodology they are accustomed to—feel them comfortable with and have everything under control. When the change is to move learning from the classroom to the outdoors, to get students to learn by moving, the challenge is even greater.

For this reason, before we start our new implementation plan, we must always keep in mind the most common challenges that can hinder the successful practice of classroom-based PAs, which we can overcome and manage well with the right preparation:

- The noise. The exaltation of playful activities or motivational challenges is undoubtedly very characteristic of this change in methodology. This can be reflected in external noise, in the knowledge that another teacher is teaching next door, or even in difficulties of communication, even to the point of shouting or making our message unheard. For PAL, it is advisable to try to hold the lesson outdoors as much as possible, always establishing rules of silence when walking through the corridors. If PAL or active break is indoors, it is important to create a silence control routine when implementing this methodology. The first few times are especially important; do not mind spending some time getting into the routine.
- The specific needs and uniqueness of each student. Each student has his or her own needs. As teachers, we need to identify them and prepare our activities to meet those needs, trying to individualize our sessions as much as possible. A practical recommendation is to try to manage the roles in the activities, play with balanced groupings, work with level groups, or look for activities where everyone can participate equally without compromising the learning of those who are at a higher level.
- Lack of experience and knowledge of how to use PAL. It is normal for a teacher who does not have a lot of experience and knowledge to lack practical strategies, so they do not feel competent and confident to use this methodology in their classroom. It is very important that the implementation process is done very slowly, with a realistic plan, in order to increase the level of experience and confidence of the teachers, as well as to provide the necessary training to improve the teachers' knowledge.
- Differences in student participation. Because of differences in the personalities of individual students, some may be more shy and reserved, while others may be more open to participation. In addition, differences in academic levels mean that students with higher levels tend to work harder than those with lower levels. To solve this limitation, we should try to (1) incorporate role-based work and collaboration to encourage all students to make an effort; (2) use smaller groups to get students more involved; (3) mix heterogeneous groups to encourage disinhibition and help pupils to support each other; and (4) propose activities that require everyone's individual participation or that require everyone in the group to participate because everyone's participation is necessary to complete the exercise.
- Lack of space. For PAL activities, the traditional classroom does not allow for many activities, so the surrounding area of the school must be taken into account. Another problem is that PE teachers may be teaching their classes. For active breaks, some classrooms do not allow for a wide range of movement, depending on the number of student rate. For the implementation of PAL, it is important to be in contact with colleagues (mainly PE teachers) to inform them when you plan to implement PAL outdoor. To overcome the lack of space in the active

break, you can choose the type of exercises that do not require a wide range of movement (e.g., exercises on the vertical axis such as squats or skipping).
- Lack of support from the school staff and other teachers. The best way for this methodology to be effective is to have a whole-school philosophy. Share your idea with teachers and staff in school meetings, describing the potential benefits of these methodologies. Try to get other teachers to follow your initiative by inviting them to a lesson and offering your time to help with the first steps.

References

1. Panahi S, Tremblay A. Sedentariness and health: is sedentary behavior more than just physical inactivity? Front Public Health. 2018;6:258.
2. Chaput JP, Willumsen J, Bull F, Chou R, Ekelund U, Firth J, Jago R, Ortega FB, Katzmarzyk PT. 2020 WHO guidelines on physical activity and sedentary behavior for children and adolescents aged 5–17 years: summary of the evidence. Int J Behav Nutr Phys Act. 2020;17(1):141.
3. Suchert V, Hanewinkel R, Isensee B, läuft Study Group. Sedentary behavior, depressed affect, and indicators of mental well-being in adolescence: does the screen only matter for girls? J Adolesc. 2015;42:50–8.
4. Der NV, Anneke G, Erik JA. Associations between daily physical activity and executive functioning in primary school-aged children. J Sci Med Sport. 2015;18:673–7.
5. Biddle SJ, Pearson N, Ross GM, Braithwaite R. Tracking of sedentary behaviors of young people: a systematic review. Prev Med. 2010;51(5):345–51.
6. Hancox RJ, Milne BJ, Poulton R. Association between child and adolescent television viewing and adult health: a longitudinal birth cohort study. Lancet. 2004;364(9430):257–62.
7. Verloigne M, Loyen A, Van Hecke L, Lakerveld J, Hendriksen I, De Bourdheaudhuij I, Deforche B, Donnelly A, Ekelund U, Brug J, van der Ploeg HP. Variation in population levels of sedentary time in European children and adolescents according to cross-European studies: a systematic literature review within DEDIPAC. Int J Behav Nutr Phys Act. 2016;13:69.
8. Erickson KI, Hillman C, Stillman CM, Ballard RM, Bloodgood B, Conroy DE, Macko R, Marquez DX, Petruzzello SJ, Powell KE. Physical activity, cognition, and brain outcomes: a review of the 2018 physical activity guidelines. Med Sci Sports Exerc. 2019;51(6):1242–51.
9. Álvarez-Bueno C, Pesce C, Cavero-Redondo I, Sánchez-López M, Martínez-Hortelano JA, Martínez-Vizcaíno V. The effect of physical activity interventions on children's cognition and metacognition: a systematic review and meta-analysis. J Am Acad Child Adolesc Psychiatry. 2017;56(9):729–38.
10. Donnelly JE, Hillman CH, Castelli D, Etnier JL, Lee S, Tomporowski P, Lambourne K, Szabo-Reed AN. Physical activity, fitness, cognitive function, and academic achievement in children: a systematic review. Med Sci Sports Exerc. 2016;48(6):1197–222.
11. Tomporowski PD, McCullick B, Pendleton DM, Pesce C. Exercise and children's cognition: the role of exercise characteristics and a place for metacognition. J Sport Health Sci. 2015;4:47–55.
12. Lubans D, Richards J, Hillman C, Faulkner G, Beauchamp M, Nilsson M, Kelly P, Smith J, Raine L, Biddle S. Physical activity for cognitive and mental health in youth: a systematic review of mechanisms. Pediatrics. 2016;138(3):e20161642.
13. Hillman CH, Erickson KI, Kramer AF. Be smart, exercise your heart: exercise effects on brain and cognition. Nat Rev Neurosci. 2008;9(1):58–65.
14. Chaddock L, Pontifex MB, Hillman CH, Kramer AF. A review of the relation of aerobic fitness and physical activity to brain structure and function in children. J Int Neuropsychol Soc. 2011;17(6):975–85.

15. Diamond A. Close interrelation of motor development and cognitive development and of the cerebellum and prefrontal cortex. Child Dev. 2000;71(1):44–56.
16. Pesce C. Shifting the focus from quantitative to qualitative exercise characteristics in exercise and cognition research. J Sport Exerc Psychol. 2012;34(6):766–86.
17. Visier-Alfonso ME, Sánchez-López M, Álvarez-Bueno C, Ruiz-Hermosa A, Nieto-López M, Martínez-Vizcaíno V. Mediators between physical activity and academic achievement: a systematic review. Scand J Med Sci Sports. 2022;32(3):452–64.
18. Fairclough SJ, Beighle A, Erwin H, Ridgers ND. School day segmented physical activity patterns of high and low active children. BMC Public Health. 2012;12:406.
19. Vetter M, O'Connor HT, O'Dwyer N, Chau J, Orr R. 'Maths on the move': effectiveness of physically active lessons for learning maths and increasing physical activity in primary school students. J Sci Med Sport. 2020;23(8):735–9.
20. Kibbe DL, Hackett J, Hurley M, McFarland A, Schubert KG, Schultz A, Harris S. Ten Years of TAKE 10!(®): integrating physical activity with academic concepts in elementary school classrooms. Prev Med. 2011;52(Suppl 1):S43–50.
21. Ma JK, Le Mare L, Gurd BJ. Four minutes of in-class high-intensity interval activity improves selective attention in 9- to 11-year-olds. Appl Physiol Nutr Metab. 2015;40(3):238–44.
22. Wilson M. Six views of embodied cognition. Psychon Bull Rev. 2002;9(4):625–36.
23. Mavilidi MF, Pesce C, Benzing V, Schmidt M, Paas F, Okely AD, Vazou S. Meta-analysis of movement-based interventions to aid academic and behavioral outcomes: a taxonomy of relevance and integration. Educ Res Rev. 2022;37:100478.
24. Mavilidi MF, Ruiter M, Schmidt M, Okely AD, Loyens S, Chandler P, Paas F. A Narrative review of school-based physical activity for enhancing cognition and learning: the importance of relevancy and integration. Front Psychol. 2018;9:2079.
25. Daly Smith AJ, Zwolinsky S, McKenna J, Tomporowski PD, Defeyter MA, Manley A. Systematic review of acute physically active learning and classroom movement breaks on children's physical activity, cognition, academic performance and classroom behavior: understanding critical design features. BMJ Open Sport Exerc Med. 2018;4(1):e000341.
26. Watson A, Timperio A, Brown H, Best K, Hesketh KD. Effect of classroom-based physical activity interventions on academic and physical activity outcomes: a systematic review and meta-analysis. Int J Behav Nutr Phys Act. 2017;14(1):114.
27. Masini A, Marini S, Gori D, Leoni E, Rochira A, Dallolio L. Evaluation of school-based interventions of active breaks in primary schools: a systematic review and meta-analysis. J Sci Med Sport. 2020;23(4):377–84.
28. Peiris DLIHK, Duan Y, Vandelanotte C, Liang W, Yang M, Baker JS. Effects of in-classroom physical activity breaks on children's academic performance, cognition, health behaviors and health outcomes: a systematic review and meta-analysis of randomized controlled trials. Int J Environ Res Public Health. 2022;19(15):9479.
29. Ruhland S, Lange KW. Effect of classroom-based physical activity interventions on attention and on-task behavior in schoolchildren: a systematic review. Sports Med Health Sci. 2021;3(3):125–33.
30. Bedard C, St John L, Bremer E, Graham JD, Cairney J. A systematic review and meta-analysis on the effects of physically active classrooms on educational and enjoyment outcomes in school age children. PLoS One. 2019;14(6):e0218633.
31. Papadopoulos N, Mantilla A, Bussey K, Emonson C, Olive L, McGillivray J, Pesce C, Lewis S, Rinehart N. Understanding the benefits of brief classroom-based physical activity interventions on primary school-aged children's enjoyment and subjective wellbeing: a systematic review. J Sch Health. 2022;92(9):916–32.
32. Robles Campos A, Zapata-Lamana R, Gutiérrez MA, Cigarroa Cuevas II, Nazar G, Salas Bravo C, Sánchez López M, Reyes Molina D. Psychological outcomes of classroom-based physical activity interventions in children 6-to 12-year-olds: a scoping review. Retos. 2023;48:388–400.

33. Liu A-L, Hu X-Q, Ma G-S, Cui Z-H, Pan Y-P, Chang S-Y, et al. Report on childhood obesity in China (6) evaluation of a classroom-based physical activity promotion program. Biomed Environ Sci. 2007;20(1):19–23.
34. de Greeff JW, Hartman E, Mullender-Wijnsma MJ, Bosker RJ, Doolaard S, Visscher C. Effect of physically active academic lessons on body mass index and physical fitness in primary school children. J Sch Health. 2016;86(5):346–52.
35. Donnelly JE, Lambourne K. Classroom-based physical activity, cognition, and academic achievement. Prev Med. 2011;52:S36–42.
36. Donnelly JE, Hillman CH, Greene JL, Hansen DM, Gibson CA, Sullivan DK, et al. Physical activity and academic achievement across the curriculum: results from a 3-year cluster-randomized trial. Prev Med. 2017;99:140–5.
37. Michael SL, Merlo CL, Basch CE, Wentzel KR, Wechsler H. Critical connections: health and academics. J Sch Health. 2015;85(11):740–58.
38. Martin R, Murtagh EM. Effect of active lessons on physical activity, academic, and health outcomes: a systematic review. Res Q Exerc Sport. 2017;88(2):149–68.
39. Thapa A, Cohen J, Guffey S, Higgins-D'Alessandro A. A review of school climate research. Rev Educ Res. 2013;83:357–85.
40. Jones M, Defever E, Letsinger A, Steele J, Mackintosh KA. A mixed-studies systematic review and meta-analysis of school-based interventions to promote physical activity and/or reduce sedentary time in children. J Sport Health Sci. 2020;9(1):3–17.
41. Chalkley AE, Mandelid MB, Thurston M, Daly Smith A, Singh A, Huiberts I, et al. "Go beyond your own comfort zone and challenge yourself": a comparison on the use of physically active learning in Norway, The Netherlands and the UK. Teach Teach Educ. 2022;118:103825.
42. Mandelid MB. Approaching physically active learning as a multi, inter, and transdisciplinary research field. Front Sports Act Living. 2023;5:1228340.
43. Norris E, Van Steen T, Direito A, Stamatakis E. Physically active lessons in schools and their impact on physical activity, educational, health and cognition outcomes: a systematic review and meta-analysis. Br J Sports Med. 2020;54(14):826–38.
44. Ottesen CL, von Seelen J. Physically active lessons in secondary school: an intervention study. 2019:1–23.
45. Daly Smith A, Ottesen C, Mandelid M, von Seelen J, Trautner N, Resaland G. ACTivate European physically active learning teacher training curriculum. Sogndal. 2021.
46. Sánchez-Oliva D, García-Calvo T, Sánchez-López M, Castro-Piñero J, Grao-Cruces A, Martins J, et al. EUMOVE Project: an Erasmus+ Project for the promotion of healthy lifestyles among children and adolescents. Eur J Pub Health. 2022;32(Supplement_2):ckac095-016.
47. Grao-Cruces A, Camiletti-Moirón D, Sánchez-Oliva D. Aprendizaje físicamente activo. Aprendizaje físicamente activo. Dykinson; 2023.
48. Sánchez-López M, Ruiz-Hermosa A, Redondo-Tébar A, Visier-Alfonso ME, Jimenez-López E, Martínez-Andres M, et al. Rationale and methods of the MOVI-da10! Study – a cluster-randomized controlled trial of the impact of classroom-based physical activity programs on children's adiposity, cognition and motor competence. BMC Public Health. 2019;19(1):417.
49. Amor-Barbosa M, Ortega-Martínez A, Carrasco-Uribarren A, Bagur-Calafat MC. Active school-based interventions to interrupt prolonged sitting improve daily physical activity: a systematic review and meta-analysis. Int J Environ Res Public Health. 2022;19(22):15409.
50. Masini A, Ceciliani A, Dallolio L, Gori D, Marini S. Evaluation of feasibility, effectiveness, and sustainability of school-based physical activity "active break" interventions in preadolescent and adolescent students: a systematic review. Can J Public Health. 2022;113(5):713–25.
51. Infantes-Paniagua Á, Silva AF, Ramirez-Campillo R, Sarmento H, González-Fernández FT, González-Víllora S, et al. Active school breaks and students' attention: a systematic review with meta-analysis. Brain Sci. 2021;11(6):675.
52. Chang YK, Labban JD, Gapin JI, Etnier JL. The effects of acute exercise on cognitive performance: a meta-analysis. Brain Res. 2012;1453:87–101.

53. Mavilidi MF, Drew R, Morgan PJ, Lubans DR, Schmidt M, Riley N. Effects of different types of classroom physical activity breaks on children's on-task behavior, academic achievement and cognition. Acta Paediatr. 2020;109(1):158–65.
54. Dl K, Cushman D, Reynolds J, Njike V, Ja T, Walker J. Putting physical activity where it fits in the school day: preliminary results of the ABC (Activity Bursts in the Classroom) for fitness program. Prev Chronic Dis. 2010;7(4):A82.
55. van den Berg V, Saliasi E, de Groot RHM, Chinapaw MJM, Singh AS. Improving cognitive performance of 9–12 years old children: Just Dance? A randomized controlled trial. Front Psychol. 2019;10:174.
56. Drummy C, Murtagh EM, McKee DP, Breslin G, Davison GW, Murphy MH. The effect of a classroom activity break on physical activity levels and adiposity in primary school children. J Paediatr Child Health. 2016;52(7):745–9.
57. Redondo-Tebar A, Ruiz-Hermosa A, Martinez-Vizcaino V, Bermejo-Cantarero A, Cavero-Redondo I, Martín-Espinosa NM, et al. Effectiveness of MOVI-KIDS programme on health-related quality of life in children: cluster-randomized controlled trial. Scand J Med Sci Sports. 2023;33(5):660–9.
58. Martínez-Vizcaíno V, Soriano-Cano A, Garrido-Miguel M, Cavero-Redondo I, de Medio EP, Madrid VM, et al. The effectiveness of a high-intensity interval games intervention in schoolchildren: a cluster-randomized trial. Scand J Med Sci Sports. 2022;32(4):765–81.
59. Sánchez-López M, Cavero-Redondo I, Álvarez-Bueno C, Ruiz-Hermosa A, Pozuelo-Carrascosa DP, Díez-Fernández A, et al. Impact of a multicomponent physical activity intervention on cognitive performance: the MOVI-KIDS study. Scand J Med Sci Sports. 2019;29(5):766–75.
60. Martínez-Vizcaíno V, Pozuelo-Carrascosa DP, García-Prieto JC, Cavero-Redondo I, Solera-Martínez M, Garrido-Miguel M, et al. Effectiveness of a school-based physical activity intervention on adiposity, fitness and blood pressure: MOVI-KIDS study. Br J Sports Med. 2020;54(5):279.
61. Sánchez-López M, Ruiz-Hermosa A, Martínez-Vizcaíno V, Redondo-Tebar A. MOVI-da 10! An active breaks programme to improve health and cognitive performance in preschool education. UCLM; 2020.

Chapter 11
Multicomponent School-Based Physical Activity Programs

Collin A. Webster

11.1 The Problem of Physical Inactivity

Regularly engaging in physical activity (PA) improves physical, mental, social, and emotional health, increases overall well-being, and constitutes an important measure in the prevention of noncommunicable diseases [1]. However, one in four adults and over 80% of adolescents worldwide do not meet PA guidelines [2]. It is anticipated that within this decade, US$ 300 billion (INT$ 524 billion) will be spent on treating diseases that PA can help to prevent [3]. In 2012, leading public health scientists deemed physical inactivity a pandemic, noting that it was the fourth leading cause of death worldwide [4]. Lack of PA may be attributed to many factors [5, 6]. Some factors, such as age, biological sex, race, and ethnicity, are considered invariant in nature (i.e., not modifiable as intervention targets), while others, such as the physical, social, and technological environments in which people live, are considered modifiable [7], and warrant prioritization in interventions designed to increase PA behavior.

11.2 Addressing Physical Inactivity Through the School System

The school system spanning primary/elementary and secondary education has garnered much attention in efforts to promote and increase PA. "System" is used in an ecological sense to refer to the multiple spheres of influence acting upon children

C. A. Webster (✉)
Department of Kinesiology, Texas A&M University – Corpus Christi, Corpus Christi, TX, USA
e-mail: collin.webster@tamucc.edu

and adolescents through schools (Fig. 11.1). Building upon previous social-ecological models [8–10], spheres of influence are envisioned here to encompass the opportunities afforded across the school day, people's intrapersonal characteristics, such as their beliefs and abilities, and the resource, social, and policy environments. The appeal of addressing physical inactivity through the school system lies largely in the understanding that this system has extensive reach and existing resources to facilitate behavior change. Each school and its constellation of community allies contribute to a collective constituting the world's largest institutionally based intervention to foster learning and influence behavior across the formative years of human development. Early intervention through the school system may lead to a generation of adults who are more physically active, given evidence that PA behavior tracks from childhood to adulthood [11].

Another reason schools can be viewed as a suitable setting for PA promotion is because there is convincing evidence that PA often supports students' academic engagement and performance, which are priorities for school leaders [12]. Participating in PA is tied to students' cognitive functioning, ability to stay on task during classroom lessons, and achievement in reading and math [13, 14]. It is thus easy to argue that the agendas of education and public health stand to gain from cross-sector collaboration to ensure all school-age youth have access to ample opportunities for PA participation. The Whole School, Whole Community, Whole Child (WSCC) model stands as an exemplar of such collaboration applied to the

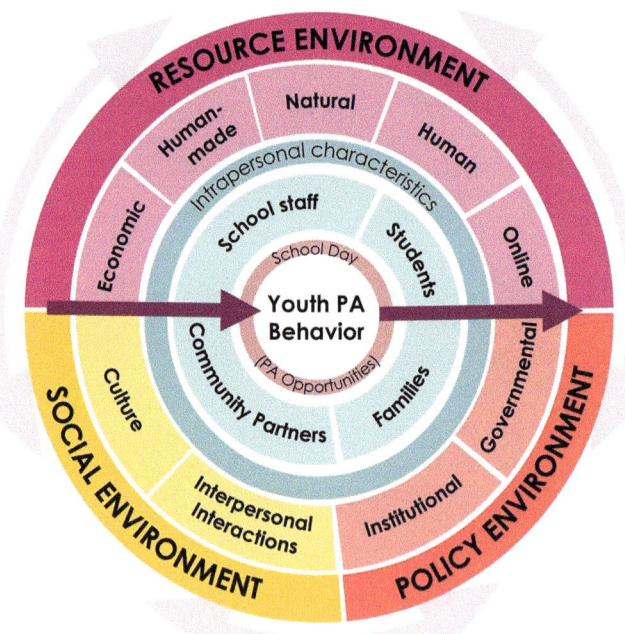

Fig. 11.1 Physical activity promotion through the school system. PA, physical activity

broader domain of school health [15]. WSCC combines elements of the Coordinated School Health (CSH) model and the Whole Child (WC) model to holistically address child health and academic success through ten components: (a) health education; (b) nutrition environment and services; (c) employee wellness; (d) social and emotional climate; (e) physical environment; (f) health services; (g) counseling, psychological, and social services; (h) community involvement; (i) family engagement; and (j) physical education (PE) and PA. The model represents a systems approach as it highlights environmental factors within the school and the community that influence these outcomes. Furthermore, the synergistic potential of the system through coordination among the model's components, between the school and the community, and across policy, process, and practice is emphasized.

The implementation of PA promotion initiatives through the school system is also cost effective [16, 17]. For example, authors of a simulation study in the United States reported that implementing a national policy that increases the amount of time elementary students spend being physically active during regularly scheduled PE lessons would reduce children's body mass index (BMI) by 0.020 units [17]. The estimated cost would be US$ 401 per BMI unit reduction after 2 years, substantially less than the estimated cost of clinical and surgical treatments for obese youth, which would be US$ 1000 to US$ 2100 per BMI unit change [17]. In a different US-based study, authors estimated that there would be no additional cost to usual school expenditures for time spent doing two daily 10-min in-class PA breaks [18].

Yet, it must also be recognized that school-based PA promotion has limitations and faces challenges. The school system does not reach all school-age youth. One in every five children ages 5–17 worldwide (303 million) are out of school, due to poverty and living in countries afflicted by war, disasters, and other humanitarian emergencies [19]. Another problem is that educational resourcing is uneven. A notable example of this is school funding, which varies greatly across income levels and race/ethnicity. Low-income countries spend US$ 53 per student, whereas upper-middle income countries spend US$ 7800 per student [20]. In the United States, the Center for American Progress reported in 2012 that schools made up of 90% or more students of color spent US$ 733 less per student annually than schools made up of 90% or more white students [21]. One of the biggest challenges to school-based PA promotion is that current educational practices tend to restrict students' PA. In a review of studies conducted in the United States, authors found that on average, students were sedentary 63% of their time at school [22]. School leaders and teachers feel pressure to produce academic results that meet the expectations and requirements of educational standards, policies, and mandates. Despite the many known benefits of PA and consequences of physical inactivity, concerns persist that PA competes with academic learning time in high stakes subjects, such as reading and math, where schools are most accountable for competitive test scores. Authors have documented a notable decline in school PE programming alongside the increased focus on academic testing. From 2000 to 2013, global averages for allocated curriculum time in primary/elementary and secondary PE dropped from 116 to 97 min per week and from 143 to 99 min per week, respectively [23].

11.3 Whole-of-School Physical Activity: Concept, National Initiatives, and Lessons Learned

An innovative approach to school-based PA programming that has emerged in recent years is what has been referred to as WOS PA. This term gained traction via a 2013 report by the Institute of Medicine (now the National Academies of Science) in the United States, in which WOS PA was defined as when "all of the school's components and resources operate in a coordinated and dynamic manner to provide access, encouragement, and programs that enable all students to engage in vigorous- or moderate-intensity PA 60 min or more each day" [24]. The IOM further explained that WOS PA expands to all segments of the school day, including the hours before, during, and after school, and draws upon the involvement of everyone within the school system, including students, school staff, and community partners. While WOS PA is not an answer to all the limitations and challenges of school-based PA promotion, it provides a systems-aligned conceptual frame for research, professional practice, and policy aimed at increasing daily PA participation among school-age youth. In 2022, the International Society for Physical Activity and Health (ISPAH) identified WOS PA as one of eight investments that work for increasing PA [25].

Several countries have implemented WOS PA initiatives. Some notable examples are Schools on the Move (Finland), Active School Flag (ASF, Ireland), Active Schools (United States), and Creating Active Schools (CAS, United Kingdom). Finland has seen much success with its initiative, as 90% of comprehensive schools nationally have been designated "Schools on the Move" since the initiative's launch in 2010 [26]. To earn this designation, schools apply for government funding (the initiative is financed by the Ministry of Education and Culture), which the schools then use to develop and evaluate their PA programming in ways that best fit their needs and goals and with the support of the Schools on the Move program. Schools are not required to meet specific criteria, but the initiative aligns with national education policy that promotes customization, creativity, risk-taking, and shared responsibility [27]. Schools have chosen to implement practices that increase organized PA opportunities beyond PE, improve PA equipment and facilities, and encourage involvement of students, teachers, school leaders, parents, and municipalities in PA planning and promotion [28].

The ASF initiative in Ireland has also had considerable success. ASF was originally designed for implementation in primary schools and has more recently expanded to the secondary school setting [29]. The initiative began in 2009 with Ireland's Department of Education and Skills as its primary funder. In 2015, Ireland's Department of Health joined as a funder, and in 2016, the initiative was added to Ireland's National Physical Activity Plan [30]. By 2020, 85% of primary schools nationally had engaged with the initiative and nearly half of all-primary schools met pre-established "success criteria" to earn a flag and be named an active school [30]. There are 47 criteria that fall within four categories, including PE (e.g., minimum of 60 min of PE each week for all children, PE staff undergo continuing professional development annually), PA (e.g., school provides two daily playground breaks for all children, every class provides short PA breaks as part of their daily routine), partnerships (e.g., school informs students and parents about PA opportunities in the community, school seeks support to ensure PE and other PA opportunities are inclusive for students with special needs), and Active School Week (e.g., schools include students in the design and organization of the event, school promotes cross-curricular PA during the event) [30]. Schools are required to self-evaluate their implementation and provide evidence of meeting the criteria to be accredited with Active School Flag. Although all criteria must be met, teacher feedback was used to develop the criteria and schools are afforded flexibility in terms of when they need to meet different criteria. Active School Flag offers workshops to aid schools in meeting the criteria and to facilitate a community of practice approach to professional development [30].

Implementation rates for the Active Schools initiative in the United States are more difficult to determine due to differences in the way an active school has been defined in national studies. While the initiative began in 2013 (originally called *Let's Move!* Active Schools), its conceptual basis can be traced to earlier work in the 1980s on comprehensive school health [31], and more specifically a 2007 publication in the *Journal of Physical Education, Recreation and Dance* [32] and then a 2008 position statement by the *American Alliance for Health, Physical Education, Recreation and Dance* (AAHPERD)—now the *Society of Health and Physical Educators* (SHAPE) America [33]. The focus of this work was on a comprehensive school PA program (CSPAP), which the *Centers for Disease Control and Prevention* (CDC) adopted as the national framework for school PE and PA in 2019 [34] and the *Physical Activity Alliance included in the National Physical Activity Plan* in 2016 [35]. The CSPAP framework includes five components: (a) PE, (b) PA during school, (c) PA before and after school, (d) staff involvement (including staff wellness programming and staff promotion of youth PA), and (e) family and community engagement. Expansions of the framework have highlighted the importance of environmental factors, both internal (e.g., a CSPAP champion, administrative support, policies, and normative beliefs that support PA promotion in the school culture) [36] and external (e.g., university support, communities of practice) to the school [37], to build capacity for program implementation. AAHPERD reported in 2011 that only 16% of elementary schools, 13% of middle schools, and 6% of high schools nationally had implemented all CSPAP components [38]. In a different national survey using 2016 data, the Centers for Disease Control and Prevention (CDC) found that the percentage of secondary schools that had implemented all CSPAP components ranged from 0.07% to 13.9% across states [39]. More recently, however, authors have argued that there should be less focus on ensuring all CSPAP components are implemented [40]. Rather, schools should be able to draw from the CSPAP framework as needed to ensure students receive quality PE and meet current PA guidelines. Using this more flexible conceptualization of a CSPAP, national surveys conducted with school principals and PE teachers indicate that around 70% of schools have adopted a CSPAP [41, 42]. The most frequently reported CSPAP-aligned school practices across elementary and secondary school levels included standards-based instruction in PE, classroom-based PA, and staff wellness programming [42]. SHAPE America, the CDC, and other organizations provide CSPAP training and resources to support schools' planning, implementation, and evaluation [43]. However, policies and funding from state and federal agencies have been inconsistent, underutilized, or lacking in many instances to help institutionalize active schools at scale.

CAS in the United Kingdom is one of the most recent examples of a national WOS PA initiative. The initiative was launched in 2019 in Leeds, United Kingdom, through a multisector collaboration of public health, education, and sport professionals and local authorities who, through an iterative process, co-designed a framework to guide planning, implementation, and evaluation [44]. Like the CSPAP framework and its conceptual expansions, the CAS framework identifies school contexts where PA can occur (e.g., PE lessons, regular classroom time, break periods, before and after school clubs), emphasizes the need for a collaborative and coordinated support system, and highlights the importance of the policy, physical, and social environments in shaping PA opportunities. A distinct feature of the framework is that it places whole-of-school practices and ethos at its center and clearly considers the role of evidence-informed initial teacher training and continuing professional development in contributing to this culture. CAS is led by a national team that includes the University of Bradford, Yorkshire Sport Foundation, and Bradford Institute for Health Research [45]. The national team works with local leadership teams to train CAS champions (mainly representatives from local schools) to support an annual cycle of self-assessment, planning, and implementation [45]. To date, no national-level data on CAS implementation have been reported, but over 200 schools have signed up to participate in the initiative [46]. Multiple organizations, including the Bradford metropolitan government, help to fund CAS [47]. However, not all schools that have adopted CAS received funding and one study found no differences in implementation between schools that received funding and those that did not [45].

The national WOS PA initiatives in Finland, Ireland, the United States, and the United Kingdom demonstrate that the school system provides a viable means for large-scale youth PA promotion. Some of the common assets among these initiatives are the inclusion of multiple components; an emphasis on a strong PE program; PA opportunities beyond PE, both during and outside of school hours; the involvement of multiple organizations and entities beyond schools themselves; a shared vision of an active school that allows for flexible implementation and teacher input; the provision of trainings, professional development, and resources for school staff; a focus on school culture; and school staff's self-assessment of the school's needs, the implementation processes, and program outcomes. Funding has clearly played an important role in most cases, although the evidence from CAS implementation suggests that not every school requires extra funds to adopt active school practices.

11.4 Implementing Whole-of-School Physical Activity: Key Factors for Consideration Within Each Sphere of Influence

Understanding what it takes to effect large-scale systems change through national WOS PA initiatives is important for achieving broad and sustainable impact on children and adolescents' PA and development toward pursuing a physically active lifestyle as adults. However, planning, implementing, and evaluating WOS PA also requires a close inspection of the various factors known to be associated with youth PA. Returning to the concept of the school system introduced earlier in this chapter (Fig. 11.1), these factors can be categorized using three spheres of influence, namely, the opportunities afforded across the school day, the intrapersonal characteristics of the individuals within the system, and the system's resource, social, and policy environments. It should be noted that intraindividual factors are likely to exert the strongest influence on behavior (e.g., whether a teacher creates a PA opportunity, whether a child chooses to engage in a PA opportunity) [42, 48, 49]. Additionally, all factors in the system have the potential to either positively or negatively influence youth PA. For example, the built environment may support or discourage PA, or school staff may use PA-promoting or PA-thwarting behaviors. Furthermore, factors within and across each sphere can influence one another (e.g., interactions between families and school staff may influence institutional policies; parents who perceive PA as important may influence human resources via volunteering to help with school PA opportunities). Comprehensively reviewing all factors linked to youth PA behavior is beyond the scope of this chapter (a recent review identified 167 facilitators and barriers that influence children and adolescents' PA from a social-ecological perspective) [50]. Therefore, examples will be provided to illustrate key areas of focus in the literature and draw implications for future research and professional practice. Consideration will be directed toward modifiable factors within the intrapersonal and environmental spheres of influence as these factors lend themselves to interventions aimed at increasing school day PA opportunities and youth PA engagement.

11.4.1 The Intrapersonal Sphere

Within the intrapersonal sphere, students' own thoughts and abilities directly impact their PA behavior. Examples include perceived competence, motivation, attitudes, physical skills, and physical fitness [51–53]. Some of these factors, such as perceived competence, physical skills, and physical fitness, strengthen in their association with PA behavior as children get older [53]. It is important to recognize the inter-play between different intrapersonal factors. For instance, students are more self-determined in their motivation to be physically active if they also perceive that they have autonomy as learners in PE [52]. Interventions to increase children and adolescents' PA should begin with assessing students' intrapersonal profiles in relation to PA participation, as this information must form the basis for decision-making about appropriate environmental supports for PA promotion.

The intrapersonal sphere also includes the perceptions and competencies of the people who are asked to promote children and adolescents' PA, including students' peers, school staff, parents, and community partners. Peer support is an evidence-based strategy for youth PA engagement [54], but the intrapersonal factors influencing such support are not well investigated. There could be value in exploring the beliefs and lived experiences of students who engage in peer support activities like volunteering to serve as PA role models, assisting with PE instruction, and helping to lead other PA opportunities. Such research could be used to better prepare and assist students in taking on peer support roles for PA promotion. A substantial amount of the evidence concerning intrapersonal factors influencing youth PA behavior centers on school staff [55]. Authors often have called upon PE teachers to serve as PA school leaders [56–58], although PE teachers do not always view WOS PA as part of their professional responsibilities [59]. Physical education teachers who perceive implementation as simple, compatible with their skills, advantageous compared to current practices, and open to multicomponent involvement from the outset may be more likely to engage in WOS PA initiatives [41]. Additionally, PE teachers' WOS PA engagement may hinge on how knowledgeable they feel about such initiatives and how innovative they perceive themselves to be as educators [60]. Adequately preparing PE teachers as school PA leaders should be an integral part of both pre-service and in-service teacher education and should focus on the development of knowledge, skills, and values aligned with promoting PA through the school system.

Given that schools typically have many more classroom teachers than PE teachers, it is critical to understand how classroom teachers can help to support WOS PA initiatives. An extensive literature describes the intrapersonal factors associated with classroom teachers' PA promotion [61–64]. Among the most frequently reported factors are classroom management skills and perceived competence or efficacy to integrate PA opportunities during regular classroom time [64]. Other factors include satisfaction with personal experiences as a student in PE, the perceived attributes of PA promotion during class time, teachers' educational innovativeness, intrinsic motivation for PA promotion, and personal health and PA behavior [64]. To increase classroom teachers' involvement in WOS PA, pre-service teacher education programs and in-service continuing professional development should prioritize explaining how classroom management and PA promotion overlap [65] and building teachers' competencies for PA promotion during class time. Teacher trainings may also aim to raise awareness of quality PE and the benefits of PE and PA for students; encourage creativity regarding PA promotion; and foster self-care through personal PA and other healthy behaviors.

Relatively little research has addressed the intrapersonal factors associated with school leaders' involvement in WOS PA. School leaders are at the helm of school change efforts, serving as gatekeepers for various initiatives, setting the pace for program implementation, and in many ways creating school culture. Therefore, school leaders' support of WOS PA is vital to its successful adoption and maintenance. In one US-based study, school leaders at the school, district, and state levels who participated in focus groups lacked an awareness and understanding of outcomes used to evaluate quality PE [66]. Another study in the United States, which drew upon survey data from a national sample of school principals, also underscored the importance of program outcomes in WOS PA [42]. Participants were more likely to report being involved with a CSPAP if they felt the program would result in positive outcomes, such as promoting whole-child learning, students' attention to academics, and students' attendance at school. Further investigation with the same sample of principals revealed that, like classroom teachers, principals' own childhood experiences in school PE predicted their current CSPAP involvement [67]. Other research in the United States using a national sample of principals indicates that modifiable intrapersonal factors, including value for PA and personal PA behaviors, play a minor role in predicting the presence of an active school compared to principals' years of experience and environmental factors [68]. Opportunities to learn about the many benefits (e.g., academic, physical, social, emotional) of WOS PA, including quality PE, should be embedded within administrator preparation programs, and continuing professional development for school leaders. The educational impact of such opportunities may be leveraged through discussions that tie school-based PA promotion to personal lifestyle choices and involve school leaders with different levels of experience who work in diverse school contexts.

Parents and community partners also play key roles in WOS PA. Only scant research exists on intrapersonal factors driving parents' involvement with WOS PA. The results of a national survey in the United States indicated that parents were more likely to advocate for and be involved in an active school if they had positive attitudes toward before and after school PA programming [69]. This suggests that schools should provide quality out-of-school time PA programs (e.g., intramurals, clubs, active transportation options), raise parents' awareness of these initiatives, and then seek parents' support for active schools. Regarding the involvement of community partners in WOS PA, the literature offers little insight from an intrapersonal perspective. In future research, scholars should investigate the role of attitudes, self-efficacy, motivation, and other intrapersonal variables in community partners' WOS PA involvement.

11.4.2 The Environmental Sphere

As shown in Fig. 11.1, the environmental sphere of the school system encompasses the resource, social, and policy environments. The resource environment consists of economic, human-made, natural, human, and online resources. Economic resources include all monetary assets to support WOS PA, such as government spending, alumni donations, family income, and other funding sources. Human-made resources refer to things that people create, such as physical structures (e.g., sports facilities, parks, sidewalks), equipment/materials (e.g., PE equipment, classroom materials, school-issued laptops for online learning), schedules (e.g., allocated curriculum time for PE, scheduled movement breaks during regular classroom time, scheduled PA time in after school programs), and plans (e.g., lesson plans, curriculum guides, school-level strategic plans). Natural resources include the geography, landscape, climate, and other relatively invariant features of the environment. Human resources have to do with the quantity (e.g., the number of parent volunteers to help with a PA promotion event) and quality of personnel (e.g., whether the person teaching PE is a certified PE teacher) who are available to support WOS PA. Online resources include Internet access and the virtual infrastructure related to WOS PA, such as the navigability of learning management system (LMS) platforms used for virtual PA programming.

In a national survey in the United States, school staff cited factors in the resource environment, such as lack of funding, lack of facilities, and school scheduling, as barriers to implementing a CSPAP [38]. Ways to modify the resource environment for PA promotion range widely in terms of their economic burden on schools and community partners. Constructing new buildings, sidewalks, bicycle lanes, and parks may not be economically feasible in many cases. However, there are also lower-cost options that can increase youth PA. For example, classrooms can be outfitted to be more movement permissive by changing classroom furniture and seating (e.g., replacing traditional desks with stand-biased desks, using exercise balls instead of chairs) and purchasing evidence-based curricula that teachers can use to infuse PA into academic lessons [70–72]. Still other options are cost-free, such as using playground markings, zoning, and portable equipment at recess, optimizing the use of outdoor space to teach PE lessons, and purposively scheduling and planning PA opportunities as part of routine practice in after school programs [73–75]. Another cost-effective approach could be the use of online resources, particularly in leveraging family and community support for PA promotion. Although WOS PA programming delivered virtually/online remains an under-researched area of focus, authors have offered considerations for online WOS PA promotion based on the CSPAP framework [76].

Social factors associated with children and adolescents' PA span the cultural norms and interpersonal interactions within the school system. With respect to school culture, it is important that teachers perceive that they have support for PA promotion from school leaders, their colleagues, and parents [49, 61]. Some evidence indicates that secondary schools are less likely to implement WOS PA than primary/elementary schools [68]. This could be due in part to differences between primary/elementary and secondary schools in normative beliefs and behaviors that make up the school culture [77]. Family culture also plays a role in youth PA engagement. Examples include parents role modeling PA and providing logistical support for their children's PA participation [78].

Interpersonal interactions within the school system occur at school, home, and in the community. These interactions can occur both within (e.g., student-student, parent-parent) and between different groups (e.g., student-teacher, principal-community partner). One type of interaction that has received considerable investigative attention is staff-child interactions. Staff can influence children's PA by enacting certain behaviors while leading activities. Examples of such behaviors include making sure to not have children wait their turn in lines, reducing team size when playing games, and actively supervising and staying engaged while children play/practice [73, 79]. During normal classroom time, teachers can provide PA breaks, teach academic lessons that involve PA opportunities, and use a variety of other strategies to reduce sitting and keep children active during school [80]. Student-student interactions also warrant careful consideration [81, 82]. Studies have identified numerous ways in which peers influence one another's PA [50, 54, 83]. In one study, for instance, displaying a desire for friends to be active, participating together in PA, and teaching each other how to play a sport increased the chances that adolescents would engage in five or more days of moderate PA and three or more days of vigorous PA per week [54].

Another key consideration related to interpersonal interactions is teacher socialization. Teachers' PA promotion behavior stems in part from their previous and current school-related social experiences, which span being a student in K-12 education, being a pre-service teacher in a formal (e.g., university-based) teacher education program, and being an in-service teacher [84]. In a recent US study, efficacy to implement WOS PA was associated with socializing factors from pre-service teacher education (e.g., implementing school-based PA opportunities with in-service teachers) and in-service teaching (e.g., seeing students enjoy participating in WOS PA opportunities and being supported by other teachers at school) in a national sample of PE teachers [85]. Other research has also highlighted the importance of teacher education and professional trainings in supporting WOS PA implementation [60, 86–90]. For example, university-facilitated field experiences focused on implementing PA during regular classroom time in elementary schools mutually benefited both pre-service and in-service teachers' PA promotion knowledge and skills [87].

Finally, the policy environment captures institutional policies and governmental policies related to WOS PA. Institutional policies are created by organizations, such as schools or community recreation centers, whereas governmental policies are created by public policymakers who work at local or higher levels (e.g., state, federal) of government. A major focus of policies related to school-based PA is time. For instance, many government policies require a certain number of minutes be provided for students to be physically active each week in school. Yet, such policies often lack the specificity and accountability needed to impact school practices and ensure children and adolescents gain the desired benefits from policy implementation [91]. Much of the research on WOS PA to date has focused on bottom-up approaches that emphasize working with teachers to increase children and adolescents' PA. Increased attention to top-down approaches that can institutionalize WOS PA at scale is needed.

11.5 Conclusions

The potential of the school system to inculcate active living in children and adolescents continues to gain interest in the education and health sectors and is increasingly underpinned by evidence to guide WOS PA implementation. Further research is needed to understand how to maximize synergies within the system, tailor implementation to secondary school contexts, strengthen accountability through the policy environment, and sustain programming. Increased attention must also be given to establishing internationally agreed upon assessments and metrics for measuring, monitoring, and evaluating WOS PA [3]. Ultimately, it must be acknowledged that PA is but one of society's many agendas for the school system and various advocacy groups vie for schools' adoption of new curricula, programs, and initiatives. Weaving PA into the fabric of school life will require a shared understanding among all stakeholders that an active school is in everyone's best interest.

References

1. World Health Organization. Physical activity. Available from: https://www.who.int/news-room/fact-sheets/detail/physical-activity.
2. Guthold R, Stevens GA, Riley LM, Bull FC. Worldwide trends in insufficient physical activity from 2001 to 2016: a pooled analysis of 358 population-based surveys with 1.9 million participants. Lancet Glob Health. 2018;6(10):e1077–86.
3. World Health Organization. Global status report on physical activity 2022. Available from: https://iris.who.int/bitstream/handle/10665/363607/9789240059153-eng.pdf?sequence=1.
4. Kohl HW, Craig CL, Lambert EV, Inoue S, Alkandari JR, Leetongin G, et al. The pandemic of physical inactivity: global action for public health. The Lancet [Internet]. 2012;380(9838):294–305. Available from: https://www.thelancet.com/journals/lancet/article/PIIS0140-6736(12)60898-8/fulltext.
5. Physical activity. Available from: https://www.physio-pedia.com/Physical_Inactivity#cite_note-p9-11.
6. Harvard TH. Chan School of Public Health. Obesity prevention source. Environmental barriers to activity. Available from: https://www.hsph.harvard.edu/obesity-prevention-source/obesity-causes/physical-activity-environment/.
7. Seefeldt V, Malina RM, Clark MA. Factors affecting levels of physical activity in adults. Sports Med. 2002;32(3):143–68.
8. McLeroy KR, Bibeau D, Steckler A, Glanz K. An ecological perspective on health promotion programs. Health Educ Q. 1988;15(4):351–77.
9. Sallis JF, Cervero RB, Ascher W, Henderson KA, Kraft MK, Kerr J. An ecological approach to creating active living communities. Annu Rev Public Health. 2006;27(1):297–322.
10. Langille JLD, Rodgers WM. Exploring the influence of a social ecological model on school-based physical activity. Health Educ Behav. 2010;37(6):879–94.
11. Telama R. Tracking of physical activity from childhood to adulthood: a review. Obes Facts. 2009;2(3):187–95.
12. Chan TC, Jiang B, Chandler M, Morris R, Rebisz S, Turan S, Shu Z, Kpeglo S. School principals' self-perceptions of their roles and responsibilities in six countries. New Waves Educ Res Dev. 2019;22(2):37–61.

13. Ruhland S, Lange KW. Effect of classroom-based physical activity interventions on attention and on-task behavior in schoolchildren: a systematic review. Sports Med Health Sci. 2021;3(3):125–33.
14. Álvarez-Bueno C, Pesce C, Cavero-Redondo I, Sánchez-López M, Garrido-Miguel M, Martínez-Vizcaíno V. Academic achievement and physical activity: a meta-analysis. Pediatr Int. 2017;140(6):e20171498. Available from: https://pediatrics.aappublications.org/content/140/6/e20171498.
15. Lewallen TC, Hunt H, Potts-Datema W, Zaza S, Giles W. The whole school, whole community, whole child model: a new approach for improving educational attainment and healthy development for students. J Sch Health [Internet]. 2015;85(11):729–39. Available from: https://onlinelibrary.wiley.com/doi/abs/10.1111/josh.12310.
16. Sutherland R, Reeves P, Campbell E, Lubans DR, Morgan PJ, Nathan N, et al. Cost effectiveness of a multi-component school-based physical activity intervention targeting adolescents: the "Physical Activity 4 Everyone" cluster randomized trial. Int J Behav Nutr Phys Act [Internet]. 2016;13(1). Available from: https://www.ncbi.nlm.nih.gov/pmc/articles/PMC4994166/.
17. Barrett JL, Gortmaker SL, Long MW, Ward ZJ, Resch SC, Moodie ML, et al. Cost effectiveness of an elementary school active physical education policy. Am J Prev Med [Internet]. 2015 [cited 2019 May 14];49(1):148–59. Available from: http://choicesproject.org/wp-content/uploads/2015/06/AMEPRE_49_1-Barrett.pdf.
18. Babey SH, Wu S, Cohen D. How can schools help youth increase physical activity? An economic analysis comparing school-based programs. Prev Med. 2014;69:S55–60.
19. UNICEF. 1 in 3 children and young people is out of school in countries affected by war or natural disasters. Available from: https://www.unicef.org/press-releases/1-3-children-and-young-people-out-school-countries-affected-war-or-natural-disasters.
20. World Bank Blogs. A call for transformative action on education financing as learning poverty soars. Available from: https://blogs.worldbank.org/education/call-transformative-action-education-financing-learning-poverty-soars.
21. Center for American Progress. Unequal education: federal loophole enables lower spending on students of color. Available from: https://cdn.uncf.org/wp-content/uploads/PDFs/UnequalEduation.pdf?_ga=2.220864088.1515144513.1705030684-278896860.1705030684.
22. Egan CA, Webster CA, Beets MW, Weaver RG, Russ LB, Michael D, Nesbitt DR, Orendorff KL. Sedentary time and behavior during school: a systematic review and meta-analysis. Am J Health Educ. 2019;50:283–90.
23. UNESCO. Worldwide survey of school physical education. Available form: https://en.unesco.org/inclusivepolicylab/e-teams/quality-physical-education-qpe-policy-project/documents/world-wide-survey-school-physical.
24. Kohl III HW, Cook HD; Committee on Physical Activity and Physical Education in the School Environment, Food and Nutrition Board, Institute of Medicine, editors. Educating the student body: taking physical activity and physical education to school. Washington, DC: National Academies Press (US); 2013.
25. ISPAH. Eight investments that work for physical activity. Available from: https://ispah.org/wp-content/uploads/2020/11/English-Eight-Investments-That-Work-FINAL.pdf.
26. Schools on the Move. Available from: https://schoolsonthemove.fi/about-us/.
27. Laakso L. Finnish schools on the move: students' physical activity and school-related social factors. 2017. Available from: https://www.researchgate.net/publication/323259365_Finnish_Schools_on_the_Move_Students%27_physical_activity_and_school-related_social_factors.
28. Blom A, Tammelin T, Laine K, Tolonen H. Bright spots, physical activity investments that work: the Finnish Schools on the Move programme. Br J Sports Med. 2017;52(13):820–2.
29. Ng KW, McHale F, Cotter K, O'Shea D, Woods C. Feasibility study of the secondary level Active School Flag programme: study protocol. J Funct Morphol Kinesiol. 2019;4(1):16.

30. Belton S, Britton Ú, Murtagh E, Meegan S, Duff C, McGann J. Ten years of "flying the flag": an overview and retrospective consideration of the active school flag physical activity initiative for children—design, development & evaluation. Children. 2020;7(12):300.
31. Allensworth DD, Kolbe LJ. The comprehensive school health program: exploring an expanded concept. J Sch Health. 2013;57(10):409–12.
32. Castelli DM, Beighle A. The physical education teacher as school activity director. J Phys Educ Recreat Dance. 2007;78(5):25–8.
33. National Association for Sport and Physical Education. Comprehensive School Physical Activity Programs. 2008. Available from: https://files.eric.ed.gov/fulltext/ED541610.pdf.
34. Centers for Disease Control and Prevention. Increasing physical education and physical activity: a framework for schools 2019. 2019. Available from: https://www.cdc.gov/healthyschools/physicalactivity/pdf/2019_04_25_PE-PA-Framework_508tagged.pdf.
35. National Physical Activity Plan. 2016. Available from: https://paamovewithus.org/wp-content/uploads/2020/07/National-PA-Plan.pdf.
36. Carson RL, Castelli DM, Beighle A, Erwin H. School-based physical activity promotion: a conceptual framework for research and practice. Child Obes. 2014;10(2):100–6.
37. Webster CA, Beets M, Weaver RG, Vazou S, Russ L. Rethinking recommendations for implementing comprehensive school physical activity programs: a partnership model. Quest. 2015;67(2):185–202.
38. American Alliance for Health, Physical Education, Recreation and Dance. Comprehensive School Physical Activity Program (CSPAP) survey report. Reston: Author; 2011.
39. Brener ND, Demissie Z, McManus T, Shanklin SL, Queen B, Kann L. School health profiles 2016: characteristics of health programs among secondary schools. Atlanta: Centers for Disease Control and Prevention; 2017. Available from: https://www.cdc.gov/healthyyouth/data/profiles/pdf/2016/2016_profiles_report.pdf.
40. Webster CA, Rink JE, Carson RL, Moon J, Gaudreault KL. The comprehensive school physical activity program model: a proposed illustrative supplement to help move the needle on youth physical activity. Kinesiol Rev. 2020;9(2):112–21.
41. Webster CA, Mîndrilă D, Moore C, Stewart G, Orendorff K, Taunton S. Measuring and comparing physical education teachers' perceived attributes of CSPAPs: an innovation adoption perspective. J Teach Phys Educ. 2020;39(1):78–90.
42. Orendorff K, Webster CA, Mîndrilă D, Cunningham KM, Doutis P, Dauenhauer B, et al. Principals' involvement in comprehensive school physical activity programmes: a social-ecological perspective. Eur Phys Educ Rev. 2020;27:1356336X2097668.
43. Centers for Disease Control and Prevention. National framework for physical activity and physical education. Available from: https://www.shapeamerica.org//Common/Uploaded%20files/uploads/pdfs/CSPAP/NationalFramework.pdf.
44. Daly-Smith A, Quarmby T, Archbold VSJ, Corrigan N, Wilson D, Resaland GK, et al. Using a multi-stakeholder experience-based design process to co-develop the Creating Active Schools Framework. Int J Behav Nutr Phys Act. 2020;17(1):13.
45. Helme ZE, Morris JL, Nichols J, Chalkley AE, Bingham DD, McLoughlin GM, et al. Assessing the impacts of creating active schools on organisational culture for physical activity. Int J Environ Res Public Health [Internet]. 2022 [cited 2023 Mar 14];19(24):16950. Available from: https://www.mdpi.com/1660-4601/19/24/16950.
46. Creating Active Schools. Available from: https://www.creatingactiveschools.org.
47. Morris JL, Chalkley A, Helme ZE, Timms O, Young E, McLoughlin GM, et al. Initial insights into the impact and implementation of Creating Active Schools in Bradford, UK. Int J Behav Nutr Phys Act. 2023;20(1):80.
48. Nam K, Kulinna PH, Mulhearn SC, Yu H, Griffo JM, Mason AJ. Social–ecological considerations in sustaining comprehensive school physical activity programs: a follow-up study. J Teach Phys Educ. 2023;42(1):144–54.

49. Webster CA, Caputi P, Perreault M, Doan R, Doutis P, Weaver RG. Elementary classroom teachers' adoption of physical activity promotion in the context of a statewide policy: an innovation diffusion and socio-ecologic perspective. J Teach Phys Educ. 2013;32(4):419–40.
50. Hu D, Zhou S, Crowley-McHattan ZJ, Liu Z. Factors that influence participation in physical activity in school-aged children and adolescents: a systematic review from the social ecological model perspective. Int J Environ Res Public Health. 2021;18(6):3147.
51. Sterdt E, Liersch S, Walter U. Correlates of physical activity of children and adolescents: a systematic review of reviews. Health Educ J. 2013;73(1):72–89.
52. Kalajas-Tilga H, Koka A, Hein V, Tilga H, Raudsepp L. Motivational processes in physical education and objectively measured physical activity among adolescents. J Sport Health Sci [Internet]. 2020;9(5):462–71. Available from: https://www.sciencedirect.com/science/article/pii/S2095254619300729.
53. den Uil AR, Janssen M, Busch V, Kat IT, Scholte RHJ. The relationships between children's motor competence, physical activity, perceived motor competence, physical fitness and weight status in relation to age. PLoS One. 2023;18(4):e0278438.
54. Haidar A, Ranjit N, Archer N, Hoelscher DM. Parental and peer social support is associated with healthier physical activity behaviors in adolescents: a cross-sectional analysis of Texas School Physical Activity and Nutrition (TX SPAN) data. BMC Public Health. 2019;19(1):640.
55. Webster CA, Hoke A, Cornett K, Goh TL, Pulling Kuhn A. Staff involvement and family and community engagement. J Phys Educ Recreat Dance. 2022;93(5):27–34.
56. Beighle A, Erwin H, Castelli D, Ernst M. Preparing physical educators for the role of physical activity director. J Phys Educ Recreat Dance. 2009;80(4):24–9.
57. Carson R. Certification and duties of a director of physical activity. J Phys Educ Recreat Dance. 2012;83(6):16–29.
58. Heidorn B, Centeio E. The director of physical activity and staff involvement. J Phys Educ Recreat Dance. 2012;83(7):13–26.
59. Carson RL, Kuhn AP, Moore JB, Castelli DM, Beighle A, Hodgin KL, et al. Implementation evaluation of a professional development program for comprehensive school physical activity leaders. Prev Med Rep. 2020;19:101109.
60. Webster CA, Mindrila D, Moore C, Stewart G, Orendorff K, Taunton S. Exploring the role of physical education teachers' domain-specific innovativeness, educational background, and perceived school support in CSPAP adoption. J Teach Phys Educ. 2020;39(1):36–47.
61. Webster CA, Russ L, Vazou S, Goh TL, Erwin H. Integrating movement in academic classrooms: understanding, applying and advancing the knowledge base. Obes Rev [Internet]. 2015;16(8):691–701. Available from: https://www.ncbi.nlm.nih.gov/pubmed/25904462.
62. Michael RD, Webster CA, Egan CA, Nilges L, Brian A, Johnson R, et al. Facilitators and barriers to movement integration in elementary classrooms: a systematic review. Res Q Exerc Sport. 2019;90(2):151–62.
63. Mulhearn SC, Kulinna PH, Webster C. Stakeholders' perceptions of implementation of a comprehensive school physical activity program: a review. Kinesiol Rev. 2020;9(2):159–69.
64. Webster CA. Toward a general theory of classroom teachers' movement integration. Kinesiol Rev. 2023:1–14.
65. Moon J, Webster CA, Herring J, Egan CA. Relationships between systematically observed movement integration and classroom management in elementary schools. J Posit Behav Interv. 2020;24(2):109830072094703.
66. Lounsbery MAF, McKenzie TL, Thompson HR. Prioritizing physical activity in schools. Transl J ACSM. 2019;4(22):248–56.
67. Orendorff K, Webster CA, Mindrila D, Cunningham KMW, Doutis P, Dauenhauer B, et al. Social-ecological and biographical perspectives of principals' involvement in comprehensive school physical activity programs: a person-centered analysis. Phys Educ Sport Pedagog. 2022;29:1–16.

68. Dauenhauer B, Ha T, Webster C, Erwin H, Centeio E, Papa J, et al. Predicting the presence of active schools: a national survey of school principals in the United States. J Phys Act Health. 2022;19(11):771–6.
69. Webster CA, McLoughlin G, Starrett A, Papa J, Erwin H, Reed JA, et al. Parents' perceptions and engagement regarding school-based physical activity promotion. Am J Health Promot [Internet]. 2021;35(8):1125–8. Available from: https://pubmed.ncbi.nlm.nih.gov/34047206/.
70. Mahar MT, Murphy SK, Rowe DA, Golden J, Tamlyn Shields A, Raedeke TD. Effects of a classroom-based program on physical activity and on-task behavior. Med Sci Sports Exerc [Internet]. 2006;38(12):2086–94. Available from: http://nycphysicaleducation.com/wp-content/uploads/2013/03/Effects-of-a-Classroom-Based-Program-on-Physical-Activity-and-On-Task-Behavior1.pdf.
71. Kibbe DL, Hackett J, Hurley M, McFarland A, Schubert KG, Schultz A, et al. Ten years of TAKE 10!(®): integrating physical activity with academic concepts in elementary school classrooms. Prev Med [Internet]. 2011 [cited 2019 Dec 5];52 Suppl 1:S43–50. Available from: https://www.ncbi.nlm.nih.gov/pubmed/21281670.
72. Hinckson E, Salmon J, Benden M, Clemes SA, Sudholz B, Barber SE, et al. Standing classrooms: research and lessons learned from around the world. Sports Med. 2015;46(7):977–87.
73. Beets MW, Glenn Weaver R, Brazendale K, Turner-McGrievy G, Saunders RP, Moore JB, et al. Statewide dissemination and implementation of physical activity standards in afterschool programs: two-year results. BMC Public Health. 2018;18(1):819.
74. Weaver RG, Webster CA, Beets MW, Brazendale K, Chandler J, Schisler L, et al. Initial outcomes of a participatory-based, competency-building approach to increasing physical education teachers' physical activity promotion and students' physical activity: a pilot study. Health Educ Behav. 2017;45(3):359–70.
75. Pfledderer CD, Kwon S, Strehli I, Byun W, Burns RD. The effects of playground interventions on accelerometer-assessed physical activity in pediatric populations: a meta-analysis. Int J Environ Res Public Health. 2022;19(6):3445.
76. Webster CA, D'Agostino E, Urtel M, McMullen J, Culp B, Egan Loiacono CA, et al. Physical education in the COVID era: considerations for online program delivery using the comprehensive school physical activity program framework. J Teach Phys Educ. 2021;40(2):327–36.
77. Fenesi B, Graham JD, Crichton M, Ogrodnik M, Skinner J. Physical activity in high school classrooms: a promising avenue for future research. Int J Environ Res Public Health. 2022;19(2):688.
78. Hutchens A, Lee RE. Parenting practices and children's physical activity: an integrative review. J Sch Nurs. 2017;34(1):68–85.
79. Brazendale K, Chandler JL, Beets MW, Weaver RG, Beighle A, Huberty JL, et al. Maximizing children's physical activity using the LET US Play principles. Prev Med. 2015;76:14–9.
80. Russ LB, Webster CA, Beets MW, Egan C, Weaver RG, Harvey R, et al. Development of the system for observing student movement in academic routines and transitions (SOSMART). Health Educ Behav. 2016;44(2):304–15.
81. Zhang T, Solmon MA, Gao Z, Kosma M. Promoting school students' physical activity: a social ecological perspective. J Appl Sport Psychol. 2012;24(1):92–105.
82. Abdelghaffar EA, Hicham EK, Siham B, Samira EF, Youness EA. Perspectives of adolescents, parents, and teachers on barriers and facilitators of physical activity among school-age adolescents: a qualitative analysis. Environ Health Prev Med. 2019;24(1):21.
83. Howie EK, Daniels BT, Guagliano JM. Promoting physical activity through youth sports programs: it's social. Am J Lifestyle Med [Internet]. 2018;14(1):155982761875484. Available from: https://www.ncbi.nlm.nih.gov/pmc/articles/PMC6933572/.
84. Richards KAR, Pennington CG, Sinelnikov OA. Teacher socialization in physical education: a scoping review of literature. Kinesiol Rev. 2019;8(2):86–99.
85. Merica CB, Egan CA, Webster CA, Mindrila D, Karp GG, Paul DR, et al. Association of Physical Educators' socialization experiences and confidence with respect to comprehensive school physical activity program implementation. Int J Environ Res Public Health. 2022;19(19):12005.

86. Webster CA, Nesbitt D, Lee H, Egan C. Preservice physical education teachers' service learning experiences related to comprehensive school physical activity programming. J Teach Phys Educ. 2017;36(4):430–44.
87. Michael RD, Webster CA, Egan CA, Stewart G, Nilges L, Brian A, et al. Viability of university service learning to support movement integration in elementary classrooms: perspectives of teachers, university students, and course instructors. Teach Teach Educ. 2018;72:122–32.
88. Kwon JY, Kulinna PH, van der Mars H, Koro-Ljungberg M, Amrein-Beardsley A, Norris J. Physical education preservice teachers' perceptions about preparation for comprehensive school physical activity programs. Res Q Exerc Sport. 2018;89(2):221–34.
89. Kuhn AP, Carson RL, Beighle A, Castelli DM. Changes in psychosocial perspectives among physical activity leaders: teacher efficacy, work engagement, and affective commitment. J Teach Phys Educ. 2020:1–9.
90. Goh TL. School–university partnered before-school physical activity program: experiences of preservice teachers, program facilitators, and students. J Teach Phys Educ. 2024;43(1):114–22.
91. McCullick BA, Baker T, Tomporowski PD, Templin TJ, Lux K, Isaac T. An analysis of state physical education policies. J Teach Phys Educ. 2012;31(2):200–10.

Chapter 12
School-Based Before-School Physical Activity Programs

Michalis Stylianou and James Woodforde

12.1 Introduction

Physical activity (PA) occurring before the start of the school day, herein described as before-school PA, is typically presented in PA promotion frameworks as part of a combined before- and after-school component. While there is abundant literature on after-school programs and their contributions to children and adolescents' physical activity, before-school literature has predominantly focused on active transport to school. This chapter focuses on school-based programs occurring before the start of the school day as another key strategy for supporting children and adolescents' PA in this segment and once they arrive at school. Such programs can capitalize on existing strengths of the school setting in facilitating PA and have the potential to meaningfully contribute to various student and school outcomes. Alongside the potential of such programs, however, complexities inherent to the specific segment and the school context need to be considered.

This chapter includes four sections. The first section sets the scene by defining the before-school segment and exploring children and adolescents' PA behaviors and efforts to promote PA in this time period. The second section considers the role and potential of schools in supporting PA in the before-school segment, including factors that make school-based physical activities opportunities appealing. The third section focuses on school-based PA programs occurring in this segment, providing an overview of their characteristics, effectiveness, and implementation considerations, as well as insights from stakeholders regarding factors potentially limiting the promise of these opportunities. Finally, the last chapter offers recommendations for both practice and research that can help enhance our understanding of relevant

---

M. Stylianou (✉) · J. Woodforde
School of Human Movement and Nutrition Sciences, The University of Queensland, St. Lucia, QLD, Australia
e-mail: m.stylianou@uq.edu.au

outcomes from school-based before-school programs and optimize such opportunities and children and adolescent's PA behaviors in this segment.

12.2 The Before-School Segment: Definition, Physical Activity Levels, and Promotion Efforts

The before-school segment can be broadly defined as the time period between waking up and the official start of the school day [1]. During this segment, children and adolescents typically spend time at home and potentially in other settings, including at school, center-based care programs, and the broader community. They also engage in various activities, including self-care, homework, transport to school, recreational screen time, and potentially physical activity, such as organized sport or unstructured play on school grounds. The duration of the before-school segment can vary substantially across contexts and even across seasons as a function of location, daylight saving time adjustments, and school systems (i.e., school start times). This, along with factors such as the weather, can influence how and where children and young people spend their time before school and the potential of this segment for PA promotion.

Available data suggest limited engagement in PA in the before-school segment by children and adolescents. For example, time use diary data from a national sample of Australian adolescents indicated about 60% of girls and 50% of boys did not report engaging in any activities classified as physical activities before school [2]. Accelerometer data from multiple countries also indicate low engagement in moderate-to-vigorous PA (MVPA) before school. This includes about 2–3 min of MVPA accumulated between 12 and 8 am in a nationally representative sample of US boys and girls aged 6–11 and 12–19 years [3]; 2.9 and 3.5 MVPA minutes between 6 am and school start time in students from 20 primary and 10 secondary schools in the Netherlands, respectively [4]; and about 6 MVPA minutes from waking up to school start time in grade 4 and 5 students from 20 randomly selected South African schools [5]. Further, studies with data for various segments of the day point to lower MVPA contributions in the before-school segment compared to other school and out-of-school segments [3, 6].

Collectively, evidence demonstrating low PA engagement in the before-school segment [3–5], along with findings that highly active children are more active in the mornings than low active children [7, 8], and high proportions of sedentary time before school [9, 10], highlight the importance of focusing PA promotion efforts on this segment. The role of the before-school segment for PA promotion in children and adolescents has been highlighted by the World Health Organization in their Global Action Plan on Physical Activity, where they advocate for partnerships and initiatives that support opportunities for PA before and after school [11].

Research examining the before-school segment has predominantly focused on active transport, which has been identified to be positively associated with PA in children and adolescents [12, 13]. However, evidence from 47 participating countries in the Global Matrix 3.0 initiative indicates only about half of children and youth (47–53%) use active transport to get to and from places [14] and various barriers [15] may make active transport to school a less feasible option for many children and adolescents. While active transport to school should continue to be a key component of PA promotion efforts for this population, it should not be viewed as the sole option for supporting PA before school. School-based initiatives can offer an alternative option for PA when active transport is not an option, or an additional opportunity for PA once children and adolescents arrive at school.

12.3 The Role and Potential of Schools in Supporting Before-School Physical Activity

The role of schools in supporting PA has been widely acknowledged [11, 16]. This includes the support of opportunities in the before-school segment, which feature in whole-of-school frameworks, such as the Centers for Disease Control and Prevention's (CDC) Comprehensive School PA Program framework [17] and the World Health Organization's (WHO) whole-of-school approach domains [18]. Both of these frameworks present before and after school opportunities as one of multiple components or domains that can help students meet the PA guidelines.

However, available data indicate limited offering of school-based PA opportunities before school. For example, in the United States, organized activities in this segment were rarely observed in a sample of 24 middle schools in Southern California [19]. Further, self-report data showed PA opportunities before school were offered in only 13% of 905 elementary schools in Georgia [20] and 36.6% of 47 public elementary, middle, and high schools in Nevada [21]. In a study examining level of implementation, only 24% of 22 Texan elementary schools reported high implementation of PA opportunities in the before-school segment [22]. Beyond the United States, data from Northern Ireland indicated only 6.8% of 59 post-primary schools provided regular in-school extra-curricular physical activities to female students before school [23]. In all these studies, PA offerings in the after-school segment were more common, provided in 33.2% of Georgia elementary schools [20], 67.2% of Nevada elementary, middle, and high schools [21], 89.9% of Northern Ireland post-primary schools [23], and highly implemented in 73% of Texas elementary schools [22]. While available evidence is limited and mostly originates from the United States, it suggests that the introduction of additional school-based opportunities for PA during the before-school segment (i.e., expansion) can help further support children and adolescents' daily PA behaviors [24].

School-based PA opportunities in the before-school segment can be viewed as meaningful and appealing options for stakeholders for several reasons. For schools, PA opportunities before school may be considered an attractive alternative to other opportunities occurring during the school day. This is because before-school opportunities do not interfere with timetabled requirements and are not seen to contribute to the time pressures frequently reported by school staff as a major barrier to PA implementation during the school day [25, 26]. This is a key argument for the appeal of school-based PA programming in the before-school segment and has been highlighted in relevant qualitative work examining stakeholders' perspectives of such opportunities [27].

Children and adolescents can benefit from school-based PA opportunities before school in multiple ways. Such opportunities can facilitate engagement in PA for many children and adolescents who already arrive at school before the official start of the school day or who tend to spend this time at home engaging in sedentary behaviors [28, 29]. Indeed, stakeholders, including parents, students, and school staff, tend to view school-based before-school PA opportunities as an extension of the school day that can facilitate inclusive and safe engagement in PA [29]. Physical activity opportunities in this segment of the day are often deemed particularly important for children and adolescents who are less active overall or less engaged in competitive sports or physical education (PE) [28, 29], as well as in locations where warm climates limit activity later in the day [29].

Participation in PA directly prior to the school day may also help support children and adolescents' classroom engagement and learning. There's a growing body of literature suggesting enhanced cognitive and academic-related outcomes following acute bouts of PA [30], including some studies that specifically examined before-school PA programs (e.g., Garnett et al. [31]; Stylianou et al. [32]). Qualitative data from parents, students, and school staff consistently highlight perceived cognitive and behavioral benefits associated with participation in PA prior to class time, which are discussed as supportive of classroom engagement and learning [27–29, 31]. Enhanced school attendance and timely arrival at school have also been identified by stakeholders as outcomes associated with before-school PA programming at school and linked to the perceived value of such opportunities [29, 31].

Parents and families also stand to benefit from before-school PA offerings on school grounds. Stakeholder reports highlight these offerings align well with many parents' work schedules and help them with their day by allowing them to drop off their children to school earlier and/or supporting supervised engagement during a time when children would otherwise be unsupervised [28, 29]. This is often discussed as an indirect benefit of school-based PA programming in the before-school segment, but an important one for many families and young people [29]. For parents with some more flexibility in the morning, school-based programming may also allow involvement in facilitating PA opportunities or may encourage their own participation, thus enhancing a whole-of-school approach to PA [27].

Despite the several appealing features of school-based before-school PA opportunities, it needs to be acknowledged that the implementation of such opportunities can be a complex task. As relevant data highlight, organizational demands, supervision requirements, and employment conditions of school staff need to be carefully considered in planning and implementing successful school-based PA opportunities in the before-school segment [22, 29]. Further, there are key barriers to the implementation, uptake, and sustainability of such opportunities that need to be addressed, some of which are presented in the next section of this chapter. Of course, benefits and challenges can depend on the type of initiative adopted to support before-school PA on school grounds, which can range from PA friendly policies and practices (e.g., allowing PA once students arrive to school, allowing access to facilities and equipment) to more structured activities and programs. The next section focuses on the latter, where we synthesize available evidence from the growing body of work on school-based programs, defined as initiatives organized within the school setting for students to participate. In particular, we consider program characteristics, effectiveness, and implementation.

12.4 School-Based Before School Physical Activity Programs: An Overview of Existing Literature

This section is largely based on the first systematic review to examine the effectiveness of school-based before-school PA programs, where it was reported that there is a limited but growing body of evidence in this area [33]. Thirteen articles from ten unique studies published between 2012 and 2020 contributed to this review, spanning various outcome domains. Since the systematic review's search date in 2021, additional studies focusing on school-based PA programs before school have been published and these will also be considered here.

12.4.1 Intervention Characteristics

The synthesis of program characteristics in the review provides insights into the design elements, such as frequency, duration, and types of activities, that characterize existing before-school PA interventions. A commonly studied and widely implemented program is *Active Kids*, formerly *Build Our Kids Success* (BOKS), run by volunteers following standardized multi-activity plans including running, skill development, and game play [34]. The studies of this program reported frequencies of 2–3 days per week, and session lengths between 40 and 60 min [35–37]. Running and walking programs delivered by volunteers or school staff are also common in this segment [38–40], having been heralded for their simplicity and resource-efficiency [41]. There is some variety among other programs that have been subject to research, including non-competitive games [42], games and dance [43], yoga [44], and endurance training exercises [45]. The review found that programs were most often run 5 days per week, and all programs following this approach were delivered by professionals external to the school [33]. The intensive nature of these programs raises questions about the practicalities of program delivery and sustainability in the absence of ongoing research support. We explore factors known to influence the provision of, and participation in, before-school PA programs later in this section.

12.4.2 Intervention Effectiveness

This part of the chapter focuses on the effectiveness of before-school PA programs across diverse outcomes that illustrate the breadth of research foci in this evolving area. The systematic review did not limit its inclusion criteria by outcome and found that despite limited numbers, studies have examined a wide range of outcomes that were organized within the domains of PA, physical health, psychosocial wellbeing, and learning-related outcomes.

12.4.2.1 Physical Activity Outcomes

Physical activity outcomes of before-school programs have rarely been reported, with three studies having contributed to the systematic review [33]. The limited reporting of PA outcomes in these programs despite their targeted focus may, in part, stem from challenges of low accelerometer wear time in the mornings [1]. As a point of comparison, a systematic review of after-school PA published 5 years prior examined 15 articles reporting outcomes of MVPA [46].

Collectively, the three studies of before-school programs offer encouraging evidence for the effectiveness of such initiatives, as demonstrated by their positive associations with PA outcomes. Cradock et al. used a quasi-experimental design to compare PA levels of BOKS participants with non-participants, finding a statistically significant mean difference of 13.4 minutes of daily MVPA [35]. Within-person analyses comparing BOKS participants' PA on days with and without programming found participants accumulated 8.8 additional MVPA minutes on program days [35]. Shorter duration before-school programs have also shown promise through preliminary evidence for their ability to meaningfully influence PA levels. Stylianou et al.'s study into before-school running/walking clubs found that children accrued substantial PA during the 15- and 20-min programs (8.5 and 10 MVPA minutes, respectively), without decreasing their PA levels during the school day on days they participated in these programs [40]. Additionally, through direct observation, Black, Menzel, and Bungum identified a significant and large-effect reduction in the number of sedentary children on days when a before-school jogging and walking program was active [38]. While the available evidence indicates that school-based before-school PA programs are positively associated with PA levels, supporting the promise of such opportunities, further research examining PA outcomes is needed in this area [33].

12.4.2.2 Health and Wellbeing Outcomes

Physical health, psychosocial health, and learning-related outcomes are more prevalent in the before-school literature than PA outcomes [33]. The physical health and psychosocial health outcome domains, discussed here, were found to have indeterminate associations with before-school PA intervention by the systematic review, meaning evidence is mixed [33]. Select studies reveal more about these associations. For example, the largest included randomized controlled trial demonstrated significantly greater improvements in both cardiorespiratory fitness and muscular fitness in Grade 4 children after having participated in a before-school PA program for 8 weeks, relative to a control group [43]. As well as this, another three included studies [36, 42, 45] that examined cardiorespiratory fitness contributed statistically significant positive associations, demonstrating the potential of before-school programs for developing children and adolescents' fitness. Since then, Kulp and Zhu found that children participating in a before-school PA program just once weekly for 45 min also underwent significant improvements in their cardiorespiratory fitness compared to non-participating children [47].

Drawing inferences about specific psychosocial outcomes is challenging, as relevant variables have only been examined in single studies [33]. While some studies have considered the impact of before-school programs on factors such as quality of peer relationships [37], others have examined sociability [42], or mood and stress [39]. Further research is needed to understand more about the role of these programs for psychosocial aspects such as mood and affect, and peer relationships and behaviors, where reviewed evidence showed a mix of positive and null effects. Building on the evidence of the reviewed studies, Goh et al. more recently found that a before-school PA program significantly improved social and emotional learning competencies among fourth and sixth-grade students, demonstrating a 7–10% increase compared to a control group with no change [48].

12.4.2.3 Cognitive and Academic Outcomes

The literature on PA for cognitive and academic outcomes is in its relative infancy compared to the literature on physical health outcomes. Nonetheless, this is a developing area that is demonstrating positive impacts of PA [49, 50]. Examining the research on before-school PA, evidence for cognitive and academic outcomes (called "learning-related outcomes" in the systematic review) is mixed, which may be due to heterogeneity in specific variables examined, program characteristics, and other study design elements [33]. These studies have examined outcomes such as academic performance [43], concentration [39, 43], selective attention [43], and on-task behavior in class [32].

An important area of distinction in the body of work on PA and cognition is between acute and chronic effects. While much of the wider literature focuses on cognitive impacts of sustained PA [51], evidence also exists for effects on cognitive outcomes following acute bouts of activity [30], which highlights a potential benefit of the before-school segment given its positioning immediately before classes. Despite this, only one reviewed study examined acute effects of before-school PA, according to which consistently higher on-task behavior was observed on program versus non-program days in the first 45 min of school [32]. Diverging from field-based studies included in the review, Kawabata et al. [52] conducted a laboratory-based randomized controlled trial exploring the acute effects of morning exercise combined with breakfast on adolescents' academic and cognitive performance. Having found improvements in mathematical scores and speed compared to fasted and sedentary adolescents, the authors identified the potential benefits of integrating PA opportunities and nutrition-focused initiatives, like breakfast clubs, in schools to support academic performance [52].

Other work conducted since the review has examined before-school PA participation and academic performance, finding that children participating in a before-school PA program once per week significantly improved their performance in reading, but not mathematics, compared to non-participating children [47]. This is not the first study to demonstrate improvements in academic performance, as García-Hermoso et al. previously found improvements in both language and mathematics performance attributable to a before-school PA program [43]. However, there are limitations associated with the measurement of these outcomes, such as non-blinding of teachers who assigned the grades used in the latter study.

12.4.2.4 Limitations

The evidence gathered from the systematic review and from work completed since the review is mixed but supports the potential of before-school PA programs to positively contribute to several important areas of children and adolescents' health and development. In particular, the growing evidence for readiness to learn and academic performance supports stakeholder perceptions of meaningful effects in the classroom and may have important implications for schools. However, results across all outcome domains examined in the systematic review need to be interpreted with caution due to factors like high risk of bias and variability in program characteristics. To develop the limited evidence base in this area, there is a need for higher-quality research that addresses persisting gaps, such as the collection and reporting of PA outcomes, and examination of programs in secondary school contexts [33].

12.4.3 Implementation Evaluations and Stakeholder Views

Implementation evaluation serves as a means of understanding factors that may bridge the gap between developing effective interventions and implementing these interventions in school settings under "real world" conditions [53]. The importance of implementation evaluation cannot be overstated; however, this evaluation component has been largely absent in studies examining school-based before-school programs. The only known structured and comprehensive implementation evaluation in this area [28] used the RE-AIM framework to examine the implementation of the BOKS before-school program, which was led by trained school staff in two low-resource elementary schools and one middle school in the United States. This evaluation showed some promising findings, including (a) high fidelity of program frequency and duration (3 times/week for 12 weeks), with schools offering 89–100%

of scheduled sessions; (b) high student attendance (77%); and (c) continuation of the program in the three schools as well as uptake of the program by an additional three schools in the following year. Findings from this study also revealed some challenges, such as: low fidelity to recommended session length, with two schools reducing sessions from 60 min to 25 and 45 min due to challenges relating to accessing facilities and school start time; moderate initial reach in the middle school (51%) and a decline in middle school enrolment over time; and program leader attrition, with 3 of 11 program leaders discontinuing their involvement in the following year because of time and administrative requirements. This evaluation provides key insights about the functioning of before-school PA programs in schools, including a need to more carefully consider the local context and the needs and interests of involved stakeholders (e.g., by developing tailored programs for adolescents). Similarly, data gathered through qualitative methods have revealed facilitators and barriers that can inform the direction of future before-school programs.

The current body of qualitative evidence specific to before-school PA is drawn from a few studies from the United States and Australia. These studies have engaged parents [28], families, teachers, principals [27], and students, external PA providers, and school health experts in addition to the groups previously mentioned [29], to gain perspectives about factors that support or limit before-school PA. Parents have described the presence of barriers relating to the early morning scheduling of some before-school offerings as influential over their children's participation [28]. Indeed, some families may find it challenging to fit any activities in their morning schedule and some adolescents' sleeping patterns may not be conducive to participation in PA before school starts [29]. Additionally, and similar to the after-school context, transport arrangements may limit or completely prohibit participation in PA at school in the before-school segment, particularly for students using buses to get to school or for families needing to coordinate transport to school for multiple children [27–29].

Barriers and facilitators of before-school PA have been mapped to various levels of social-ecological influence [29]. Focusing on the school level, resource allocation and availability have been identified as key determinants [27, 29]. For example, the active engagement of champions has been described as pivotal for implementing and sustaining before-school programs, and the implementation of incentive-based systems has been identified as a strategy that may support children's participation in these programs [27]. Elsewhere, stakeholders highlighted the influence of structured PA opportunities, noting that their absence signified a loss of potential in what was described as an "untapped" segment [29]. However, this was said to rely on the availability of supervising staff, the feasibility of which is influenced by "teachers' goodwill, expertise and experience, increasing workload, and competing school priorities" [29, p15]. Examples were also shared where program sustainability faced challenges due to staff turnover, especially when reliant on a single teacher [29]. Despite these challenges, stakeholders provided several suggestions for strategies that could support the implementation and sustainability of before school programs, including facilitator training and recognition, broader community engagement, and development of partnerships [29]. Key recommendations are further explored in the final section of this chapter.

12.5 Recommendations

12.5.1 *Practice*

Given the unique nature of the before-school segment as a discretionary time period for PA that occurs early in the day and outside the official school day, specific considerations are needed for school-based programs taking place in this segment. Accordingly, this section offers four key recommendations that can support successful implementation and sustainability of before-school school-based PA programs. These recommendations should be considered alongside broader recommendations for the promotion of PA through school and the development, implementation, and evaluation of whole-of-school PA programs (e.g., CDC [17]; WHO [18]), as well as existing recommendations for before-school PA programs (e.g., Dauenhauer et al.) [54].

(1) *Create a working group or use an existing PA or wellness committee to undertake a consultation process with key stakeholder groups.* For a before-school program, these stakeholder groups need to—at a minimum—include school staff, students, and parents, all of which can uniquely contribute to decisions around the feasibility and design of a before-school program. Students, for instance, can help inform decisions around the type of activities to implement, whereas parents, students, and teachers can collectively offer key insight into the practicalities of scheduling, such as frequency, start times, and transport arrangements. As an example, input from a group of Australian stakeholders highlighted various strategies to enhance the uptake and success of school-based programs before school, including providing additional transport options and providing snacks or access to food (e.g., canteen opening earlier) on program days [29].

(2) *Invest time in developing partnerships that can help support the program.* These partnerships can involve community businesses or groups, the school's parent association or parents more broadly, sporting clubs and organizations, or local universities; and can help support the purchase of necessary equipment, facilitation of activities, training and development of facilitators, or the development and evaluation of theoretically informed programs [29, 55–57]. Examples of school—university partnerships specifically focusing on before-school programs demonstrate benefits for both children and adolescents, who have additional opportunities for PA participation, and pre-service teachers, who have practical experiences to help support their competencies as future school PA leaders [55–57]. Given time and administrative burden is a key reason facilitators discontinue their involvement in before-school programs [28], partnerships that help build capacity and/or divide responsibilities can be critical for sustained program implementation.

(3) *Consider strategies that can support curriculum integration and broader student development outcomes.* For example, the design of a before-school pro-

gram, including the types of activities used, can be informed by curriculum work within Health and PE. This can involve students collecting and evaluating relevant data from their peers and communities to identify factors at various levels that could influence participation in a before-school program and explore ways to optimize inclusion and regular participation. Broader student development outcomes may involve leadership and decision-making skills [29], which can be authentically fostered when offering opportunities for different student roles in PA programs and are embedded in school curricula around the world in different ways. To illustrate, the Australian F-10 curriculum focuses on general capabilities, including a personal and social capability with elements such as social management (e.g., communication, collaboration, leadership, decision-making).

(4) *Establish an ongoing monitoring and evaluation plan* early that considers both set objectives/expected outcomes and the process of implementation. The data collected through this process can help assess the impact of the program on students and the school and can also be used to communicate benefits to the broader community, a strategy perceived as key to enhance buy in across stakeholders [29]. Collected data can also inform potentially necessary adjustments in resourcing and implementation to ensure programs continue to meet the needs and interests of stakeholders and are able to be implemented in a sustainable manner.

12.5.2 Research

The research and evidence on PA in schools during the before-school segment is considerably limited relative to other time periods (e.g., after school) and even other domains of before-school PA (i.e., active transport). Therefore, future research is needed to increase certainty of evidence about the effectiveness of school-based before-school PA programs and to deepen understanding of their implementation. One aspect of this is the need to conduct research that minimizes risk of bias (e.g., from potential confounding) where possible, as concerns regarding this contributed to the low certainty of intervention evidence identified in the Woodforde et al. [33] systematic review. Several recommendations for the future of school-based before-school PA intervention research were made in this review, which has informed the three recommendations below.

(1) *Design theory-informed and contextually relevant programs.* Future research may benefit from theory-informed program design to support PA behavior change [58]. Additionally, programs that are designed with "end-users" (e.g., students, school staff) may result in features and strategies that align with the given school context and therefore support implementation and sustainability [59]. Research has acknowledged the importance of offering culturally relevant

activities that are viewed by students as meaningful beyond school [60], reflecting students' calls for relevant and context-specific offerings in the before-school segment, such as an open gym or Pilates [29]. An approach that solicits for student voice in program design has been suggested by stakeholders [29] and may result in greater diversity of activity types than have currently been evaluated in the before-school segment. Another factor to consider in design of activity type may be the program's goals, in light of literature indicating that different types of PA may benefit different aspects of cognition [61], and similarly, specific social outcomes may be targeted through intentional design [62].

(2) *Examine impact on youth PA levels and in adolescent populations.* Examination of all relevant outcome variables should continue; however, given that PA outcomes are particularly scarce in relevant literature, heightened attention to these outcomes is needed to better understand the potential influence of before-school programs on youth PA levels. Further, no identified studies examined the contributions of before-school programs to secondary school students' PA, and given declining PA in adolescence [63] and calls for novel interventions in education settings [59], this is a population that warrants consideration in the before school segment.

(3) *Collect implementation data and stakeholder perspectives.* Future studies should collect program implementation data and data regarding stakeholder perspectives. For instance, it is important to understand implementation outcomes, such as program reach (i.e., number of participants) and sustainability (i.e., whether the program continues) [64], which can be facilitated through follow-up data collected after intervention completion. Collection of implementation data should extend to consider determinants that influence implementation, such as program adaptability—the degree to which a program can be adapted to suit the specific requirements of a local context [64].

12.6 Conclusion

School-based PA programs represent a key strategy for supporting children and adolescents' PA behaviors in the before-school segment. They are appealing for multiple stakeholder groups and for different reasons, and a growing body of evidence suggests various positive outcomes associated with participation in such programs. Acknowledging the limitations of existing research and the complexities inherent in before-school school-based PA programming, this chapter offers recommendations for research and practice to help enrich our understanding of program implementation and effectiveness and maximize the impact on students and broader school communities. Figure 12.1 presents a summary of the key messages from this chapter.

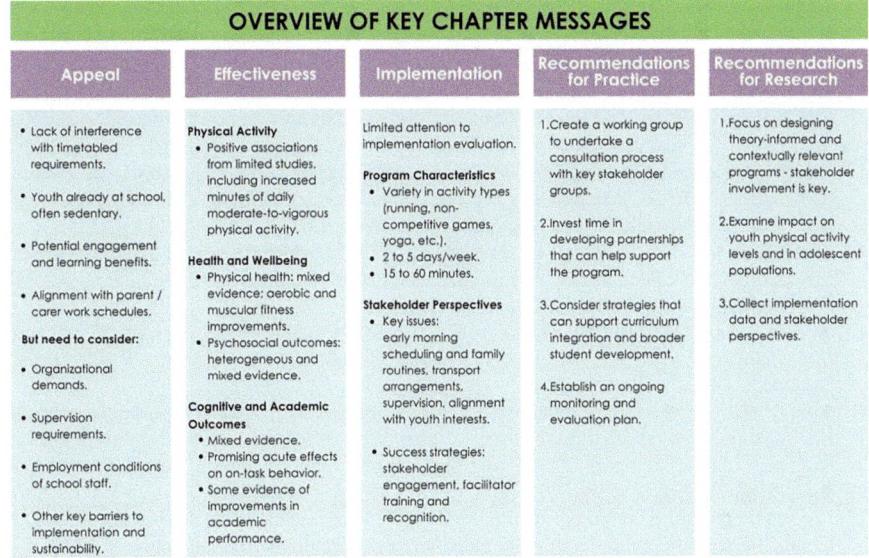

Fig. 12.1 Summary of key messages from the chapter

References

1. Woodforde J, Gomersall S, Timperio A, Loh V, Browning H, Perales F, Salmon J, Stylianou M. Conceptualizing, defining, and measuring before-school physical activity: a review with exploratory analysis of adolescent data. J Meas Phys Behav. 2023;6(2):101–14.
2. Woodforde J, Perales F, Salmon J, Gomersall S, Stylianou M. Before-school physical activity levels and sociodemographic correlates among Australian adolescents. J Sport Sci. 2024;42:1–10.
3. Long MW, Sobol AM, Cradock AL, Subramanian SV, Blendon RJ, Gortmaker SL. School-day and overall physical activity among youth. Am J Prev Med. 2013;45(2):150–7.
4. Remmers T, Van Kann D, Kremers S, Ettema D, De Vries SI, Vos S, Thijs C. Investigating longitudinal context-specific physical activity patterns in transition from primary to secondary school using accelerometers, GPS, and GIS. Int J Behav Nutr Phys Act. 2020;17:66.
5. Uys M, Broyles ST, Draper C E, Hendricks S, Rae D, Naidoo N, Katzmarzyk PT, Lambert EV. Perceived and objective neighborhood support for outside of school physical activity in South African children. BMC Public Health. 2016;16:1–9.
6. Saint-Maurice PF, Bai Y, Vazou S, Welk G. Youth physical activity patterns during school and out-of-school time. Children. 2018;5(9):118.
7. Fairclough SJ, Beighle A, Erwin H, Ridgers ND. School day segmented physical activity patterns of high and low active children. BMC Public Health. 2012;12:406.
8. Garriguet D, Colley RC. Daily patterns of physical activity among Canadians. Health Rep. 2012;23(2):B1.
9. Beck J, Chard CA, Hilzendegen C, Hill J, Stroebele-Benschop N. In-school versus out-of-school sedentary behavior patterns in US children. BMC Obesity. 2016;3:1–9.
10. Wiersma R, Lu C, Hartman E, Corpeleijn E. Physical activity around the clock: objectively measured activity patterns in young children of the GECKO Drenthe cohort. BMC Public Health. 2019;19:1647.

11. World Health Organization. Global action plan on physical activity 2018–2030: more active people for a healthier world. Geneva: World Health Organization; 2018. Licence: CC BY-NC-SA 3.0 IGO
12. Denstel KD, Broyles ST, Larouche R, Sarmiento OL, Barreira TV, Chaput JP, Church TS, Fogelholm M, Hu G, Kuriyan R, Kurpad A. Active school transport and weekday physical activity in 9–11-year-old children from 12 countries. Int J Obesity Suppl. 2015;5(2):S100–6.
13. Prince SA, Lancione S, Lang JJ, Amankwah N, de Groh M, Garcia AJ, Merucci K, Geneau R. Are people who use active modes of transportation more physically active? An overview of reviews across the life course. Transplant Rev. 2022;42(5):645–71.
14. González SA, Aubert S, Barnes JD, Larouche R, Tremblay MS. Profiles of active transportation among children and adolescents in the global matrix 3.0 initiative: a 49-country comparison. Int J Environ Res Public Health. 2020;17(16):5997
15. Aranda-Balboa MJ, Huertas-Delgado FJ, Herrador-Colmenero M, Cardon G, Chillón P. Parental barriers to active transport to school: a systematic review. Int J Public Health. 2020;65:87–98.
16. Kohl HW III, Cook HD, Committee on Physical Activity and Physical Education in the School Environment, Food and Nutrition Board, & Institute of Medicine, editors. Educating the student body: taking physical activity and physical education to school. National Academies Press (US); 2013.
17. Centers for Disease Control and Prevention. Comprehensive school physical activity programs: a guide for schools. Atlanta, GA: U.S. Department of Health and Human Services; 2013.
18. World Health Organization. Promoting physical activity through schools: a toolkit. Geneva: World Health Organization; 2021. Licence: CC BY-NC-SA 3.0 IGO
19. McKenzie TL, Marshall SJ, Sallis JF, Conway TL. Leisure-time physical activity in school environments: an observational study using SOPLAY. Prev Med. 2000;30(1):70–7.
20. Cheung PC, Franks PA, Kramer MR, Kay CM, Drews-Botsch CD, Welsh JA, Gazmararian JA. Elementary school physical activity opportunities and physical fitness of students: a statewide cross-sectional study of schools. PloS One. 2019;14(1):e0210444.
21. Monnat SM, Lounsbery MA, McKenzie TL, Chandler RF. Associations between demographic characteristics and physical activity practices in Nevada schools. Prev Med. 2017;95:S4–9.
22. Walker TJ, Pfledderer CD, Craig DW, Robertson MC, Heredia NI, Bartholomew JB. Elementary school staff perspectives on the implementation of physical activity approaches in practice: an exploratory sequential mixed methods study. Frontiers. Public Health. 2023;11:11.
23. Carlin A, Murphy MH, Gallagher AM. Using the school environment to promote walking amongst adolescent females: a mixed-method study. Children. 2019;6(3):49.
24. Beets MW, Okely A, Weaver RG, Webster C, Lubans D, Brusseau T, Carson R, Cliff DP. The theory of expanded, extended, and enhanced opportunities for youth physical activity promotion. Int J Behav Nutr Phys Act. 2016;13(1):1–5.
25. Nathan N, Elton B, Babic M, McCarthy N, Sutherland R, Presseau J, Seward K, Hodder R, Booth D, Yoong SL, Wolfenden L. Barriers and facilitators to the implementation of physical activity policies in schools: a systematic review. Prev Med. 2018;107:45–53.
26. Naylor PJ, Nettlefold L, Race D, Hoy C, Ashe MC, Higgins JW, McKay HA. Implementation of school based physical activity interventions: a systematic review. Prev Med. 2015;72:95–115.
27. Schirmer T, Bailey A, Kerr N, Walton A, Ferrington L, Cecilio ME. Start small and let it build; a mixed-method evaluation of a school-based physical activity program, Kilometre Club. BMC Public Health. 2023;23(1):137.
28. Whooten RC, Horan C, Cordes J, Dartley AN, Aguirre A, Taveras EM. Evaluating the implementation of a before-school physical activity program: a mixed-methods approach in Massachusetts, 2018. Prev Chronic Dis. 2020;17:E116.
29. Woodforde J, Kuswara K, Perales F, Salmon J, Gomersall S, Stylianou M. A qualitative exploration of multi-stakeholder perspectives of before-school physical activity. Int J Behav Nutr Phys Act. 2024;21:25.

30. De Greeff JW, Bosker RJ, Oosterlaan J, Visscher C, Hartman E. Effects of physical activity on executive functions, attention and academic performance in preadolescent children: a meta-analysis. J Sci Med Sport. 2018;21(5):501–7.
31. Garnett BR, Becker K, Vierling D, Gleason C, DiCenzo D, Mongeon L. A mixed-methods evaluation of the Move it Move it! before-school incentive-based physical activity programme. Health Educ J. 2017;76(1):89–101.
32. Stylianou M, Kulinna PH, Van Der Mars H, Mahar MT, Adams MA, Amazeen E. Before-school running/walking club: effects on student on-task behavior. Prev Med Rep. 2016;3:196–202.
33. Woodforde J, Alsop T, Salmon J, Gomersall S, Stylianou M. Effects of school-based before-school physical activity programmes on children's physical activity levels, health and learning-related outcomes: a systematic review. Br J Sports Med. 2022;56(13):740–54.
34. Active Kids Programming [Internet]. [Place unknown: Active Kids and Minds]; 2023 [cited 2023 Nov 27]. Available from: https://activekids.org/program/
35. Cradock AL, Barrett JL, Taveras EM, Peabody S, Flax CN, Giles CM, Gortmaker SL. Effects of a before-school program on student physical activity levels. Prev Med Rep. 2019;15:100940.
36. Westcott WL, Puhala K, Colligan A, Loud RL, Cobbett R. Physiological effects of the BOKS before-school physical activity program for preadolescent youth. J Ex Sports Orthoped. 2015;2(2):1–17.
37. Whooten RC, Perkins ME, Gerber MW, Taveras EM. Effects of before-school physical activity on obesity prevention and wellness. Am J Prev Med. 2018;54(4):510–8.
38. Black IE, Menzel NN, Bungum TJ. The relationship among playground areas and physical activity levels in children. J Pediatr Health Care. 2015;29(2):156–68.
39. Kalak N, Gerber M, Kirov R, Mikoteit T, Yordanova J, Pühse U, Holsboer-Trachsler E, Brand S. Daily morning running for 3 weeks improved sleep and psychological functioning in healthy adolescents compared with controls. J Adolesc Health. 2012;51(6):615–22.
40. Stylianou M, Van Der Mars H, Kulinna PH, Adams MA, Mahar M, Amazeen E. Before-school running/walking club and student physical activity levels: an efficacy study. Res Q Exerc Sport. 2016;87(4):342–53.
41. Chesham RA, Booth JN, Sweeney EL, Ryde GC, Gorely T, Brooks NE, Moran CN. The Daily Mile makes primary school children more active, less sedentary and improves their fitness and body composition: a quasi-experimental pilot study. BMC Med. 2018;16:64.
42. Park Y, Moon J. Effects of early morning physical activity on elementary school students' physical fitness and sociality. Int Electron J Elemen Educ. 2018;10(4):441–7.
43. García-Hermoso A, Hormazábal-Aguayo I, Fernández-Vergara O, González-Calderón N, Russell-Guzmán J, Vicencio-Rojas F, Chacana-Cañas C, Ramírez-Vélez R. A before-school physical activity intervention to improve cognitive parameters in children: the Active-Start study. Scand J Med Sci Sports. 2020;30(1):108–16.
44. Verma A, Shete SU. Effect of yoga practices on general mental ability in urban residential school children. J Complement Integr Med. 2020;17(4):20190238.
45. Jung DK, Lee J, Kim SY, Kang BY. Effects of morning exercise on blood BDNF level and its associated factors in elementary school students. Gazzetta Medica Italiana Archivio per le Scienze Mediche. 2014;173(9):447–56.
46. Mears R, Jago R. Effectiveness of after-school interventions at increasing moderate-to-vigorous physical activity levels in 5-to 18-year olds: a systematic review and meta-analysis. Br J Sports Med. 2016;50(21):1315–24.
47. Kulp AJ, Zhu X. Before school exercise effects on fitness and academic performance in schoolchildren: a retrospective case-controlled study. J Teach Phys Educ. 2021;41(4):738–43.
48. Goh TL, Leong CH, Fede M, Ciotto C. Before-school physical activity program's impact on social and emotional learning. J Sch Health. 2022;92(7):674–80.
49. Donnelly JE, Hillman CH, Castelli D, Etnier JL, Lee S, Tomporowski P, Lambourne K, Szabo-Reed AN. Physical activity, fitness, cognitive function, and academic achievement in children: a systematic review. Med Sci Sports Exerc. 2016;48(6):1197–222.

50. Biddle SJ, Ciaccioni S, Thomas G, Vergeer I. Physical activity and mental health in children and adolescents: an updated review of reviews and an analysis of causality. Psychol Sport Exerc. 2019;42:146–55.
51. Álvarez-Bueno C, Pesce C, Cavero-Redondo I, Sanchez-Lopez M, Martínez-Hortelano JA, Martinez-Vizcaino V. The effect of physical activity interventions on children's cognition and metacognition: a systematic review and meta-analysis. J Am Acad Child Adolesc Psychiatry. 2017;56(9):729–38.
52. Kawabata M, Lee K, Choo HC, Burns SF. Breakfast and exercise improve academic and cognitive performance in adolescents. Nutrients. 2021;13(4):1278.
53. Durlak JA, DuPre EP. Implementation matters: a review of research on the influence of implementation on program outcomes and the factors affecting implementation. Am J Community Psychol. 2008;41:327–50.
54. Dauenhauer B, Kulinna P, Marttinen R, Stellino MB. Before-and after-school physical activity: programs and best practices. J Phys Educ Recreat Dance. 2022;93(5):20–6.
55. Brusseau TA, Bulger SM, Elliott E, Hannon JC, Jones E. University and community partnerships to implement comprehensive school physical activity programs: insights and impacts for kinesiology departments. Kinesiol Rev. 2015;4(4):370–7.
56. Goh TL. School–university partnered before-school physical activity program: experiences of preservice teachers, program facilitators, and students. J Teach Phys Educ. 2023;1(aop):1–9.
57. McMullen J, van der Mars H, Jahn JA. Creating a before-school physical activity program: pre-service physical educators' experiences and implications for PETE. J Teach Phys Educ. 2014;33(4):449–66.
58. McEwan D, Beauchamp MR, Kouvousis C, Ray CM, Wyrough A, Rhodes RE. Examining the active ingredients of physical activity interventions underpinned by theory versus no stated theory: a meta-analysis. Health Psychol Rev. 2019;13(1):1–7.
59. van Sluijs EM, Ekelund U, Crochemore-Silva I, Guthold R, Ha A, Lubans D, Oyeyemi AL, Ding D, Katzmarzyk PT. Physical activity behaviours in adolescence: current evidence and opportunities for intervention. Lancet. 2021;398(10298):429–42.
60. Garn AC, McCaughtry N, Kulik NL, Kaseta M, Maljak K, Whalen L, Shen B, Martin JJ, Fahlman M. Successful after-school physical activity clubs in urban high schools: perspectives of adult leaders and student participants. J Teach Phys Educ. 2014;33(1):112–33.
61. Vasilopoulos F, Jeffrey H, Wu Y, Dumontheil I. Multi-level meta-analysis of physical activity interventions during childhood: effects of physical activity on cognition and academic achievement. Educ Psychol Rev. 2023;35(2):59.
62. Weiss MR, Kipp LE, Reichter AP, Espinoza SM, Bolter ND. Girls on the run: impact of a physical activity youth development program on psychosocial and behavioral outcomes. Pediatr Exerc Sci. 2019;31(3):330–40.
63. Brooke HL, Atkin AJ, Corder K, Ekelund U, van Sluijs EM. Changes in time-segment specific physical activity between ages 10 and 14 years: a longitudinal observational study. J Sci Med Sport. 2016;19(1):29–34.
64. McKay H, Naylor PJ, Lau E, Gray SM, Wolfenden L, Milat A, Bauman A, Race D, Nettlefold L, Sims-Gould J. Implementation and scale-up of physical activity and behavioural nutrition interventions: an evaluation roadmap. Int J Behav Nutr Phys Act. 2019;16(102):1–12.

Chapter 13
School-Based After-School Physical Activity and Sports Programs

Hyungsik Min, Donetta Cothran, and Pamela Hodges Kulinna

13.1 Introduction

As has been described multiple times throughout this book, physical activity (PA) has been shown to have numerous benefits for physical, cognitive, social, and emotional health. It can improve cardiovascular health, bone and muscle strength, and reduce the risk of certain cancers [1, 2]. In terms of cognitive benefits, PA can enhance memory and cognitive function, improve executive function and academic achievement [3, 4]. Socially, PA can increase social support, improve communication skills, reduce isolation, and provide opportunities for social interaction [5, 6]. Additionally, PA has been shown to reduce symptoms of anxiety and depression, improve mood and overall well-being, and reduce stress levels [7, 8].

Despite the benefits of PA for children and youth, the World Health Organization [9] reported that more than 80% of adolescents all around the world do not meet the recommended daily PA levels (e.g., 60 min per day in the United States). PA patterns (measured using accelerometry) of children from 10 countries showed similar patterns of less than desirable PA levels. After age five, an average decrease of 4.2% in PA was observed each year. Boys are also more active and less sedentary than girls at all ages, highlighting the need for after-school programs (ASPs) to target girls' participation in particular [10]. Younger children fare only slightly better as 72.2% of children aged 6–12 vs. 81.8% of youth aged 7–17 fail to meet the recommended daily goals for PA in the United States [11].

H. Min · P. H. Kulinna (✉)
Mary Lou Fulton Teachers College, Arizona State University, Tempe, AZ, USA
e-mail: hmin14@asu.edu; pkulinna@asu.edu

D. Cothran
Department of Kinesiology, School of Public Health, Indiana University Bloomington, Bloomington, IN, USA
e-mail: dcothran@indiana.edu

Globally, schools provide high rates of access to youth with enrollment in schools estimated at primary education reaching 87% of children, while lower secondary education reaches 77%, and upper secondary education serves 59% of youth (United Nations Educational, Scientific and Cultural Organization) [12]. Therefore, the school setting is considered crucial for promoting PA [13, 14]. Traditionally schools' primary PA delivery mechanism has been Physical Education (PE) during the school day with recess contributing to PA for younger students. Several studies, however, point out that PE alone in not enough to fulfill students' daily recommended PA levels [15–17], and there is limited evidence to ensure that PE guarantees an active lifestyle beyond adolescence [18]. Furthermore, due to various factors such as academic pressures, budget constraints, and underestimation of the importance of PE, the time allotted to PE classes has been gradually decreasing [19, 20]. As a result, there have been creative efforts to promote PA outside PE during, before, and after school hours [21]. This chapter focuses on those efforts devoted to ASPs.

13.2 Whole-of-School Approaches

Given the importance of PA and increasing efforts to use after-school time more effectively, numerous models and programs have been proposed to increase student PA, often as part of a broader mission to increase student wellness in general. The most comprehensive of these models are "whole-of-school" approaches that involve pre-, during-, and after-school programming, and also include the local community, and families [26].

The Healthy and Physically Active Schools (HEPAS) Model is one example of a comprehensive model. It is described as "a framework for investigating the realization of a school environment in which PA is fully integrated and promoted" [27]. The multi-pronged initiative includes PA and school sport in addition to broader dimensions of health in school and community. The HEPAS model includes an activity leader (or champion) who may be the PE teacher. Two promising, but often underutilized ideas in their PA dimension worth noting are active homework (assignments to be active on their own or with family and friends) and active commuting to schools. The studies have shown active commuting to schools (e.g., walking, biking) may provide more PA participation than all other types of daily PA combined in the United States.

In nations with more centralized education systems, some countries have developed national active school initiatives (whole-of-school approaches) that include after-school programming. For example, Ireland's Active School Flag (ASF) initiative to create an active school culture has enrolled nearly 50% of the primary schools in efforts to increase PA through a variety of school offerings. Similarly, the Finnish Schools on the Move program to increase PA has expanded to 90% of the basic schools in Finland. These programs share a bottom-up approach that emphasizes the school's own planning, implementation, and evaluation.

Another example of a whole school approach to overall student health in general and PA in particular, is the Comprehensive School Physical Activity Program (CSPAP) model [28] that supports the framework of the United States national initiative Active Schools (formerly Let's Move Active Schools). Both HEPAS and CSPAP approach increased opportunity for PA as part of a broader concept of health that includes family and community. Both also suggest utilizing time throughout the school day as well as before/after school programming to meet their goals. In addition, the Whole School, Whole Community, Whole Child model was developed in the United States considering the development of the whole child with a holistic approach [29]. It expands the role of a comprehensive school-based approach in improving students' health and education through the integration of multiple components including: (a) PE and PA, (b) nutrition environment and services, (c) health education, (d) social and emotional climate, (e) physical environment, (f) health services, (g) counseling psychological and social services, (h) employee wellness, (i) community involvement, and (j) family engagement.

13.3 After-School Programs

ASPs are not a new development with the first United States programs developed in the late 1800s as a function of changing child labor laws, mandatory education requirements, and labor workforce changes which creates a mismatch between the hours children are in school and the hours their parents work [22]. Plantenga and Remery [23] explored ASPs across European Union countries and found that nearly all countries offered some form of ASPs, but the infrastructure and quality varied widely. Within the Organization for Economic Cooperation and Development countries of Europe, approximately 30% of children participate in before and/or after school programs, but those participation rates vary from 5 to 7% (e.g., Hungary, Italy, Spain) to over 60% (e.g., Denmark, Slovenia, Sweden) [24]. In the United States, over ten million youth participate in ASPs with another 19 million who would participate if an ASP was available [25]. Elementary school students make up the largest age group in ASPs (60%), followed by middle school students (21%) and high school students (19%) [25]. These programs vary widely in time, provider, funding, focus, and access.

13.3.1 *Guidelines for After-School Programming*

There are program guidelines focused more specifically on the after-school hours opportunities to increase student PA and wellness. The National Physical Activity Plan [30] in the United States suggest that children in ASPs engage in a variety of PA formats for 60 min for each full day in the setting, a goal that parallels the recommended PA for a day for children aged 6–17 [31]. In 2011, the National

After-School Association (NAA) in the United States adopted standards for healthy eating and PA (HEPA) in Out-of-School (OST) time. Those standards focus on a broad range of healthy behaviors including PA. Specifically, the NAAHEPA standards suggest at least 10 min of PA for every 60 OST minutes be spent in PA and 50% of the PA time should be of at least moderate intensity. The standards also suggest that a wide range of activities be offered including outdoor time. Similarly, Canada has ASP guidelines that include offering at least 30 min of daily active play that is developmentally appropriate, fitness level appropriate, and interesting for children [32]. Please see Fig. 13.1 for components of effective ASPs.

13.4 After-School Program Examples

Given the wide variety of school structures, funding models, and community values around the world, it is not surprising that a wide variety of ASPs have been developed. A full review of those programs is beyond the scope of this chapter, but the programs described in this section are a representative sample of the types of programs offered.

13.4.1 Physical Activity and Leaders

The whole-of-school approach often relies on classroom and PE teachers to lead PA during the school day while other staff are critical to OST initiatives. Leaders were crucial factors in positively impacting the effectiveness of the interventions in ASPs.

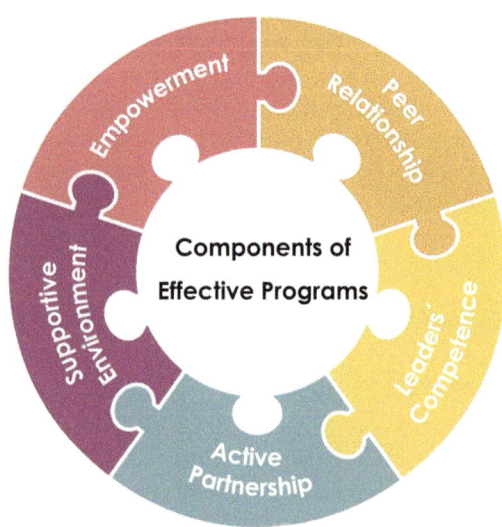

Fig. 13.1 Components of effective programs

Training and supporting leaders were effective, feasible, and acceptable ways to increase the time spent in moderate to vigorous PA (MVPA) and improve executive functioning. For after-school programming, one model is to involve trained teaching assistants and staff as PA leaders.

One example of trained PA leaders in ASPs from the UK is the Action 3:30 intervention, led by trained teaching assistants (TAs), and designed to promote PA among primary school students after school [33, 34]. The TAs provided after-school interventions twice a week for 60 min each, for a total of 20 weeks for students in Year 5 and 6 from 10 primary schools (There were also 10 control schools). When compared to the control schools, students in the intervention schools showed increased levels of PA, confidence, and self-esteem among many children, especially those who were previously inactive. In addition, elements of intervention related to these outcomes included the enjoyment of the session, opportunities to build teamwork, a range of choices across all activities (especially child-led sessions), and an appealing and empowering TA leadership style. This research demonstrates that it is possible to provide an enjoyable and effective PA program after school through the use of TAs.

Another program that relied on after-school leaders or staff for implementation was Norway's Active Play in ASP, which built on the foundation of another program, Health Promoting ASP. A central facet of the program was building the capacity of ASP staff to provide a supportive environment for PA and motivation, and by encouraging children to take action and assume responsibility [35]. In addition, providing a safe environment from leaders during PA interventions for children was identified as essential. Students were more likely to participate actively in PAs when they felt comfortable in the activity environment supported from leaders [36].

13.4.2 Physical Activity and Nutrition Focus

In the very de-centralized education system of the United States, a variety of optional programs have developed and some of those have expanded globally. One example is the Build Our Kids' Success (BOKS) program inspired by and built on the book *Spark: The Revolutionary New Science of Exercise and the Brain* [37]. Originating as a before school pilot program in a single public elementary school [38], it has since expanded globally to reach over 500,000 students. The free program has also expanded in focus to include free resources for PA throughout the school day and nutrition programming as well as expanding to all age groups through high school. Activities include games, physical skills, running, and exercises. The development of the BOKS program is significantly supported by Reebok, a fitness footwear and clothing brand company.

The effectiveness of BOKS in an after-school setting was explored by Caldwell et al. [39, 40] in a series of studies in Canada. They reported that participation in BOKS positively impacted children's overall well-being, including physical health through increased PA, and cognitive and psychological health benefits such as improved concentration and boosted self-confidence.

In contrast to the funding/development model of the BOKS program, researchers from San Diego State University in the United States received federal funding to develop and evaluate a series of PA programs, the first of which was Project SPARK (Sports, Play, and Active Recreation for Kids) [41–43], a curriculum that later expanded into after-school, active classroom, and early childhood programming. Based on successful intervention in elementary schools and additional federal funding, a middle school program for PA and nutrition education called Middle School Physical Activity and Nutrition (MSPAN) was developed. The program includes components for pre-K (ages 3–5) to high school students (i.e., grades 9–12) and adults [43].

Research on SPARK in the after-school environment has shown that it has a positive impact on improving students' MVPA and nutrition education [44–47]. The Fun 5 project in Hawaii incorporated SPARK into the state's after-school programming with a goal of daily PA and nutrition education funded by Hawaii Medical Services Association [48, 49]. Herrick et al. [50] reported on SPARK as an after-school framework and found limited impact of the program in the schools studied. The authors suggest that the amount of time allocated for PA in ASPs is as important as the curricular content of those programs.

Another program with dual goals of increased PA and nutrition knowledge is the Child and Adolescent Trial for Cardiovascular Health (CATCH) program (Later versions of the program are known as Coordinated Approach to Child Health) that aims to create a comprehensive environment for promoting PA and improving healthy eating habits among children [51]. It includes the CATCH Kids Club (CKC), an ASP designed to promote PA and nutrition education for students (grades K-8) [52]. CKC consists of three components: a) educational lessons, b) hands-on snack preparation, and c) structured PAs.

Numerous studies have supported the efficacy of CKC to improve participants' MVPA levels and food knowledge [53, 54]. CKC was also offered inside and outside schools through community organizations like the YMCA and Boys and Girls Clubs in Ontario, Canada. A related study reported that CKC implemented in these two institutions provided an average of 25 min of MVPA to students, and the time to reach this was reported to be faster than in other studies. Importantly, Sharpe et al. [52] reported a significant difference in the fidelity of implementing CKC interventions in the after-school environment depending on staff education and interest, suggesting the need for ongoing staff training and regular observations. Therefore, continuous management of staff capacity maintenance and development is necessary for successful CKC intervention in the after-school environment [52].

13.4.3 Physical Activity and Other Program Goals

SPARK, MSPAN, and CATCH share a focus on PA and nutrition education. Other programs, however, often combine PA with goals other than nutrition. Other program goals might include literacy, social-emotional learning, outdoor learning, and supporting boys or girls.

Reflective Educational Approach to Character and Health (REACH) represents another type of afterschool multiple goal program with its focus on PA and literacy enhancement among marginalized students [59]. REACH derives inspiration from the Positive Youth Development (PYD) framework, focusing primarily on fostering a positive environment to develop student competencies [60]. The competencies include critical thinking, literacy development, character molding, and advocating a salubrious lifestyle. Sessions within the REACH, typically scheduled from 4 PM to 6 PM, are designed by PA segments—encompassing warm-ups, fitness and training, and skill and game challenges—with dialogue-centric segments like team conversations, open discussions, and concluding directives [60]. In New York City, REACH has progressed through three-phases targeted at at-risk youths, underpinned by evidence-based studies [59]. Starting with a pilot phase, the second-year project focused on male students, and the third-year focused on female students.

Marttinen et al. [61] conducted a study focusing on the barriers that hinder low income male students participation in PA and outcomes from REACH through their lived experiences attending public schools in New York City. Their findings highlighted the intervention not only alleviated barriers these students faced regarding PA but also successfully offered them a safe environment. Furthermore, this program fostered the development of positive life skills through active peer interactions and the influence of role models.

Recognizing the need for ASPs to specifically address the needs of different student groups and building on the success of REACH, Marttinen et al. [62] expanded the intervention for female students by introducing and evaluating the GIRL (Gaining Insight through Reflective Learning), an adaptation of the REACH program designed for 5th- and 6th-grade girls. The researchers discovered persistent barriers that hindered these girls from participating in PA. They also underscored the need to create a more equitable and inclusive environment for these girls. Notably, they proposed that social media and other digital platforms hold the potential to offer spaces for giving positive and encouraging messages about body image.

Philosophically grounded in Self-Determination Theory (SDT) and Social Cognitive Theory (SCT), the Get Outside: After School Activity Program (GO-ASAP) is an outdoor ASP developed by the team at Eastern Oregon University. It aims to enhance students' PA through diverse and non-competitive outdoor activities. A distinctive feature is that the activities are planned and conducted by undergraduate and graduate students from various majors, who also evaluate youth health and engagement. Their roles and activities serve as models and mentors for students. The program content is divided into activities and health-related topics. Activities include skiing, snowboarding, rock climbing, yoga, kayaking, and hiking.

The health-related topics encompass nutrition, stress, sleep, resilience, and drug use. This program spans 10 weeks, offering 90- to 180-min sessions twice a week, either involving outdoor activities or teaching health-related subjects.

Barfield et al. [64] utilized a qualitative design to investigate the outcomes of intervention through 26 physically inactive 7th- and 8th-grade students (those not participating in extracurricular or organized sports activities) who joined the 2018/2019 GO-ASAP program. Their findings provided evidence of physical benefits (increased PA and improved sleep), psychological effects (reduced stress, enhanced self-confidence, and motivation), and improved social relationships (making friends, increased bonding). The research demonstrated that outdoor nature-based activities could be an effective approach to overall well-being promotion and disease prevention. The GO-ASAP program serves as a model for university-community collaborations as well as programming that might be a good fit for rural communities whose resources include outdoor space.

Also based on outdoor play, but specific to the equipment and after-school time available in many elementary school settings, the PLAYground (Play and Learning Activities for Youth) project is a program that enhances children's physical, social, and emotional skills using playground equipment in an after-school setting [65]. This program, utilizing non-competitive activities and playground equipment, is another model for improving ASPs for the overall well-being and health of children. Please see Fig. 13.2 for after-school PA programs across foci.

13.4.4 Physical Activity and Girls

Engaging girls in regular PA still remains a significant challenge. In efforts to solve this, there are ASPs specifically designed to support girls' participation in PA within after-school settings. For example, Girls on the Run (GOTR) is a school-based

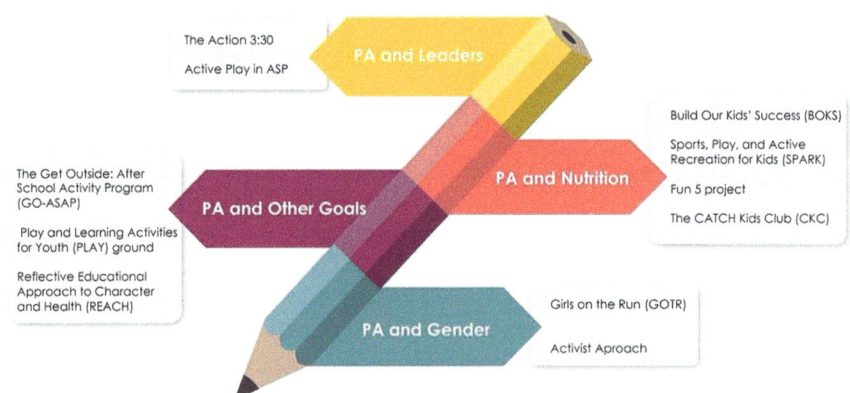

Fig. 13.2 After-school physical activity programs with different foci. PA, physical activity

after-school intervention focused on PA and PYD outcomes. Since its inception in 1996, GOTR has served over 200,000 girls annually. This program offers a platform to promote healthy behaviors, life skills, and core values (inclusive, diverse, equitable, accessible) to female students from grades 3 to 12 through running and other PAs. The 10-week curriculum plan, combining PA and skill training (two 90-minute sessions per week), focuses on relevant concepts for the girls including self-management and self-awareness, connectivity related to harmonious relationships, and empowerment [55]. The program culminates in a 5K running event. The program relies on trained coaches who focus on relationship building and providing a positive, motivational climate.

In a study conducted by Weiss and colleagues in 2019 [55], they evaluated the impact of GOTR on 203 female students from grades 3 to 5. Through surveys and focused interviews held before and after the program, and a follow-up 3 months post-program, they aimed to determine changes in PA, sedentary behavior, and the six aspects related to PYD (known as Five C + 1: Competence, Confidence, Connection, Character, Care, and Contribution). Their findings suggested an increase in the girls' PA levels from an average of 3.0 days to 4.4 days a week of at least 60 min daily, marking a 42% improvement, which persisted at the 3-month follow-up. Importantly, those who initially scored below the preseason average showed significant post-season enhancements in areas like perceived social capabilities, self-awareness, and overall self-worth lasting up to 3 months. Weiss et al. [56] integrated a comparative group who only participated in PE. They compared the post-season outcomes of this group against the intervention group involved in GOTR, focusing on the transfer of life skills and social processes. The findings revealed that the intervention group exhibited a pronounced tendency to rank higher in aspects like emotion management, conflict resolution, altruism, and decision-making skills. A noteworthy finding was the intervention group's robust ability to generalize the skills they acquired in other contexts, such as in classroom settings or at home, compared to the control group. This underscores the pivotal role of GOTR in reinforcing and generalizing psychosocial and behavioral skills and promoting a positive attitude among girls. Running programs like GOTR are a common focus of ASPs and several studies have demonstrated the value of running programs to positively influence self-concept [57], aerobic capacity [58], MVPA, and other psychological outcomes [14].

Another ASP is an extended version of the activist approach from PE to after-school setting to working with girls. Nuñez Enriquez and Oliver [63] worked with students to critically examine current PA offerings and to create more meaningful programming in ASPs in co-educational setting at the middle school level. Through a student-centered approach that negotiated the curriculum with students, the 22-week after-school intervention encouraged students' interest, motivation, and learning about PA. Key factors identified during this process included: a) recruiting resource leaders, b) internalizing common rules, and c) the actual sports' limitations for the challenge and a) providing sample work groups, b) co-creating methods and rules, and c) introducing new sports for the success. Through this, students' took the lead in promoting student PA participation and constructing a program that all students could enjoy.

13.4.5 Youth Sport

Another common type of ASP that provides PA are those focused specifically on youth involvement in sport. According to a study conducted in 38 countries worldwide, approximately half of children and youth participate in organized sports [66]. Depending on the sport as well as the nation's school and sport structure, sport offerings might be community or school based, or a mix of the two. The previously described HEPAS initiative has sport, both competitive and non-competitive, as one of the four domains of their whole school approach [67]. After-school sport does seem to positively influence PA levels and sustained participation, but that participation does not appear to be related to body composition [68].

Specific to the after-school hours, the Active After School Communities (AASC) was a government initiative in Australia that provided free sport and PA opportunities to two million primary school age children from 6000 schools or community partners during after-school hours. It was developed by The Australian Sports Commission and delivered by schools or community organizations. The program incorporated the "Playing for Life" (P4L) philosophy. P4L offers specific sports or structured PAs ensuring that all children can participate in PA regardless of their skill level, favoring games over drills. Ling et al. [69] investigated children's experiences with the AASC where the P4L was applied, using qualitative methods. They found that children experienced physical (motor development), cognitive (knowledge acquisition, creativity), social (teamwork, social interaction), and psychological (confidence, identity) benefits when participating in sports-related activities in an autonomy-supportive environment. These findings suggest that applying the P4L philosophy to PA interventions during after-school hours plays a crucial role in children's holistic development and understanding of the value of a physically active life. It has now been integrated into the Sporting Schools program which operates as a comprehensive school-based program to promote PA among students.

In the United States, sport teams are often linked to extracurricular programming in schools during the after-school hours. In the 2022–2023 academic year, more than 7.8 million secondary students participated in interscholastic sports in the United States according to the National Federation of State High School Association (NFHS, 2023). Interscholastic sports provide benefits not only in physical skills but also in areas such as confidence, mental resilience, and academic achievements [70]. Interscholastic sports often involve competition against teams at other schools. However, these sports often demand significant time, skills (e.g., usually selection for team membership), and financial expenses, which can discourage many adolescents from participating [71].

In contrast, intramural sports, which are offered within schools, often provide a broader range of activities and are open to all students, distinguishing them fundamentally from interscholastic sports [72]. Although intramurals can be offered, they are less common. Middle school students' participation levels are higher in intramural sports compared to interscholastic sports, with students participating in more diverse sports within intramural sports [71]. Given the increased participation rates of intramurals versus interscholastic sport, some experts have called for schools to reframe their offerings to prioritize intramurals [71, 73]. The issue of sport offerings, however, is not either or as with creative programming from administrators and sport leaders, both can be offered to meet the needs of students at all skill and interest levels [74].

Equitable access is an issue for all ASP programs, but particularly so for sport in the United States. For example, the Aspen Institute [75] reported that 15% of schools in higher income areas offered no school sport, but in low-income areas 34% of schools did not offer sport opportunities. For those schools that do offer sports, or other ASPs on campus, lack of transportation is a major barrier for some children [76]. Other types of ASPs can level the playing field for enrichment activities that have been previously unavailable to some students due to the expense of the activity and transportation to it.

13.5 Conclusion

This brief overview of the current landscape of ASPs suggests that it is possible for ASPs to positively impact PA and other goals in cognitive, social, and psychological domains. That landscape is one of variety which offers models and insights into potential approaches around the world. This review also described some of the evaluation mechanisms that researchers have used to investigate the efficacy of the program and their varied goals. Variety in context as well as both program and assessment makes it difficult to make comparisons across settings or to develop best practices. As Kahan and McKenzie [14] note, ASPs have limited evaluative data to guide those interested in designing and implementing effective PA programs. These results also suggest that there is no single best practice with regard to program content, but there are likely guiding principles that can be used to frame local programming. One attempt to provide a list of best practices is offered by Dauenhauer et al. [16]. That same wide variety that makes comparisons and evaluation problematic, however, allows schools to maximize their individual resources to meet their context specific needs and goals.

One consistent finding across programs is that leadership and staffing knowledge and support matter. Wiecha et al. [77] reported that just having a program leader aware of the HEPA guidelines increased the likelihood of PA being included in ASPs. Perhaps the individual best prepared to be a school's PA leader is the PE teacher and increasingly preservice and inservice teachers are learning how to approach PA beyond their class and influence the whole school's PA programming

[78]. Program implementers also need training and support. Greater PA student engagement occurs when staff engage in PA with students, verbally promote PA participation, and offer a variety of movement choices for students [79, 80]. Without training, however, those behaviors are less likely to occur [81]. Multiple researchers [82, 83] report that ongoing professional development and support for program staff are key to increasing student PA levels.

Another consistent principle found in successful programs is the importance of collaborations whether that be collaborations among school staff, community partners, funding agencies, or the students and their families to name but a few of the players involved in ASPs. Chen and Gu [84] report that the CSPAP model calls for engagement of multiple parties, but that component of the model (e.g., family and community involvement) has been the least researched of the model components. A collaborator rarely explored in the current literature is that of students' families. Choudhry et al. [85] created the Power Up program that included content for both children and their parents in an ASP focused on PA and nutrition. The investigators, however, noted the challenges of inconsistent engagement of adult family members. Programs that strengthen the school-home link will increase their chance of success.

The opportunity to review so many different kinds of programs also reveals some interesting, unanswered questions. One of those important questions is to better understand why unstructured play tends to produce more MVPA than does structured movement opportunities, at least for some students in some settings. To investigate the impact of structured curriculum implementation on children's PA levels, West et al. [13] employed a pre-post intervention design. The research findings showed that though students' moderate PA (MPA) levels improved in structured educational settings, the levels of vigorous PA (VPA) relatively decreased. Interestingly, in unstructured activities, students exhibited higher levels of MVPA. Chandler et al. [86] explored the effects of different interventions' structural types (free play, organized activities, mixed) and gender on children's PA levels in ASPs. Male students showed higher MVPA levels in free play compared to organized activities and in mixed activities compared to organized activities. Female students exhibited slightly higher PA levels in free play than in organized and mixed activities. In addition, Kinder et al. [36] investigated children's PA levels and perceptions based on interventions combining four structures (free time, PA games, nutrition games, and behavioral activities). Unstructured environments showed the highest step counts and activity durations compared to structured PA environments. However, the structured PA opportunities were preferred by children, primarily due to the social context of participating with friends.

These results suggest the recommendation of a mixed approach involving both structured and unstructured activities. However, it is crucial to be aware that factors beyond program structure, related to curriculum implementation, can influence the outcomes. PA levels in structured environments were higher indoors than outdoors [87], and they increased during spring compared to fall [88]. Therefore, practitioners should not view structured and unstructured PA as an either/or decision and should build into their programs a variety of these activity types to maximize outcomes and motivation depending on the situation and context [36].

Another movement opportunity in ASP time that needs more emphasis and understanding is that of active transportation. Sirard et al. [89] reports that up to 1/3 of a child's recommended PA could be attained by active transport. Larouche et al.'s [90] review of active transport studies found that in over 80% of the 68 reviewed studies, active transport resulted in students with significantly more PA during their day. Many national policies call for more active transport for adults and children, but fewer initiatives in this area are reported in the literature. The HEPAS proposal to consider active homework is another intriguing yet underutilized strategy for ASP PA.

Whether as part of a whole school program or as a stand-alone ASP, PA in students can be positively impacted with effective programming. That programming needs strong leaders and collaborations, but the specific format and content should reflect the goals and resources of the local community. With that freedom more children can move more often in meaningful ways in their school years and those positive experiences will carry forward into healthier adulthood.

References

1. Warburton DER. Health benefits of physical activity: the evidence. CMAJ. 2006;174:801–9.
2. Blair SN, Morris JN. Healthy hearts—and the universal benefits of being physically active: physical activity and health. Ann Epidemiol. 2009;19:253–6.
3. Hillman CH, Erickson KI, Kramer AF. Be smart, exercise your heart: exercise effects on brain and cognition. Nat Rev Neurosci. 2008;9:58–65.
4. Donnelly JE, Hillman CH, Castelli D, Etnier JL, Lee S, Tomporowski P, et al. Physical activity, fitness, cognitive function, and academic achievement in children: a systematic review. Med Sci Sports Exerc. 2016;48:1197–222.
5. Duncan MJ, Spence JC, Mummery WK. Perceived environment and physical activity: a meta-analysis of selected environmental characteristics. Int J Behav Nutr Phys Act. 2005;2:11.
6. Holt-Lunstad J, Robles TF, Sbarra DA. Advancing social connection as a public health priority in the United States. Am Psychol. 2017;72:517–30.
7. Stathopoulou G, Powers MB, Berry AC, Smits JAJ, Otto MW. Exercise interventions for mental health: a quantitative and qualitative review. Clin Psychol Sci. 2006;13:179–93.
8. Craft LL, Perna FM. The benefits of exercise for the clinically depressed. Prim Care Companion CNS Disord [Internet]. 2004 [citado 12 de febrero de 2024];6. Disponible en: https://www.psychiatrist.com/pcc/benefits-exercise-clinically-depressed
9. World Health Organization (WHO). Global status report on physical activity 2022: country profiles [Internet]. [citado 28 de febrero de 2024]. Disponible en: https://www.who.int/publications/i/item/9789240064119
10. Cooper AR, Goodman A, Page AS, Sherar LB, Esliger DW, Van Sluijs EM, et al. Objectively measured physical activity and sedentary time in youth: the international children's accelerometry database (ICAD). Int J Behav Nutr Phys Act. 2015;12:113.
11. Friel CP, Duran AT, Shechter A, Diaz KM. U.S. children meeting physical activity, screen time, and sleep guidelines. Am J Prev Med. 2020;59:513–21.
12. GEM Report UNESCO. Global Education Monitoring Report 2023: Technology in education: A tool on whose terms? [Internet]. 1.a ed. GEM Report UNESCO; 2023 [citado 26 de febrero de 2024]. Disponible en: https://unesdoc.unesco.org/ark:/48223/pf0000385723

13. West T, Boyd M, Holeva-Eklund W, Liebert M, Schuna J, Behrens T. Implementing structured curriculum in an after-school physical activity program. TPE [Internet]. 2021 [citado 12 de febrero de 2024];78. Disponible en: https://js.sagamorepub.com/pe/article/view/10773
14. Kahan D, McKenzie TL. Physical activity and psychological correlates during an after-school running club. Am J Health Educ. 2018;49:113–23.
15. Hollis JL, Sutherland R, Williams AJ, Campbell E, Nathan N, Wolfenden L, et al. A systematic review and meta-analysis of moderate-to-vigorous physical activity levels in secondary school physical education lessons. Int J Behav Nutr Phys Act. 2017;14:52.
16. Dauenhauer B, Kulinna P, Marttinen R, Stellino MB. Before- and after-school physical activity: programs and best practices. J Phys Educ Recreat Dance. 2022;93:20–6.
17. Demetriou Y, Gillison F, McKenzie TL. After-school physical activity interventions on child and adolescent physical activity and health: a review of reviews. APE. 2017;07:191–215.
18. Kirk D. Physical education, youth sport and lifelong participation: the importance of early learning experiences. Eur Phys Educ Rev. 2005;11:239–55.
19. Jones R. Why is physical education being cut in schools: the top reasons behind the trend [Internet]. CollegeUSCom; 2023. Disponible en: https://college.us.com/why-is-physical-education-being-cut-in-schools/
20. Nancy M. Quality physical education. UNESCO; 2015.
21. Centeio EE, Erwin H, Barcelona J, McKown H. Implementing before-and after-school physical activity programs within the whole school, whole community, whole child framework. In: Before and after school physical activity programs [Internet]. Routledge; 2020. [citado 19 de marzo de 2024]. pp. 9–21. Disponible en: https://www.taylorfrancis.com/chapters/edit/10.4324/9781003051909-1/implementing-school-physical-activity-programs-within-whole-school-whole-community-whole-child-framework-erin-centeio-heather-erwin-jeanne-barcelona-hayley-mckown.
22. Mahoney JL, Parente ME, Zigler EF. Afterschool programs in America: origins, growth, popularity, and politics. JYD. 2009;4:23–42.
23. Plantenga J, Remery C. Out-of-school childcare: exploring availability and quality in EU member states. J Eur Soc Policy. 2017;27:25–39.
24. OECD Family Database. Out-of-school-hours services [Internet] 2024. Disponible en: https://www.oecd.org/els/family/PF4-3-Out-of-school-hours-care.pdf
25. Afterschool Alliance. America after 3PM: demand grows, opportunity shrinks. Washington, DC: Afterschool Alliance; 2020.
26. McMullen J, Ní Chróinín D, Tammelin T, Pogorzelska M, Van Der Mars H. International approaches to whole-of-school physical activity promotion. Quest. 2015;67:384–99.
27. Bailey R, Adamakis M, Boronyai Z, Vašíčková J, Raya Demidoff A, Repond R, Heck S, Scheuer C. The HEPAS Model: a healthy and physically active school model promoting physical activity and healthy lifestyles in school settings. Physical education and physical activities of children, youth and adults and healthy active living research—best practices—Situation. p. 229–38.
28. Comprehensive School Physical Activity Program (CSPAP) [Internet]. [citado 19 de marzo de 2024]. Disponible en: https://www.shapeamerica.org/MemberPortal/cspap/default.aspx
29. Center For Disease Control and Prevention. Whole school, whole community, whole child (WSCC). [Internet] CDC Healthy Schools 2023. Disponible en: https://www.cdc.gov/healthy-schools/wscc/index.htm
30. National Physical Activity Plan [Internet]. PAA. [citado 19 de marzo de 2024]. Disponible en: https://paamovewithus.org/national-physical-activity-plan/
31. Piercy KL, Troiano RP, Ballard RM, Carlson SA, Fulton JE, Galuska DA, et al. The physical activity guidelines for Americans. JAMA. 2018;320:2020.
32. Canadian Ministry of Education. Before and afterschool programs kindergarten to grade 6: policies and guidelines for school boards. Ministry of Education Canada; 2019.

33. Jago R, Edwards MJ, Cooper AR, Fox KR, Powell J, Sebire SJ, et al. Action 3:30: protocol for a randomized feasibility trial of a teaching assistant led extracurricular physical activity intervention. Trials. 2013;14:122.
34. Jago R, Sebire SJ, Davies B, Wood L, Banfield K, Edwards MJ, et al. Increasing children's physical activity through a teaching-assistant led extracurricular intervention: process evaluation of the action 3: 30 randomised feasibility trial. BMC Public Health. 2015;15:1–15.
35. Riiser K, Helseth S, Ellingsen H, Fallang B, Løndal K. Active play in after-school programmes: development of an intervention and description of a matched-pair cluster-randomised trial assessing physical activity play in after-school programmes. BMJ Open. 2017;7:e016585.
36. Kinder CJ, Gaudreault KL, Jenkins JM, Wade CE, Woods AM. At-risk youth in an after-school program: structured vs. unstructured physical activity. Phys Educ. 2019;76:1157–80.
37. Ratey JJ, Hagerman EC. Spark: The revolutionary new science of exercise and the brain. 2008 [citado 19 de marzo de 2024]; Disponible en: https://psycnet.apa.org/record/2008-02933-000?trk=public_post_comment-text
38. Hall G, Poston KF, Harris S. Before the school bell rings. 2015
39. Caldwell HAT, Miller MB, Tweedie C, Zahavich JBL, Cockett E, Rehman L. The effect of an after-school physical activity program on children's cognitive, social, and emotional health during the COVID-19 pandemic in Nova Scotia. IJERPH. 2022;19:2401.
40. Caldwell HAT, Miller MB, Tweedie C, Zahavich JBL, Cockett E, Rehman L. The impact of an after-school physical activity program on children's physical activity and well-being during the COVID-19 pandemic: a mixed-methods evaluation study. IJERPH. 2022;19:5640.
41. Sallis JF, McKenzie TL, Kolody B, Lewis M, Marshall S, Rosengard P. Effects of health-related physical education on academic achievement: project SPARK. Res Q Exerc Sport. 1999;70:127–34.
42. McKenzie TL, Sallis JF, Rosengard P. Beyond the stucco tower: design, development, and dissemination of the SPARK physical education programs. Quest. 2009;61:114–27.
43. McKenzie TL, Sallis JF, Rosengard P, Ballard K. The SPARK programs: a public health model of physical education research and dissemination. J Teach Phys Educ. 2016;35:381–9.
44. Strelow JS, Larsen JS, Sallis JF, Conway TL, Powers HS, McKenzie TL. Factors influencing the performance of volunteers who provide physical activity in middle schools. J Sch Health. 2002;72:147–51.
45. Cardon GM, Haerens LL, Verstraete S, De Bourdeaudhuij I. Perceptions of a school-based self-management program promoting an active lifestyle among elementary school children, teachers, and parents. J Teach Phys Educ. 2009;28:141–54.
46. Messiah SE, Diego A, Kardys J, Kirwin K, Hanson E, Nottage R, et al. Effect of a park-based after-school program on participant obesity-related health outcomes. Am J Health Promot. 2015;29:217–25.
47. Sallis JF, McKenzie TL, Conway TL, Elder JP, Prochaska JJ, Brown M, et al. Environmental interventions for eating and physical activity. Am J Prev Med. 2003;24:209–17.
48. Nigg C, Geller K, Adams P, Hamada M, Hwang P, Chung R. Successful dissemination of fun 5 — a physical activity and nutrition program for children. Behav Med Pract Policy Res. 2012;2:276–85.
49. Iversen CSS, Nigg C, Titchenal CA. The impact of an elementary after-school nutrition and physical activity program on children's fruit and vegetable intake, physical activity, and body mass index: fun 5. Hawaii Med J. 2011;70:37–41.
50. Herrick H, Thompson H, Kinder J, Madsen KA. Use of SPARK to promote after-school physical activity. J Sch Health. 2012;82:457–61.
51. Franks A, Kelder SH, Dino GA, Horn KA, Gortmaker SL, Wiecha JL, et al. School-based programs: lessons learned from CATCH, planet health, and not-on-tobacco. Prev Chronic Dis. 2007;4:A33.
52. Sharpe EK, Forrester S, Mandigo J. Engaging community providers to create more active after-school environments: results from the Ontario CATCH kids club implementation project. J Phys Act Health. 2011;8:S26–31.

53. Werner D, Teufel J, Holtgrave PL, Brown SL. Active generations: an intergenerational approach to preventing childhood obesity. J Sch Health. 2012;82:380–6.
54. Dzewaltowski DA, Rosenkranz RR, Geller KS, Coleman KJ, Welk GJ, Hastmann TJ, et al. HOP'N after-school project: an obesity prevention randomized controlled trial. Int J Behav Nutr Phys Act. 2010;7:90.
55. Weiss MR, Kipp LE, Phillips Reichter A, Espinoza SM, Bolter ND. Girls on the run: impact of a physical activity youth development program on psychosocial and behavioral outcomes. Pediatr Exerc Sci. 2019;31:330–40.
56. Weiss MR, Kipp LE, Phillips Reichter A, Bolter ND. Evaluating girls on the run in promoting positive youth development: group comparisons on life skills transfer and social processes. Pediatr Exerc Sci. 2020;32:172–82.
57. Baghurst T, Tapps T, Adib N. Effects of a youth running program on self-concept and running. J Sport Pedagogy Res. 2015;1:4–10.
58. Wanless E, Judge LW, Dieringer ST, Bellar D, Johnson J, Plummer S. Pedometers and aerobic capacity: evaluating an elementary after-school running program. Sci World J. 2014;2014:1–6.
59. Fredrick RN, Marttinen R, Johnston KC. REACH after-school: integrating literacy and PA in under-served communities. In: Before and after school physical activity programs [Internet]. Routledge; 2020. [citado 19 de marzo de 2024]. p. 96–107. Disponible en: https://www.taylorfrancis.com/chapters/edit/10.4324/9781003051909-8/reach-school-ray-fredrick-risto-marttinen-kelly-johnston.
60. Marttinen R, Fredrick RN. R.E.A.C.H: an after-school approach to physical education. Strategies. 2017;30:8–14.
61. Marttinen R, Johnston K, Phillips S, Fredrick RN, Meza B. REACH Harlem: young urban boys' experiences in an after-school PA positive youth development program. Phys Educ Sport Pedagogy. 2019;24:373–89.
62. Marttinen R, Meza B, Flory SB. Stereotypical views of beauty and boys STILL not letting girls play: a student-centered curriculum for young girls through an after-school activist approach. J Teach Phys Educ. 2021;40:442–9.
63. Nuñez Enriquez O, Oliver KL. 'Can we play the real sport?' Co-creating a student-centered after-school sports club. Phys Educ Sport Pedagogy. 2022;27:231–46.
64. Barfield PA, Ridder K, Hughes J, Rice-McNeil K. Get outside! Promoting adolescent health through outdoor after-school activity. IJERPH. 2021;18:7223.
65. Poulos A, Kulinna PH. A cluster randomized controlled trial of an after-school playground curriculum intervention to improve children's physical, social, and emotional health: study protocol for the PLAYground project. BMC Public Health. 2022;22:1658.
66. Tremblay MS, Barnes JD, González SA, Katzmarzyk PT, Onywera VO, Reilly JJ, et al. Global matrix 2.0: report card grades on the physical activity of children and youth comparing 38 countries. J Phys Act Health. 2016;13:S343–66.
67. Boronyai Z, Bailey R, Heck S, Raya Demidoff A, Repond RM, Vašíčková J, et al. Healthy and physically active schools in Europe: Framework and guidelines for implementation. 2022 [citado 25 de febrero de 2024]; Disponible en: https://zenodo.org/record/5909636
68. Lee JE, Pope Z, Gao Z. The role of youth sports in promoting children's physical activity and preventing pediatric obesity: a systematic review. Behav Med. 2018;44:62–76.
69. Ling FC, Farrow A, Farrow D, Berry J, Polman RC. Children's perspectives on the effectiveness of the playing for life philosophy in an afterschool sports program. Int J Sports Sci. 2016;11:780–8.
70. Lumpkin A, Stokowski S. Interscholastic sports: a character-building privilege. KDP Record. 2011;47:124–8.
71. Edwards MB, Kanters MA, Bocarro JN. Opportunities for extracurricular physical activity in North Carolina middle schools. J Phys Act Health. 2011;8:597–605.
72. Edwards MB, Kanters MA, Bocarro JN. Policy changes to implement intramural sports in North Carolina middle schools: simulated effects on sports participation rates and physical activity intensity, 2008–2009. Prev Chronic Dis. 2014;11:130195.

73. Bocarro J, Kanters MA, Casper J, Forrester S. School physical education, extracurricular sports, and lifelong active living. J Teach Phys Educ. 2008;27:155–66.
74. Pantzer J, Dorwart CE, Woodson-Smith A. Importance of bonding in middle school intramural sports participation: psychosocial outcomes based on gender and grade-level differences. Phys Educ. 2018;75:661–82.
75. Aspen. Reimagining school sports in America [Internet]. The Aspen institute; 2020. [citado 19 de marzo de 2024]. Disponible en: https://www.aspeninstitute.org/videos/reimagining-school-sports-in-america/
76. Maljak K, Garn A, McCaughtry N, Kulik N, Martin J, Shen B, et al. Challenges in offering inner-city after-school physical activity clubs. Am J Health Educ. 2014;45:297–307.
77. Wiecha JL, Hall G, Barnes M. Uptake of national after-school association physical activity standards among US after-school sites. Prev Med. 2014;69:S61–5.
78. Castelli DM, Carson RL, Kulinna PH. PETE programs creating teacher leaders to integrate comprehensive school physical activity programs. J Phys Educ Recreat Dance. 2017;88:8–10.
79. Weaver RG, Webster C, Beets MW. LET US play: maximizing physical activity in physical education. Strategies. 2013;26:33–7.
80. Huberty JL, Beets MW, Beighle A, Mckenzie TL. Association of staff behaviors and after-school program features to physical activity: findings from movin' after school. J Phys Act Health. 2013;10:423–9.
81. Weaver RG, Beets MW, Huberty J, Freedman D, Turner-Mcgrievy G, Ward D. Physical activity opportunities in afterschool programs. Health Promot Pract. 2015;16:371–82.
82. Weaver RG, Moore JB, Turner-McGrievy B, Saunders R, Beighle A, Khan MM, et al. Identifying strategies programs adopt to meet healthy eating and physical activity standards in afterschool programs. Health Educ Behav. 2017;44:536–47.
83. Beets MW, Weaver RG, Moore JB, Turner-McGrievy G, Pate RR, Webster C, et al. From policy to practice: strategies to meet physical activity standards in YMCA afterschool programs. Am J Prev Med. 2014;46:281–8.
84. Chen S, Gu X. Toward active living: comprehensive school physical activity program research and implications. Quest. 2018;70:191–212.
85. Choudhry S, McClinton-Powell L, Solomon M, Davis D, Lipton R, Darukhanavala A, et al. Power-up: a collaborative after-school program to prevent obesity in African American children. Prog Community Health Partnersh. 2011;5:363–73.
86. Chandler JL, Brazendale K, Drenowatz C, Moore JB, Sui X, Weaver RG, et al. Structure of physical activity opportunities contribution to children's physical activity levels in after-school programs. J Phys Act Health. 2019;16:512–7.
87. Trost SG, Rosenkranz RR, Dzewaltowski D. Physical activity levels among children attending after-school programs. Med Sci Sports Exerc. 2008;40:622–9.
88. Crouter SE, De Ferranti SD, Whiteley J, Steltz SK, Osganian SK, Feldman HA, et al. Effect on physical activity of a randomized afterschool intervention for inner city children in 3rd to 5th grade. Buchowski M, editor. PLoS One. 2015;10:e0141584.
89. Sirard JR, Alhassan S, Spencer TR, Robinson TN. Changes in physical activity from walking to school. J Nutr Educ Behav. 2008;40:324–6.
90. Larouche R, Saunders TJ, John Faulkner GE, Colley R, Tremblay M. Associations between active school transport and physical activity, body composition, and cardiovascular fitness: a systematic review of 68 studies. J Phys Act Health. 2014;11:206–27.

Chapter 14
Integrating High-Intensity Interval Training (HIIT) into the School Setting: Benefits, Criticisms, and Recommendations

Angus A. Leahy, Jordan J. Smith, Narelle Eather, Nigel Harris, and David R. Lubans

14.1 Introduction

Over the past two decades, there has been a surge of scientific interest in the effectiveness of high-intensity interval training (HIIT) as a health promotion strategy [1]. HIIT has also been popular among the health and fitness community, ranking within the top five fitness trends globally from 2014 to 2020 (number one in 2014 and 2018). HIIT remains in the top 10 most popular trends in many regions around the world [2]. There is an accumulating body of research demonstrating that HIIT produces comparable and in some cases superior health benefits to longer continuous bouts of lower intensity exercise (e.g., moderate-intensity continuous training) [3, 4]. As a result, it has been suggested that HIIT may be a viable alternative to traditional forms of exercise, especially those that require more overall time commitment, given perceived lack of time is a common cited barrier to exercise [5, 6].

A. A. Leahy (✉) · J. J. Smith · N. Eather
Centre for Active Living and Learning, College of Human and Social Futures, University of Newcastle, Callaghan, NSW, Australia

Active Living Research Program, Hunter Medical Research Institute,
New Lambton Heights, NSW, Australia
e-mail: angus.leahy@newcastle.edu.au

N. Harris
Human Potential Centre, Auckland University of Technology, Auckland, New Zealand

D. R. Lubans
Centre for Active Living and Learning, College of Human and Social Futures, University of Newcastle, Callaghan, NSW, Australia

Active Living Research Program, Hunter Medical Research Institute,
New Lambton Heights, NSW, Australia

Faculty of Sport and Health Sciences, University of Jyväskylä, Jyväskylä, Finland

© The Author(s), under exclusive license to Springer Nature Switzerland AG 2024
A. García-Hermoso (ed.), *Promotion of Physical Activity and Health in the School Setting*, https://doi.org/10.1007/978-3-031-65595-1_14

With the growing recognition of HIIT as a potential health promotion strategy, school-based HIIT programs have gained traction as a strategy to promote physical activity (PA) among youth. As such, the primary aim of our chapter is to provide an overview of the benefits, criticisms, and recommendations for integrating HIIT into the school setting. First, we provide a general introduction, discussing the criticisms of HIIT as a public health approach, and the importance of school settings in HIIT promotion. Following this, we provide a summary of the effects of HIIT programs on a range of physical, mental, and cognitive health outcomes. Then we outline a conceptual model for scaling up HIIT programs for population health. We conclude with recommendations and limitations of delivering HIIT in schools.

14.1.1 What Is HIIT?

The practice of interval training dates back to the early twentieth century and was used by elite athletes and coaches to improve performance of long and middle distance runners [7]. HIIT can be broadly defined as a form of interval training, that alternates periods of high-intensity activity (referred to as work bouts), with periods of rest or low-intensity activity (referred to as recovery bouts) [8]. Among the scientific literature (and in practice), HIIT protocols vary substantially. While there is no universal protocol, HIIT sessions typically involve short work bouts (between a few seconds and several minutes in duration) at a greater intensity than typical steady-state exercise, interspersed with periods of low-intensity activity or rest [8]. At the upper end of the intensity spectrum, sprint interval training (SIT) involves supra-maximal efforts (i.e., all-out maximal sprinting), interspersed by longer periods of active recovery or rest. This specific form of training was first popularized by a classic study conducted by Tabata and colleagues in the 1990s [9]. This protocol involved 8×20 s work bouts at an intensity corresponding to 170% of VO_{2max}, interspersed with 10 s recovery bouts, which equated to an exercise duration of 4 min (excluding a sufficient warm-up or cool-down). Participants repeated this protocol five times per week, for 6 weeks. After 6 weeks of training, significant improvements were found for participants' VO_{2max} and anaerobic capacity. Since the seminal work of Tabata, several other notable studies have been conducted utilizing SIT protocols, resulting in similar physiological adaptations [10–12].

It is important to acknowledge that a rapidly growing body of research has examined the efficacy of a broad range of HIIT protocols. Indeed, the prescription of HIIT can involve the interplay of up to nine parameters, including: (i) work bout duration, (ii) work bout intensity, (iii) recovery bout duration, (iv) recovery bout intensity, (v) exercise modality, (vi) number of intervals, (vii) number of series/sets, (viii) between series/sets recovery duration, and (ix) between series/sets recovery intensity [13].

14.1.2 Criticisms of HIIT

Despite its popularity, HIIT is a polarizing form of exercise [1]. Critics have argued that it has limited utility as a health promotion strategy, as it is a complex form of exercise that requires high levels of self-regulation to be effective [1]. One of the core arguments against HIIT is that exercising at an intensity above the aerobic/ventilatory threshold is known to lead to feelings of displeasure, and therefore, this will lead to lower exercise adherence [14]. The argument of negative affect during high-intensity exercise is not disputed. Indeed, affective responses during and immediately following high intensity/strenuous exercise are almost universally negative [15]. However, this appears to be more relevant to protocols that involve supramaximal efforts (i.e., SIT) [16]. Despite negative feelings "during" exercise, there is evidence from adult [17] and adolescent [18] studies highlighting an affective rebound "following" HIIT. This effect is not exclusive to HIIT, and similar (and sometimes superior) improvements in affect have been found following lower intensity exercise. For example, in a recent review, acute moderate intensity continuous training elicited more positively balanced post-exercise affect than HIIT; however, self-reported enjoyment was greater following HIIT [19].

Another criticism of HIIT is that many protocols have required the use of specialized equipment to monitor and adhere to the intensity prescribed. Indeed, seminal studies that have demonstrated the potency of HIIT have been conducted in highly controlled laboratory settings and have required participants to utilize equipment such as research-grade stationary cycling ergometers [9–11]. From a population-wide health promotion perspective, relying on specialized equipment to perform HIIT may be difficult in real world settings, such as schools. On the other hand, HIIT protocols that involve running (without the use of treadmills) have demonstrated significant physiological benefits in both adults [20] and youth [21]. Another criticism of HIIT is that individuals will fail to adhere to the high prescribed intensity when external support is removed. This has been observed in studies with protocols involving one singular mode of exercise [22, 23]. However, it is important to note that evidence used to support these claims stems from the adult literature [24]. While the majority of early HIIT studies prescribe protocols involving a singular form of exercise, researchers are now exploring more creative HIIT protocols that include a variety of engaging exercises to maximize variety, enjoyment, motivation, and adherence [25–28].

14.1.3 School-Based HIIT Programs

Among youth, schools are the most common non-laboratory setting for the delivery of HIIT programs [29]. Indeed, schools are important settings for the delivery of HIIT programs as they can reach a large proportion of children and adolescents and have existing infrastructure and personnel (e.g., teachers) to support intervention delivery, and HIIT programs delivered in the school setting have the potential to be scalable. Given the popularity of HIIT in the last decade, it is no surprise that there is growing interest in the design and evaluation of school-based HIIT programs. A recent systematic review identified 42 unique HIIT programs that have been delivered in schools, with 71% of these studies published in the last decade [30]. Typically, school HIIT programs were delivered three times per week over a period of 8–12 weeks. Of note, this aligns with current global PA recommendations that specify "vigorous-intensity PA, as well as those that strengthen muscle and bone, at least three days per week" [31]. To date, the most common HIIT modality is running; however, some programs have adopted more contemporary approaches that include body-weight resistance exercise, dance movements, and sport-specific skills [28, 32]. Unsurprisingly, most school-based HIIT programs have been delivered during physical education, although HIIT has also been performed as a "classroom activity break" during academic lessons [33, 34].

In summary, HIIT appears to be a promising health promotion strategy for children and adolescents. It is important to acknowledge that HIIT should be promoted as an exercise option, and other forms of exercise (e.g., resistance training, yoga, or team sports) should continue to be promoted among pediatric populations. In the next section, we provide a summary of the physical, mental, and cognitive health benefits of school-based HIIT programs.

14.2 Overview of Health Benefits

Systematic review evidence supports that school-based HIIT is an enjoyable and time-efficient PA option that can positively impact a range of important physical, mental, and cognitive health benefits amongst children and adolescents [30, 35–37]. While most school-based HIIT research has examined physical health outcomes (e.g., fitness), studies examining cognitive and mental health outcomes are becoming more common. Indeed, providing evidence for the effects of HIIT on affective and educational outcomes may help implement policies promoting PA within the school setting. School-based HIIT intervention studies have adopted a range of protocols, with work to rest ratios, exercise modalities, intervention duration, and dose highly varied. Despite the difficulties of comparing the effectiveness of HIIT in all its forms, there continues to be strong and consistent evidence demonstrating the array of health benefits of HIIT when implemented in the school setting for children and adolescents.

14.2.1 Physical Health Benefits

14.2.1.1 Cardiorespiratory Fitness (CRF)

A recent systematic review and meta-analysis conducted by Eather et al. [36] included 30 HIIT studies implemented in school-based physical education or sport and demonstrated that HIIT is effective for improving CRF amongst children and adolescents (effect size [ES] = 0.27). Notably, study duration significantly moderated the effects, with shorter duration studies yielding larger effects. Similarly, a review of 42 school-based HIIT studies using 10 s to 4-min exercise bouts of varied modalities (including running, cycling, dance, resistance training, circuits, games, strength training, and sports drills) was conducted by Duncombe and colleagues [30]. Duncombe's review supports with moderate certainty that school-based HIIT can increase CRF compared with a control or comparison group (ES = 1.0), despite great variation in dose and duration of HIIT programs included in the review. These results are comparable to the findings of earlier meta-analyses that have examined HIIT involving healthy adolescents in all settings (ES = 1.05) [4] and adolescents classified as obese or overweight (ES = 1.11) [38].

HIIT also appears to be effective for improving CRF in students with special educational needs. To date, only one review has examined the effects of HIIT programs among this population (in all settings) [39]. The results provide preliminary evidence that HIIT can facilitate improvements in CRF among students living with disability. However, improvements were not observed in all studies, with effect sizes ranging from −0.02 [40] to 1.25 [41], therefore firm conclusions cannot be drawn. Further, the majority of included studies were classified as having "high" or "serious" risk of bias, and future high-quality randomized controlled trials are warranted [42].

14.2.1.2 Muscular Fitness

There are limited number of studies reporting on the benefits of school-based HIIT for muscular fitness outcomes (e.g., power, strength, endurance), however, such studies are becoming more popular. Indeed, emerging HIIT protocols have included a range of exercises suitable for improving muscular fitness, such as body weight and plyometric exercises [43, 44]. Eather and colleagues' systematic review and meta-analysis of HIIT delivered in school-based physical education or sport examined 12 studies reporting on muscular fitness outcomes [36]. The results indicate that HIIT can significantly improve both lower and upper body muscular fitness (ES = 0.49 and 0.37, respectively) when compared to usual practice or alternate programs implemented in physical education or sport. On the other hand, Duncombe and colleagues found no significant difference between HIIT and control or comparison groups for reported measures of muscular fitness (i.e., jumping, handgrip strength, or sit-ups) [30]. Due to the lack of eligible studies, the authors were only able to conduct meta-analyses for lower body muscular fitness as assessed by standing long jump and countermovement jump measures, with small and non-significant effects reported [30]. Similarly, Costigan and colleagues [4] reported a small non-significant effect of HIIT interventions (conducted in all settings) on adolescents' muscular fitness (ES = 0.21) across five studies.

The effects of HIIT on muscular fitness outcomes among children and adolescents with special educational needs are inconclusive with contrasting findings reported (effect sizes ranging from −0.22 to 0.99) [39]. In their review, Poon and colleagues identified four unique studies that assessed muscular fitness outcomes. Of note, a variety of muscular fitness measures have been assessed including grip strength, sit-to-stand, push-up, standing broad jump, and muscle power sprint tests. From the limited evidence base, HIIT appears to have negligible effects on upper body muscular power, small-to-moderate effects on lower body muscular power, and mixed findings for upper/lower body muscular endurance. Overall, mixed findings have been reported for the effects of school-based HIIT programs on muscular fitness outcomes. This may be due to (a) the array of HIIT protocols available (especially regarding the included exercises, and intervention dose and duration) and (b) the skills, exposure, and repetition needed to improve muscular fitness outcomes in children and adolescents.

14.2.1.3 Body Composition

School-based HIIT programs appear to be effective for improving body composition, however, a variety of body composition measures (e.g., BMI, BMI z scores, waist circumference, body weight, and body fat percentage) have been utilised, making direct comparisons of results challenging. In the review by Duncombe and colleagues, HIIT was significantly favored in meta-analyses for waist circumference, body fat percentage, and BMI, but not for muscle mass or lean mass when compared to non-exercise control groups; however, results were much less conclusive relative to comparative exercise protocols [30]. Duncombe also reported that study protocols with a greater volume of HIIT reported greater decrease in body fat percentage and BMI, studies of longer duration had a greater decrease in body fat percentage, and girls demonstrated the largest reductions in body fat percentage and BMI [30]. Similarly, Eather et al. found HIIT significantly reduced BMI in comparison to control groups (ES = −0.27), however no significant moderators were observed. Two previous systematic reviews and meta-analyses also support the potential of HIIT for improving body composition in healthy [4], and overweight and obese [38] children and adolescents. In contrast, one review conducted by Eddolls et al. found little evidence to suggest HIIT can improve body composition in healthy children and/or adolescents [45]. Although research studies are limited for students with special education needs, a systematic review conducted by Poon et al. [39] found that HIIT can facilitate improvements in measures of body composition in this population, including body mass index (BMI) ($n = 6$; ES = − 0.55 to

0.02), waist circumference ($n = 3$; ES = − 0.33 to 0.01), body fat percentage ($n = 3$; ES = − 0.55 to − 0.14), and fat mass ($n = 4$; ES = − 0.51 to 0.00).

14.2.1.4 Other Fitness Components

There have been a multitude of school-based HIIT intervention studies that have measured changes in fitness, with both health-related and skill-related fitness components evaluated. Eather's systematic review included HIIT studies reporting on changes in speed ($n = 4$), agility ($n = 3$), coordination ($n = 4$), flexibility ($n = 3$), and balance ($n = 1$) [36]. However, due to the heterogeneity of measures and limited studies evaluating each fitness component, meta-analyses were unable to be performed. Similarly, Bond and colleagues were only able to provide a narrative synthesis regarding the effects of school-based HIIT on skill-related fitness measures [35]. Significant improvements favoring HIIT were found in 2/3 studies that assessed speed, but not for flexibility (0/3 studies), or balance (0/2 studies).

14.2.1.5 Cardiometabolic Health

Five school-based HIIT studies were included in the meta-analyses examining the effect of HIIT on blood pressure published by Eather et al. [36]. Overall, the effects of HIIT on systolic blood pressure and diastolic blood pressure were non-significant (ES = −0.13 and − 0.07, respectively). Similarly, Duncombe and colleagues found a non-significant effect on blood pressure, however found HIIT significantly improved resting heart rate in comparison to non-exercise control [30]. Duncombe et al. also reported significant improvements in HIIT conditions compared to control conditions for insulin resistance (HOMA-IR), and low-density lipoprotein (LDL), but not for other blood profile indicators (e.g., glucose triglycerides and cholesterol) [30]. Regarding students with special education needs, the only consistent findings were observed for improving insulin and insulin resistance [39].

14.2.2 Cognitive Benefits

Over the last decade, a growing body of research has examined the link between PA, physical fitness, and cognitive function in children and adolescents [46]. Given that schools, teachers, and parents continue to prioritize academic outcomes for children and adolescents throughout their schooling years, building evidence for the impact of school-based HIIT on cognitive and academic outcomes is warranted. We recently conducted a systematic review and meta-analysis [18] that evaluated the effect of HIIT on cognitive function (operationalized as basic information processing and executive function) in children and adolescents. We found a moderate effect for executive function following acute HIIT (ES = 0.50) and a small effect for chronic HIIT (ES = 0.31). Although our review did not exclusively examine school-based HIIT, 10/11 studies reporting on cognitive function were conducted in school settings. Our findings are similar to those reported in a more recent review, with positive effects of HIIT following both acute and chronic delivery for a range of cognitive outcomes (e.g., executive function, concentration, and selective attention) [47]. In the only school-based HIIT review to examine cognitive outcomes, significant effects favoring HIIT were found for inhibition (a subdomain of executive function) in 3/4 studies and for memory in 2/4 studies. As such, the authors concluded that school-based HIIT programs may improve cognitive function; however due to the limited number of studies (and heterogeneity of cognitive measures), more research was needed to confirm these findings.

Neurobiological mechanisms may help explain the positive effect of HIIT on cognitive performance (e.g., structural and functional changes in the brain). For example, in a recent cluster randomized controlled trial, a 6-month HIIT program, known as Burn 2 Learn (B2L) improved older adolescents' hippocampal metabolism. Of note, changes in hippocampal metabolism were associated with improvements in cardiorespiratory and muscular fitness, as well as working memory [48]. In another notable study from the B2L trial, significant improvements in students' on-task behavior (e.g., classroom engagement) were found following acute HIIT. Interestingly, although differences were not statistically significant, the largest improvements in on-task behavior were observed among students who were classified in the highest intensity group based on heart rate data collected during HIIT sessions.

To date, only two HIIT studies have examined cognitive outcomes in children and adolescents living with disability, neither of which were conducted in the school setting. One study observed improved inhibition response efficiency following a single 12-min HIIT bout among adolescents hospitalized for mental illness [49]. Conversely, no significant effects of HIIT were observed for academic productivity among children with ADHD, and detrimental effects were found for behavior following HIIT [50]. We cannot yet draw firm conclusions regarding the efficacy of HIIT for improving cognitive outcomes among youth living with disability. There is some promising early evidence suggesting HIIT is beneficial for a range of cognitive outcomes among children and adolescents without disability, which may have implications for the scheduling and the inclusion of HIIT on school curricula/programs.

14.2.3 Mental Health Benefits

There is a growing body of research supporting the beneficial effects of HIIT for mental health outcomes in youth populations. Evidence from both acute and chronic HIIT studies (conducted in a variety of settings) support this claim [18]. Acute HIIT has been found to benefit adolescents' affect (ES = 0.33), while chronic HIIT can benefit indicators of well-being (e.g., self-concept, quality of life), and ill-being (e.g., psychological distress, anxiety) with small to moderate effect sizes (ES = 0.22 and − 0.35, respectively) [18]. These findings are supported by Alves and colleagues who reviewed three HIIT studies involving youth and reported improvements in mental health outcomes [47]. While findings from these studies are promising, the effects of school-based HIIT interventions on mental health outcomes are less consistent. Duncombe and colleagues identified three studies that assessed wellbeing outcomes in their review of the school-based HIIT literature [30]. In comparison to a stretching control condition, 12 weeks of HIIT performed for 16 min twice a week resulted in significant improvements in adolescents' wellbeing [27]. Non-significant effects were observed in the other two studies [26, 51]. Similar findings were observed in recent cluster randomized controlled trial conducted in New Zealand, which embedded Indigenous narratives within HIIT [25]. Specifically, no intervention effects were observed for wellbeing or psychological difficulties among a sample of adolescents; however, significant improvements in self-perceived fitness and HIIT self-efficacy were observed for those participating in HIIT relative to usual physical education classes [25].

Although limited, there is some evidence to suggest that HIIT has a beneficial effect for mental health outcomes among students with special education needs [39]. Poon and colleagues reported that HIIT significantly improved a range of mental health outcomes including mood, quality of life, well-being, and social behavior. Just one study involving children with ADHD reported lower mood immediately after HIIT [50]. Because of the small number of school-based HIIT studies reporting on mental health outcomes, more high-quality research is needed to confirm these findings.

14.3 Introduction to Conceptual Model

Our previously published conceptual framework [52], guided by evidence from exercise psychology, physical education, exercise science, and implementation science, consists of four complementary, yet overlapping tenets (Fig. 14.1). These tenets serve as key considerations for the design and implementation of school-based HIIT programs. Firstly, we recommend the integration of HIIT into existing PA opportunities to optimize time efficiency and reduce reliance on children and adolescents' self-regulation. Secondly, we suggest that HIIT interventions should be carefully crafted to enhance students' physical literacy (i.e., motivation, confidence, competence, and knowledge). Thirdly, we emphasize the significance of delivering HIIT in an engaging manner to enhance participation and adherence. Finally, we advocate for the utilization of an implementation framework to guide and support youth HIIT programs.

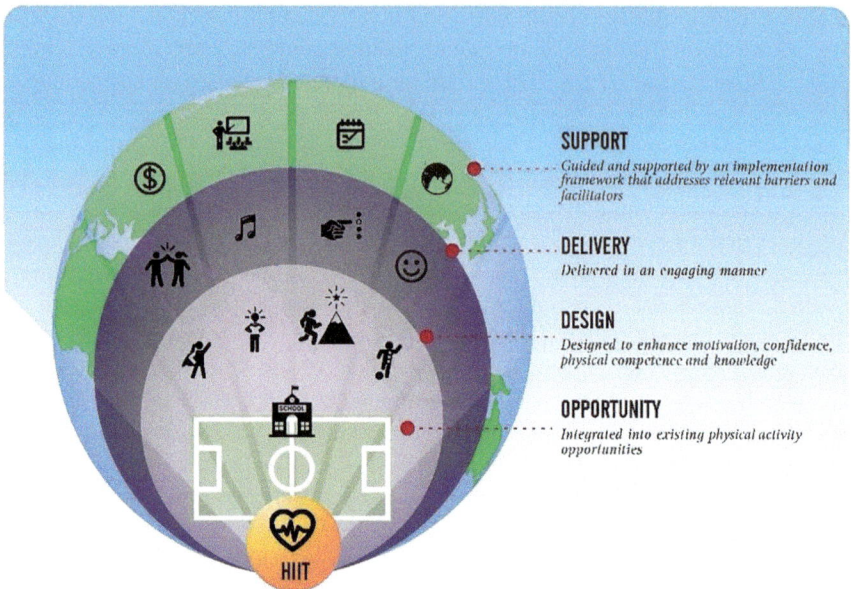

Fig. 14.1 Conceptual model outlining key considerations for the design, delivery, and scale-up of youth high-intensity interval training (HIIT) programs [52]. (Reprinted with permission from Lubans DR, Eather N, Smith JJ, Beets MW, Harris NK. Scaling-up adolescent high-intensity interval training programs for population health. Exercise and Sport Sciences Reviews. 2022;50 [3]:128–36. DOI: 10.1249/JES.0000000000000287. Copyright © 2022 by the American College of Sports Medicine)

14.3.1 Integrated into Existing Opportunities

Despite considerable research efforts spanning several decades, interventions aimed at increasing PA levels in school-aged youth have demonstrated limited effectiveness. Past interventions have relied on intrapersonal and interpersonal factors, such as motivation and social support, as catalysts for behavioral change. However, empirical evidence demonstrating significant effects on these hypothesized mediators remains scarce, and even when observed, the desired increase in PA often fails to materialize. Considering these challenges, contemporary discourse has advocated for a pragmatic shift towards prioritizing "opportunities" for PA participation as a fundamental approach for enhancing PA among youth.

The Theory of Expanded, Extended, and Enhanced Opportunities (TEO) [53] emphasizes the importance of regular, structured opportunities for PA engagement. These opportunities encompass various facets of the school day, such as physical education lessons, school recess breaks, curricular time, and out-of-school time (i.e., before and after school). Recognizing the inherent complexities in expecting youth to self-regulate their PA, the TEO philosophy holds relevance in promoting vigorous PA among school-aged youth. As previously noted, evidence from exercise psychology highlights a consistent decline in affective valence (i.e., feelings of displeasure) when individuals transition from moderate to vigorous intensity during an acute exercise bout [54]. Consequently, public health researchers have voiced skepticism regarding HIIT for public health [1], citing concerns over individuals' ability or willingness to engage in HIIT.

To address these concerns and achieve a meaningful impact on a larger scale, a reliance on HIIT opportunities that do not solely depend on young peoples' motivation and self-regulation is important. This necessitates the integration of engaging HIIT sessions within structured, regularly occurring periods, strategically implemented in settings with broad accessibility, such as that provided by schools. This time-efficient approach not only addresses previous criticisms directed at physical education and organized sports, which noted low levels of moderate-to-vigorous PA [55] but also optimizes the public health potential of these opportunities.

The TEO framework offers a compelling and pragmatic perspective for promoting PA among school-aged youth. By emphasizing the provision of regular, structured opportunities within settings that facilitate substantive reach into the youth population, this approach addresses the challenges of relying solely on youths' intrinsic motivation and self-regulation.

14.3.2 Designed to Support Students' Physical Literacy

Program design is a crucial consideration for the effective scale-up of youth HIIT programs. In this regard, we contend HIIT should be more than a means to deliver a "dose" of health-enhancing PA. Instead, we suggest HIIT programs for school-aged youth should be designed explicitly to foster "physical literacy." Whitehead [56] defines physical literacy as the "motivation, confidence, physical competence, knowledge, and understanding to value and take responsibility for engagement in PAs for life." By framing the design of HIIT programs through the lens of physical literacy, a more meaningful experience for youth may be achieved. If so, this may support short-term enjoyment and by consequence longer-term adherence to HIIT.

Although HIIT has demonstrated promise as an effective exercise modality, its distinctive nature, characterized by highly strenuous intermittent bouts, sets it apart from many other school-based PA programs. Activities like the "daily mile" program [57], where students run or walk outside each day for approximately 15 min (~1 mile) at a self-selected pace, may be easier to implement. For this intervention, there is no requirement for students to engage in (potentially aversive) high-intensity activity and the instructional and movement skill demands are minimal, but this means that the health benefits achieved through participation may also be limited. By contrast, school HIIT programs typically require some level of instruction and supervision to ensure safety and effectiveness, and students' motivation may be a barrier to overcome.

There is certainly a health rationale for prioritizing HIIT given the latent benefits, but to address the barriers to implementation, HIIT programs should be thoughtfully designed to: (a) support the development of new exercise skills, (b) instill confidence in performing such skills and a desire to apply them in the future, and (c) impart knowledge about the associated health and performance benefits to promote a sense of relevance. Students should also be encouraged to participate in the design and execution of their own HIIT sessions, as this is an authentic educational experience and one that provides a concrete skill young people can utilize throughout and beyond their schooling.

Focusing on the critical elements of physical literacy serves three key purposes. Firstly, decision makers, such as school principals and departmental administrators, are more likely to embrace school HIIT programs if they align with the core objectives of learning. Secondly, teachers and parents will view such initiatives more favorably if they address affective and educational outcomes, including motor skill competency, rather than focusing solely on fitness enhancement. Finally, students themselves are more likely to perceive HIIT as meaningful if it proves enjoyable and contributes to their acquisition of new knowledge, skills, and confidence. In conclusion, a thoughtful emphasis on physical literacy within the design of youth HIIT programs holds significant potential for facilitating effective scale-up. By aligning with core educational and engagement objectives, attending to affective and educational outcomes, and fostering an enjoyable and development-oriented experience, HIIT programs can better support the holistic well-being of young individuals.

14.3.3 Delivered in an Engaging Manner

As proponents of HIIT, we recognize the importance of delivering youth HIIT programs in a thoughtful manner. We firmly believe that while opportunity is necessary, it is not sufficient for the effective scale-up of HIIT for youth. This position is both practical and ethical, as we understand that imposing exercise on young people is not an effective strategy for promoting adherence, nor is it morally justifiable due to the potential for psychological harm [58]. Negative childhood experiences in physical education classes, for example, can have lasting effects on individuals' attitudes toward PA even into adulthood [59]. Consequently, individuals may be more inclined to avoid negative emotional states rather than actively seeking to "feel good [60]."

This has direct implications for promoting HIIT to youth, as the types of HIIT described in much of the research literature (e.g., repeated maximal sprints on exercise bikes or running tracks) may be aversive to most children and adolescents. However, there are evidence-based strategies that can be employed to mitigate the negative affective states that this mode of exercise might evoke, such as incorporating carefully selected music [61]. To begin with, this involves offering alternative versions of HIIT that differ from those used in laboratory-based research, which primarily aimed to understand the acute and chronic physiological effects. Secondly, it requires careful consideration of how HIIT can be packaged in a way that appeals to youth who are typically not motivated by the cardiovascular and metabolic benefits of exercise. For example, reminding students about the benefits of HIIT for stress reduction and cognitive function may help motivate students, especially older adolescents [18]. The design and delivery of health promotion interventions often overlook the importance of pedagogy [62], but we believe that pedagogy, which refers to the "how" of delivery, is just as crucial to the effectiveness of an intervention as its content and format.

Self-Determination Theory [63, 64] and Achievement Goal Theory [65] are two widely used psychological theories of motivation that have been applied to PA interventions in school settings [66, 67]. The former recognizes the significance of satisfying individuals' basic psychological needs for autonomy, competence, and relatedness will enhance autonomous motivation, engagement, and psychological well-being. Alternatively, Achievement Goal Theory acknowledges the importance of framing goals based on personal mastery rather than comparative performance to foster long-term motivation and commitment. While we do not expect that incorporating these concepts of basic psychological needs satisfaction or mastery goal framing into HIIT interventions will immediately result in all young people willingly engaging in HIIT during their leisure-time, it does not diminish the relevance of these concepts to the delivery of HIIT programs. Thoughtful consideration of these psychological constructs can make a difference in how young people perceive school-based HIIT, turning it from something to be avoided, to something they may consider worthwhile.

14.3.4 Guided and Supported by an Implementation Framework That Addresses Relevant Barriers and Facilitators

Finally, we emphasize the significance of using implementation science to guide and support the design, delivery, and scale-up of youth HIIT programs. HIIT is a relatively complex form of exercise, and program drift [68], which refers to deviations from intervention protocols during real-world delivery, poses a challenge to the successful scale-up of school-based HIIT programs. "Scale-up" or "scaling-up" has been defined as a "deliberate effort to increase the impact of successfully tested health interventions to benefit more people" (p. 2) [69]. It is well-known that school-based PA interventions often do not progress beyond the efficacy stage [70], and we are not aware of any HIIT-based interventions that have been implemented at scale. Indeed, most youth HIIT studies have been conducted by researchers and focused on establishing efficacy, with little consideration of real-world implementation.

To have a population health impact, youth HIIT interventions must be designed with scale-up in mind. This approach helps prevent the reduction in intervention effects, known as "voltage drop," that typically occurs when interventions transition from efficacy to effectiveness to dissemination [71, 72]. For instance, a recent systematic review found that scaled-up community-based PA interventions achieved less than 60% of their pre-scale effect size. As noted by Beets and colleagues [71], two major factors that influence intervention fidelity and effectiveness are the delivery agents (individuals responsible for delivering the intervention) and the level of implementation support. While teachers are well-suited to deliver school-based HIIT programs, they need to receive adequate training and ongoing support. Changes in delivery agents, such as the shift from researchers to teachers, and the removal of implementation support as interventions progress from small-scale pilot studies to larger-scale effectiveness trials, are significant contributors to "voltage drop."

It is not our intention to provide an exhaustive discussion on implementation and scale-up considerations, we recommend readers consult existing guidelines [73], reviews [74, 75], and conceptual articles [76] on this topic. For example, the PRACTIS guide (PRACTical planning for Implementation and Scale-up) [76] offers researchers four steps to effectively plan the dissemination, implementation, and scale-up of interventions. These steps include characterizing the parameters of the implementation settings (e.g., schools or sports clubs), identifying and engaging key stakeholders at multiple levels within the delivery system, identifying contextual barriers and facilitators to implementation using an implementation framework (e.g., Consolidated Framework for Implementation Research) [77], and addressing potential barriers to effective implementation.

In summary, HIIT holds potential as a population-level PA strategy, particularly if it can be integrated formally into existing opportunities and delivered by existing personnel, such as teachers and coaches. To realize the full potential of youth HIIT programs, they should be designed with scale-up in mind, involving partnerships with stakeholders that can identify barriers, develop resources, provide training, and offer support packages that acknowledge the real-world challenges and constraints faced by teachers when delivering HIIT.

14.4 Summary

The provision of structured opportunities for young people to be active is a reliable way to achieve improvements in PA levels. Schools represent an ideal setting to provide such opportunities. HIIT is one exercise modality that appears to be effective for improving a range of health outcomes in children and adolescent populations, and the efficacy of HIIT delivered in schools is increasingly emerging. HIIT could be applied to achieve the expansion, extension, or enhancement of PA opportunities in schools. Given its known efficacy, the design and delivery of HIIT in schools should focus on close consideration of sustainability and scalability to produce meaningful longer-term and widespread population effect. It should not be considered the panacea to the issue of physical inactivity, neither should it be considered a pariah simply owing to the known negative affective responses associated with high effort exercise.

The limitations of school-based HIIT, and their associated attenuating recommendations are summarized below. Our recommendations are underpinned by an approach that integrates HIIT into existing physical education where possible (enhances existing opportunities); or offers HIIT during other lessons (expansion of opportunity); or provides HIIT as activity between curriculum sessions times such as break/recess times (extends opportunities).

All our recommendations are predicated on the real-world setting of schools to enhance the motivation and confidence of participants through engaging delivery; include relevance to broader curricula and outcomes including but not limited to physical competence and physical fitness, and be guided in general by an implementation framework addressing relevant barriers and facilitators. Our recommendations each give consideration to SAAFE principles (Supportive, Active, Autonomous, Fair, and Enjoyable) [78]. The recommendations are for either schoolteachers, or for external providers advising on delivering HIIT in schools. We urge that external provision is designed specifically to facilitate in-school delivery by teachers or student leaders, rather than promote the ongoing need for the resourcing of non-school provision.

14.4.1 Limitation: Affective Response

The requisite intensity of HIIT can result in negative affective responses in some participants, potentially influencing enjoyment and potentially compromising intention and willingness to participate in future HIIT sessions.

Our recommendations:

- Do not prescribe or communicate expectations of the need to reach maximum HIIT intensity in early sessions. Progress the stated intensity "target" incrementally and conservatively for the first 2–4 weeks. These early sessions should be formative for exercise techniques and customized to incrementally increasing effort levels.
- Effort is best prescribed and monitored with heart-rate monitoring if available, but basic rating of perceived exertion (RPE) can be utilized as a self-monitoring tool.
- The stated intensity threshold ($\geq 85\%$ of age-predicted maximum heart rate, or 8–10 on a 1–10 RPE scale) need not be adhered to for the entire work interval duration, nor for all work intervals. Encourage participants to reach HIIT intensity target as work intervals and sessions ensue (particularly given typical work interval durations in a school setting of <60 s).
- The facility for participants to view their own heart rate in real-time will provide both motivation and an educational opportunity.

14.4.2 Limitation: Time

Lack of time is a barrier in most schools due to multiple competing priorities (e.g., academic workload).

Our recommendations:

- Choose HIIT protocols that are time efficient. Many options can be completed in 8–15 min in total.
- Minimize pre- and post-session transition time. Traditional extended "warm-up" and "cool-down" components need not be conducted to the extent of some traditional exercise sessions, particularly where the HIIT sessions are preceded and proceeded by general PA (e.g., HIIT embedded within physical education or sport). Depending on the preceding activity, a structured period of movement and physiological "warm-up" of at least 2–3 min at incrementally increasing effort is advised. The "cool-down" is not critical, provided general movement is occurring for another 2–3 min (e.g., simply re-organizing classroom furniture back to normal) before passivity. Structured post-exercise stretching is not at all critical.

14.4.3 Limitation: Space

Schools may not regularly have access to dedicated space such as gymnasia or courts, and spaces may be weather dependent.

Our recommendations:

- Consider the availability of space by discussion with the school leader responsible for the HIIT delivery. Do not assume access to dedicated specialist space.
- HIIT can be conducted in a standard school classroom in very limited space.
- Where space is particularly constrained, limit exercises requiring horizontal floor space such as push-ups and burpees.

14.4.4 Limitation: Equipment Resources

Dedicated HIIT equipment might be cost prohibitive and require ongoing logistical management.

Our recommendations:

- HIIT can be performed in schools with no equipment needed.
- Equipment ordinarily available as part of school physical education could be utilized for a variety of HIIT options.

14.4.5 Limitation: Exercise Complexity

The movement ability of youth is variable, and exercises requiring greater coordination can compromise perceived self-efficacy and short-term success.

Our recommendations:

- Accommodate the full range of learners in class, keeping movements achievable.
- Many exercises such as bodyweight resistance training will serve as physical ability learning tools, neuromuscular development, and cardiorespiratory response stimuli concurrently.
- Include exercise options specifically designed to enhance physical ability, such as formative foundational movements. This will depend on the availability and expertise of deliverers to provide ongoing coaching, so in general the less input or expertise available for program delivery, the simpler the movements should be, or the more guidance a program should provide in the form of instructional material such as videos and technique cues.

14.4.6 Limitation: Variety

Enthusiasm and interest may be compromised where boredom or monotony is perceived by youth participants.

Our recommendations:

- HIIT programs are well-suited to a defined duration within a school calendar rather than as an exclusive ongoing exercise option. For example, 6–10 weeks of HIIT represents a time frame within which a progressive, incremental approach can be applied to prescription parameters, and is known to elicit positive physiological adaptations such as improvements in the all-important cardiorespiratory fitness. A "block" such as this allows progression and variety but generally should not exhaust exercise options and the enthusiasm associated with a novel approach.
- Incorporate activities extracted as distinctive components from popular PAs, such as specific sporting actions (e.g., sprinting while bouncing a basketball), or simple cultural dance movements (singular simple movements performed repetitively rather than a choreographed series).
- Provide students with the opportunity to choose their own exercise options as a program progresses, thereby enhancing autonomy and buy-in.

14.4.7 Limitation: Curriculum Relevance

Exercise sessions may be viewed as singularly meeting physical fitness outcomes and therefore perceived as offering lower priority value than traditional academic aspects.

Our recommendations:

- Frame HIIT as complementary to curricula, including potential cross-curricula connections to mathematics, writing, cultural learning, and health education. For example (subject to age group),
  - Tracking and calculating a variety of metrics associated with recorded heart rate and RPE can be used in mathematics lessons.
  - Reflective written journals regarding personal experiences and responses to performing HIIT over the prescribed program period.
  - Connecting exercises to culturally meaningful narratives.
  - Recording and reviewing personal assessed outcomes (change in fitness, etc.).

14.4.8 Limitation: Teacher Self-Perceived Competence

Despite willingness, non-specialist physical education teachers (such as generalist classroom teachers in primary schools) may not feel confident to deliver HIIT, consequently presenting as a barrier to its use.

Our recommendations:

- Provide appropriate, expedient, accessible training, and resources to facilitate teacher delivery.
- Elicit from teachers their own identification of barriers to success and provide direct suggestions of facilitators to attenuate these.
- Ensure lesson planning requirements are minimal by providing ready to deliver session plans.

14.5 Conclusion

In summary, schools are a viable setting for the delivery of HIIT programs targeting youth. School-based HIIT programs can improve a range of physical, mental, and cognitive health outcomes among children and adolescents. To maximize the potential population health benefits, HIIT programs should be designed with scale-up in mind. The design of HIIT programs to be delivered in schools should closely consider contextually specific, pragmatic factors to best account for the inherent limitations in such a real-world setting. We recognize the importance of incorporating well-designed HIIT programs as part of a smorgasbord of PA offerings in schools.

This approach aims to improve the physical literacy of children and adolescents, equipping them with the skills and motivation to participate in a range of PAs throughout their lives.

References

1. Biddle SJH, Batterham AM. High-intensity interval exercise training for public health: a big HIT or shall we HIT it on the head? Int J Behav Nutr Phys Act. 2015;12:95.
2. Kercher VM, Kercher K, Levy P, Bennion T, Alexander C, Amaral PC, et al. 2023 fitness trends from around the globe. ACSMs Health Fit J. 2023;27(1):19–30.
3. Batacan RB, Duncan MJ, Dalbo VJ, Tucker PS, Fenning AS. Effects of high-intensity interval training on cardiometabolic health: a systematic review and meta-analysis of intervention studies. Br J Sports Med. 2017;51(6):494–503.
4. Costigan SA, Eather N, Plotnikoff RC, Taaffe DR, Lubans DR. High-intensity interval training for improving health-related fitness in adolescents: a systematic review and meta-analysis. Br J Sports Med. 2015;49(19):1253–61.
5. Biddle SJH, Atkin AJ, Cavill N, Foster C. Correlates of physical activity in youth: a review of quantitative systematic reviews. Int Rev Sport Exerc Psychol. 2011;4(1):25–49.
6. Martins J, Marques A, Sarmento H, Carreiro da Costa F. Adolescents' perspectives on the barriers and facilitators of physical activity: a systematic review of qualitative studies. Health Educ Res. 2015;30(5):742–55.
7. Gibala MJ, Hawley JA. Sprinting toward fitness. Cell Metab. 2017;25(5):988–90.
8. Laursen PB, Jenkins DG. The scientific basis for high-intensity interval training. Sports Med. 2002;32(1):53–73.
9. Tabata I, Nishimura K, Kouzaki M, Hirai Y, Ogita F, Miyachi M, Yamamoto K. Effects of moderate-intensity endurance and high-intensity intermittent training on anaerobic capacity and VO2max. Med Sci Sports Exerc. 1996;28(10):1327–30.
10. Burgomaster KA, Howarth KR, Phillips SM, Rakobowchuk M, Macdonald MJ, McGee SL, Gibala MJ. Similar metabolic adaptations during exercise after low volume sprint interval and traditional endurance training in humans. J Physiol. 2008;586(1):151–60.
11. Gibala MJ, Little JP, van Essen M, Wilkin GP, Burgomaster KA, Safdar A, et al. Short-term sprint interval versus traditional endurance training: similar initial adaptations in human skeletal muscle and exercise performance. J Physiol. 2006;575(Pt 3):901–11.
12. Little JP, Safdar A, Wilkin GP, Tarnopolsky MA, Gibala MJ. A practical model of low-volume high-intensity interval training induces mitochondrial biogenesis in human skeletal muscle: potential mechanisms. J Physiol. 2010;588(6):1011–22.
13. Viana RB, de Lira CAB, Naves JPA, Coswig VS, Del Vecchio FB, Ramirez-Campillo R, et al. Can we draw general conclusions from interval training studies? Sports Med. 2018;48:2001–9.
14. Ekkekakis P. Pleasure and displeasure from the body: perspectives from exercise. Cognit Emot. 2003;17(2):213–39.
15. Ekkekakis P, Parfitt G, Petruzzello SJ. The pleasure and displeasure people feel when they exercise at different intensities: decennial update and progress towards a tripartite rationale for exercise intensity prescription. Sports Med. 2011;41:641–71.
16. Hardcastle SJ, Ray H, Beale L, Hagger MS. Why sprint interval training is inappropriate for a largely sedentary population. Front Psychol. 2014;5:1505.
17. Oliveira BRR, Santos TM, Kilpatrick M, Pires FO, Deslandes AC. Affective and enjoyment responses in high intensity interval training and continuous training: a systematic review and meta-analysis. PLoS One. 2018;13(6):e0197124.

18. Leahy AA, Mavilidi MF, Smith JJ, Hillman CH, Eather N, Barker D, Lubans DR. Review of high-intensity interval training for cognitive and mental health in youth. Med Sci Sports Exerc. 2020;52(10):2224–34.
19. Tavares VDO, Schuch FB, Tempest G, Parfitt G, Oliveira Neto L, Galvao-Coelho NL, Hackett D. Exercisers' affective and enjoyment responses: a meta-analytic and meta-regression review. Percept Mot Skills. 2021;128(5):2211–36.
20. Sandvei M, Jeppesen PB, Støen L, Litleskare S, Johansen E, Stensrud T, et al. Sprint interval running increases insulin sensitivity in young healthy subjects. Arch Physiol Biochem. 2012;118(3):139–47.
21. Buchan DS, Ollis S, Thomas NE, Buchanan N, Cooper SM, Malina RM, Baker JS. Physical activity interventions: effects of duration and intensity. Scand J Med Sci Sports. 2011;21(6):e341–e50.
22. King AC, Haskell WL, Young DR, Oka RK, Stefanick ML. Long-term effects of varying intensities and formats of physical activity on participation rates, fitness, and lipoproteins in men and women aged 50 to 65 years. Circulation. 1995;91(10):2596–604.
23. Perri MG, Anton SD, Durning PE, Ketterson TU, Sydeman SJ, Berlant NE, et al. Adherence to exercise prescriptions: effects of prescribing moderate versus higher levels of intensity and frequency. Health Psychol. 2002;21(5):452.
24. Ekkekakis P, Biddle SH. Extraordinary claims in the literature on high-intensity interval training (HIIT): IV. Is HIIT associated with higher long-term exercise adherence? Psychol Sport Exerc. 2022:102295.
25. Harris N, Warbrick I, Fleming T, Borotkanics R, Atkins D, Lubans D. Impact of high-intensity interval training including indigenous narratives on adolescents' mental health: a cluster-randomised controlled trial. Aust N Z J Public Health. 2022;46(6):794–9.
26. Lubans DR, Smith JJ, Eather N, Leahy AA, Morgan PJ, Lonsdale C, et al. Time-efficient intervention to improve older adolescents' cardiorespiratory fitness: findings from the 'Burn 2 Learn' cluster randomized controlled trial. Br J Sports Med. 2021;55(13):751–8.
27. Ruiz-Ariza A, Suárez-Manzano S, Lopez S, Martínez-López EJ. The effect of cooperative high-intensity interval training on creativity and emotional intelligence in secondary school: a randomised controlled trial. Eur Phys Educ Rev. 2019;25(2):355–73.
28. Weston KL, Azevedo LB, Bock S, Weston M, George KP, Batterham AM. Effect of novel, school-based high-intensity interval training (HIT) on cardiometabolic health in adolescents: project FFAB (Fun Fast Activity Blasts)—an exploratory controlled before-and-after trial. PLoS One. 2016;11(8):e0159116.
29. Weston K, Barker AR, Bond B, Costigan S, Ingul C, Williams C. The BASES expert statement on the role of high-intensity interval exercise for health and fitness promotion in young people. Sport Exerc Sci. 2020;64:8–9.
30. Duncombe SL, Barker AR, Bond B, Earle R, Varley-Campbell J, Vlachopoulos D, et al. School-based high-intensity interval training programs in children and adolescents: a systematic review and meta-analysis. PLoS One. 2022;17(5):e0266427.
31. Bull FC, Al-Ansari SS, Biddle S, Borodulin K, Buman MP, Cardon G, et al. World Health Organization 2020 guidelines on physical activity and sedentary behaviour. Br J Sports Med. 2020;54(24):1451–62.
32. Leahy AA, Eather N, Smith JJ, Hillman CH, Morgan PJ, Nilsson M, et al. School-based physical activity intervention for older adolescents: rationale and study protocol for the Burn 2 Learn cluster randomised controlled trial. BMJ Open. 2019;9(5):e026029.
33. Mavilidi MF, Mason C, Leahy AA, Kennedy SG, Eather N, Hillman CH, et al. Effect of a time-efficient physical activity intervention on senior school students' on-task behaviour and subjective vitality: the 'Burn 2 Learn' cluster randomised controlled trial. Educ Psychol Rev. 2021;33(1):299–323.
34. Ma JK, Le Mare L, Gurd BJ. Four minutes of in-class high-intensity interval activity improves selective attention in 9- to 11-year olds. Appl Physiol Nutr Metab. 2015;40(3):238–44.

35. Bond B, Weston KL, Williams CA, Barker AR. Perspectives on high-intensity interval exercise for health promotion in children and adolescents. Open Access J Sports Med. 2017;8:243–65.
36. Eather N, Babic M, Riley N, Costigan SA, Lubans DR. Impact of embedding high-intensity interval training in schools and sports training on children and adolescent's cardiometabolic health and health-related fitness: systematic review and meta-analysis. J Teach Phys Educ. 2023;42(2):243–55.
37. Zapata-Lamana R, Cigarroa Cuevas I, Fuentes V, Soto Espindola C, Parrado Romero E, Sepulveda C, Monsalves-Alvarez M. HIITing health in school: can high intensity interval training be a useful and reliable tool for health on a school-based environment? A systematic review. International Journal of School Health. 2019;6(3):1–10.
38. Thivel D, Masurier J, Baquet G, Timmons BW, Pereira B, Berthoin S, et al. High-intensity interval training in overweight and obese children and adolescents: systematic review and meta-analysis. J Sports Med Phys Fitness. 2019;59(2):310–24.
39. Poon ET-C, Wongpipit W, Sun F, Tse AC-Y, Sit CH-P. High-intensity interval training in children and adolescents with special educational needs: a systematic review and narrative synthesis. Int J Behav Nutr Phys Act. 2023;20(1):1–14.
40. Boer PH, Meeus M, Terblanche E, Rombaut L, Wandele ID, Hermans L, et al. The influence of sprint interval training on body composition, physical and metabolic fitness in adolescents and young adults with intellectual disability: a randomized controlled trial. Clin Rehabil. 2014;28(3):221–31.
41. Leahy AA, Kennedy SG, Smith JJ, Eather N, Boyer J, Thomas M, et al. Feasibility of a school-based physical activity intervention for adolescents with disability. Pilot Feasibility Stud. 2021;7(1):120.
42. Kable TJ, Leahy AA, Smith JJ, Eather N, Shields N, Noetel M, et al. Time-efficient physical activity intervention for older adolescents with disability: rationale and study protocol for the Burn 2 Learn adapted (B2La) cluster randomised controlled trial. BMJ Open. 2022;12(8):e065321.
43. Costigan SA, Eather N, Plotnikoff RC, Taaffe DR, Pollock E, Kennedy SG, Lubans DR. Preliminary efficacy and feasibility of embedding high intensity interval training into the school day: a pilot randomized controlled trial. Prev Med Rep. 2015;2:973–9.
44. Leahy AA, Eather N, Smith JJ, Hillman CH, Morgan PJ, Plotnikoff RC, et al. Feasibility and preliminary efficacy of a teacher-facilitated high-intensity interval training intervention for older adolescents. Pediatr Exerc Sci. 2019;31(1):107–17.
45. Eddolls WTB, McNarry MA, Stratton G, Winn CON, Mackintosh KA. High-intensity interval training interventions in children and adolescents: a systematic review. Sports Med. 2017;47(11):2363–74.
46. Lubans DR, Leahy AA, Mavilidi MF, Valkenborghs SR. Physical activity, fitness, and executive functions in youth: effects, moderators, and mechanisms. Curr Top Behav Neurosci. 2021;53:103–30.
47. Alves AR, Dias R, Neiva HP, Marinho DA, Marques MC, Sousa AC, et al. High-intensity interval training upon cognitive and psychological outcomes in youth: a systematic review. Int J Environ Res Public Health. 2021;18(10):5344.
48. Valkenborghs SR, Hillman CH, Al-Iedani O, Nilsson M, Smith JJ, Leahy AA, et al. Effect of high-intensity interval training on hippocampal metabolism in older adolescents. Psychophysiology. 2022:e14090.
49. Lee JS, Boafo A, Greenham S, Longmuir PE. The effect of high-intensity interval training on inhibitory control in adolescents hospitalized for a mental illness. Ment Health Phys Act. 2019;17:100298.
50. Wymbs FA, Wymbs B, Margherio S, Burd K. The effects of high intensity versus low intensity exercise on academic productivity, mood, and behavior among youth with and without ADHD. J Child Fam Stud. 2021;30(2):460–73.
51. Costigan SA, Eather N, Plotnikoff RC, Hillman CH, Lubans DR. High-intensity interval training for cognitive and mental health in adolescents. Med Sci Sports Exerc. 2016;48(10):1985–93.

52. Lubans DR, Eather N, Smith JJ, Beets MW, Harris NK. Scaling-up adolescent high-intensity interval training programs for population health. Exerc Sport Sci Rev. 2022;50(3):128–36.
53. Beets MW, Okely A, Weaver RG, Webster C, Lubans D, Brusseau T, et al. The theory of expanded, extended, and enhanced opportunities for youth physical activity promotion. Int J Behav Nutr Phys Act. 2016;13(1):120.
54. Ekkekakis P, Parfitt G, Petruzzello SJ. The pleasure and displeasure people feel when they exercise at different intensities. Sports Med. 2011;41(8):641–71.
55. Hollis JL, Sutherland R, Williams AJ, Campbell E, Nathan N, Wolfenden L, et al. A systematic review and meta-analysis of moderate-to-vigorous physical activity levels in secondary school physical education lessons. Int J Behav Nutr Phys Act. 2017;14(1):52.
56. Whitehead M. Definition of physical literacy and clarification of related issues. ICSSPE. Bulletin. 2013;65(1.2)
57. Chesham RA, Booth JN, Sweeney EL, Ryde GC, Gorely T, Brooks NE, Moran CN. The Daily Mile makes primary school children more active, less sedentary and improves their fitness and body composition: a quasi-experimental pilot study. BMC Med. 2018;16(1):64.
58. Vella SA, Aidman E, Teychenne M, Smith JJ, Swann C, Rosenbaum S, et al. Optimising the effects of physical activity on mental health and wellbeing: a joint consensus statement from sports medicine Australia and the Australian Psychological Society. J Sci Med Sport. 2023;26(2):132–9.
59. Ladwig MA, Vazou S, Ekkekakis P. "My best memory is when I was done with it": PE memories are associated with adult sedentary behavior. Transl J Am College Sports Med. 2018;3(16):119–29.
60. Baumeister RF, Bratslavsky E, Finkenauer C, Vohs KD. Bad is stronger than good. Rev Gen Psychol. 2001;5(4):323–70.
61. Karageorghis CI, Priest D-L. Music in the exercise domain: a review and synthesis (part I). Int Rev Sport Exerc Psychol. 2012;5(1):44–66.
62. Morgan PJ, Young MD, Smith JJ, Lubans DR. Targeted health behavior interventions promoting physical activity: a conceptual model. Exerc Sport Sci Rev. 2016;44(2):71–80.
63. Deci EL, Ryan RM. The "what" and "why" of goal pursuits: human needs and the self-determination of behavior. Psychol Inq. 2000;11(4):227–68.
64. Ryan RM, Deci EL. Self-determination theory and the facilitation of intrinsic motivation, social development, and well-being. Am Psychol. 2000;55(1):68.
65. Nicholls JG. Achievement motivation: conceptions of ability, subjective experience, task choice, and performance. Psychol Rev. 1984;91(3):328.
66. Lonsdale C, Lester A, Owen KB, White RL, Peralta L, Kirwan M, et al. An internet-supported school physical activity intervention in low socioeconomic status communities: results from the Activity and Motivation in Physical Education (AMPED) cluster randomised controlled trial. Br J Sports Med. 2019;53(6):341–7.
67. Saugy JJ, Drouet O, Millet GP, Lentillon-Kaestner V. A systematic review on self-determination theory in physical education. Transl Sport Med. 2020;3(2):134–47.
68. Chambers DA, Glasgow RE, Stange KC. The dynamic sustainability framework: addressing the paradox of sustainment amid ongoing change. Implement Sci. 2013;8(1):117.
69. Milat AJ, Newson R, King L, Rissel C, Wolfenden L, Bauman A, et al. A guide to scaling up population health interventions. Public Health Res Pract. 2016;26(1):e2611604.
70. Kennedy SG, Sanders T, Estabrooks PA, Smith JJ, Lonsdale C, Foster C, Lubans DR. Implementation at-scale of school-based physical activity interventions: a systematic review utilizing the RE-AIM framework. Obes Rev. 2021;22(7):e13184.
71. Beets MW, Weaver RG, Ioannidis JPA, Geraci M, Brazendale K, Decker L, et al. Identification and evaluation of risk of generalizability biases in pilot versus efficacy/effectiveness trials: a systematic review and meta-analysis. Int J Behav Nutr Phys Act. 2020;17(1):19.
72. Lane C, McCrabb S, Nathan N, Naylor P-J, Bauman A, Milat A, et al. How effective are physical activity interventions when they are scaled-up: a systematic review. Int J Behav Nutr Phys Act. 2021;18(1):16.

73. Pinnock H, Barwick M, Carpenter CR, Eldridge S, Grandes G, Griffiths CJ, et al. Standards for Reporting Implementation Studies (StaRI) Statement. Br Med J. 2017;356:i6795.
74. McKay H, Naylor PJ, Lau E, Gray SM, Wolfenden L, Milat A, et al. Implementation and scale-up of physical activity and behavioural nutrition interventions: an evaluation roadmap. Int J Behav Nutr Phys Act. 2019;16(1):102.
75. Wolfenden L, McCrabb S, Barnes C, O'Brien KM, Ng KW, Nathan NK, et al. Strategies for enhancing the implementation of school-based policies or practices targeting diet, physical activity, obesity, tobacco or alcohol use. Cochrane Database Syst Rev. 2022;8(8):Cd011677
76. Koorts H, Eakin E, Estabrooks P, Timperio A, Salmon J, Bauman A. Implementation and scale up of population physical activity interventions for clinical and community settings: the PRACTIS guide. Int J Behav Nutr Phys Act. 2018;15(1):51.
77. Damschroder LJ, Aron DC, Keith RE, Kirsh SR, Alexander JA, Lowery JC. Fostering implementation of health services research findings into practice: a consolidated framework for advancing implementation science. Implement Sci. 2009;4(1):50.
78. Lubans DR, Lonsdale C, Cohen K, Eather N, Beauchamp MR, Morgan PJ, et al. Framework for the design and delivery of organized physical activity sessions for children and adolescents: rationale and description of the 'SAAFE' teaching principles. Int J Behav Nutr Phys Act. 2017;14(1):24.

Chapter 15
How Can Muscle-Strengthening Activities Be Promoted in School Settings?

Ashley Cox

15.1 Defining Muscular Fitness

Throughout the last 50 years, there has been a downward trend in muscular fitness among youth across most developed countries [1]. The physical and mental health benefits of muscular fitness are well recognized [2, 3]. However, it is acknowledged that muscular fitness has been an overlooked element of physical activity (PA) guidelines [4]. Low muscular fitness levels in children are associated with poor motor competence, functional limitations, and adverse health outcomes [1, 3, 5]. Worryingly, measures of muscular fitness are declining in modern-day youths, which may indicate declining health status and physical function [1, 6–8]. Ubiquitous measures of muscular fitness have demonstrated declines in standing long jump performance [9], handgrip strength [8], and leg power [10].

Muscular fitness is a multi-dimensional construct comprising the integrated function of muscle strength, muscle endurance, and muscle power [11]. Muscular strength is the maximum force a muscle group can exert against resistance, measured absolutely (1 RM, One-repetition maximum) or relative to body weight. Muscular endurance refers to a muscle group's capacity to maintain sub-maximal force over time. Muscular power incorporates speed and strength and captures work per unit of time [11–13]. The development of all muscular fitness attributes depends on the type of muscular fitness activity and the loading parameters prescribed [14]. Traditional aerobic moderate-to-vigorous PA (MVPA) can improve strength, endurance, and power. However, for more targeted muscle development, consider specific intensity (loading) and repetition ranges (volume) when designing muscular fitness activities [11–13]. While it is acknowledged that specificity of muscular fitness

---

A. Cox (✉)
Division of Musculoskeletal and Dermatological Sciences, Faculty of Biology, Medicine and Health, The University of Manchester, Manchester, UK
e-mail: ashley.cox@manchester.ac.uk

activity is required to elicit the desired outcome (i.e., higher volume and lower intensity for muscular strength development), the existing literature and indeed the general public often erroneously categorize all muscular fitness activity as "strength" [15].

Schools provide an established setting to deliver PA interventions [16], which may include muscular fitness interventions [17]. Most school PA interventions have focused on aerobic MVPA with limited success [18]. Indeed, a significant challenge in integrating muscular fitness activities in schools is the lack of clear, defined terminology. This hinders the interpretation of academic literature and makes it difficult for teachers to effectively implement these activities, often finding the task daunting due to this ambiguity [19].

15.2 Muscular Fitness and Aerobic Physical Activity

The role of muscular fitness in enhancing MVPA levels is recognized as a synergistic relationship. It is considered crucial to overcoming exercise deficit disorder, defined as not meeting the international guidelines of an average of 60 min of MVPA per day across a week [20]. In recognition of the interrelated components that drive physical inactivity in youth, the pediatric inactivity triad (PIT) was proposed [21] (Fig. 15.1).

The PIT acknowledges three separate but interrelated components that contribute to physical inactivity: (1) exercise deficit disorder (EDD), (2) pediatric dynapenia, and (3) physical illiteracy [21]. The PIT proposes that these three elements interact and should be viewed collectively to better effect change in PA levels among youth [21]. It should be noted that all components of the PIT are interrelated and modifiable through exposure to a variety of PA, which aligns with current international PA guideline recommendations. Despite many current national and international

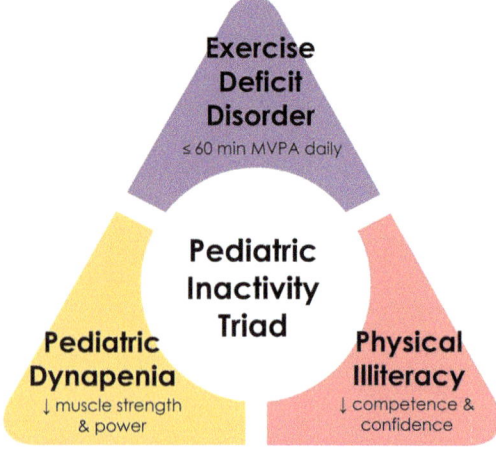

Fig. 15.1 Pediatric Inactivity Triad [21]. (Source: Faigenbaum et al. [21]. © 2018 by the American College of Sports Medicine. Used with permission)

guidelines implicitly acknowledging the interrelated components that affect change in overall PA, there remains an overarching focus on aerobic MVPA from a health policy and, subsequently, school delivery perspective [22].

While the proposed PIT framework attempts to help understand and address the pandemic of physical inactivity in modern-day youth, it has yet to be validated, and some elements lack empirical evidence. In particular, the term "pediatric dynapenia" lacks supporting evidence for its conception, context, and cut-off points for a subsequent diagnosis. Indeed, it is acknowledged that muscular fitness is declining among some young people [1, 6–8]. However, dynapenia is typically defined as age-associated muscle strength that does not result from neurological or muscular disease [23]. While the PIT attempts to address the interplay of decreased MVPA, poor muscular fitness, and a lack of physical literacy, more work is required to fully align with appropriate and contemporary terminology to support its use.

Despite the links between muscular fitness and habitual PA, there is a paucity of interventions. One study investigating links between muscular fitness development and habitual PA was conducted with 102 participants (42 girls and 60 boys) in Switzerland [24]. The participants conducted two muscular fitness sessions per week for 19 weeks. The study concluded that muscular fitness activity significantly increased daily habitual PA behavior in boys. The less active children showed the greatest increase in spontaneous PA. However, girls showed a similar increase in strength measured through leg and arm strength but not in spontaneous PA [24]. The maximum strength of the lower body in this study was determined on a seated leg press (Teca, Rom Prestige, Ortona, Italy) and for the upper body on a Cybex smith press (Cybex; Owatonna, mn) by one repetition maximum testing. While the study investigated the strength element of muscular fitness, it failed to recognize muscular power and endurance and may have missed other adaptations that contribute toward muscular fitness. When reviewing the exercise prescription, there is a possibility that elements of muscular endurance may have increased due to the nature of high repetition ranges (15 repetitions), yet this was not acknowledged in this study. A further study investigating the link between PA and muscular fitness was conducted with 46 adolescent boys from an ice hockey team in Switzerland, which reported increases in PA after a 12-week muscular fitness activity intervention [25]. The boys who participated in the twice-weekly program had significant increases in PA levels compared to the control group. These findings demonstrate the interrelated aspects of muscular fitness and device-based PA measures.

While there is growing interest and investigation into the delivery of muscular fitness in schools, it should be noted that the literature is still relatively sparse, and often, study findings lack consistency [5]. However, the literature suggests that adolescent boys may be particularly receptive to muscular fitness activity interventions if the aim is to increase device-based measures of PA and further supports the need to investigate the role muscular fitness plays in adolescent boys' overall PA levels [26, 27]. Additionally, younger children have improved muscular fitness following the delivery of muscular fitness activities during timetabled PE [28], which also supports the potential for successful muscular fitness interventions in younger children.

15.3 Assessing Muscular Fitness

The assessment of muscular fitness is a complex and multifaceted area of investigation where the specificity of measurement is as important as the prescription of muscular fitness activity itself [13, 29]. Given that muscular fitness assessments are specific to the muscle group, type of muscle action, muscle contraction, contraction velocity, equipment, joint and muscle range of motion [1], this chapter will cover three of the most common measures for power, strength, and endurance that are appropriate to be used in a school environment. The efficacy of muscular fitness activity is underpinned by appropriate testing and assessment to progress individuals safely [17]. Therefore, understanding muscular fitness testing and assessments may increase the quantity and quality of muscular fitness activity and provide a non-invasive objective assessment of the impact of school-based muscular fitness interventions [30, 31]. However, in schools, tests and assessments in PE have been highly contested [31, 32]. Youth sports experience similar problems, whereby coaches' expertise in measurements of muscular fitness and their ability to interpret them is key to muscular fitness assessment's usefulness, application, and necessity [13].

Many challenges surrounding muscular fitness assessments are centered around the complexities of youth growth and maturation [33]. These challenges are further exacerbated when working with adolescents, as the timing of puberty can differ by up to 5 years between individuals of the same sex [13, 33]. However, during adolescence, an opportunity exists for neural and architectural adaptations in the development of muscular fitness due to increases in anabolic and hormonal concentrations centered around peak height velocity (PHV) [34, 35]. Available literature suggests that children demonstrate improved muscular fitness activity ability as they age across a range of muscular fitness outcomes indicative of increased type 2 muscle fiber recruitment capability, aligning with PHV and peak strength velocity [34, 36–39].

Much of the research surrounding muscular fitness and muscular fitness assessments has focused on bodyweight movements, counting the increase in repetitions as a marker of progression and improvement in muscular fitness. However, performing bodyweight assessments may only provide an assessment of relative strength and overlook other areas of muscular fitness, such as absolute strength and power [40]. Furthermore, the assessment of relative strength alone does not provide an opportunity for overweight or obese children and adolescents to demonstrate their superior levels of absolute strength when compared to their normal-weight counterparts [41]. It is understood that overweight and obese individuals may display higher levels of absolute strength and power over their leaner counterparts, which should be assessed through power output, which accounts for body mass [40]. Such opportunities can be derived from assessing power, including the vertical jump, specifically, the counter-movement jump [42]. However, the vertical jump is often reported as the value in height and fails to report the power generated by the individual to conduct the movement [42]. Children and adolescents who are overweight or obese may evoke a higher power output for a similar vertical jump height compared to leaner peers [40, 43]. Therefore, lower-limb power output and the achieved vertical jump height may provide a better understanding of the relationship between body mass and absolute and relative strength in adolescents. Other common measures of muscular fitness include hand grip strength and variations of a sit-up test to measure strength and muscular endurance, both of which can be conducted in field-based settings such as schools.

15.3.1 Assessing Lower Limb Power

The standing long jump (SLJ) and the vertical jump (VJ) are field tests that are commonly used to assess lower-body explosive muscular strength in children and adolescents, especially in field-based settings such as schools [44]. Research conducted in 6- to 17-year-olds suggests the SLJ was strongly associated with other lower body muscular strength tests (r^2 = 0.829–0.864) and with upper body muscular strength tests (r^2 = 0.694–0.851) [44]. The SLJ (also called the Sargent jump and broad jump) may, therefore, be a reasonable assessment of lower limb muscular fitness and even an indication of upper limb muscular fitness among this age group. While this approach to assessing lower limb muscular fitness may provide a simple and accessible approach, research is evolving to acknowledge the differences in age and the specificity that may be required when assessing muscular fitness throughout growth and maturation.

To assess lower limb power, the counter-movement jump may be used in a school setting, relying on the height of the jump as a proxy measure of power [13, 42]. From a standing position, with the feet slightly apart and the hands placed on the hips, the individual would perform a counter movement with the legs before jumping. To estimate peak muscle power more accurately, a simple calculation validated with adolescents can be applied [42]. Power can be calculated by taking the vertical jump height and body mass of the individual, placing the raw scores into the following format: power (w) = 54.2 × VJH (cm) + 34.4 × body mass (kg) − 1520.4. This will allow the practitioner to account for body mass and accurately represent lower limb power output. However, it should be acknowledged that the researcher or practitioner should know how to conduct and interpret the protocol, which requires training and understanding. How the research will develop and account for the nuances of growth and maturation in children and young people has yet to be seen. However, such emerging specificity in assessment is promising and may help teachers identify young people who require further support in developing muscular fitness.

15.3.2 Assessing Abdominal Endurance

Common measures of abdominal muscular endurance are reported in the literature and consist of three main protocols [45]. The three commonly used tests of abdominal endurance are: (a) "timed" protocols, which consist of performing the maximum number of abdominal flexions possible (e.g., curl-ups, cross-curl-ups, or sit-ups) in a given time (30–120 s) [46–49]; (b) "cadence" protocols, consisting in the maintenance of a certain cadence while executing trunk flexion or extension motions for as long as possible [50]; and (c) "isometric" protocols, consisting of maintaining a prone, supine, or lateral posture against gravity until exhaustion [51–53].

Although measures of trunk strength are simple to conduct in a field-based setting, researchers and practitioners may be discouraged by the lengthy familiarization process required for accurate reproducibility and standardization [46]. Indeed, many international test batteries used to assess health-related fitness include normative data stratified by age and gender to assist in interpretation [54, 55]. Accompanying many of the test batteries are various videos, audio clips, and protocols to help teachers deliver and interpret the results.

15.3.3 Assessing Handgrip Strength

Hand grip strength testing using a dynamometer is deemed an inexpensive and effective measure of overall strength recommended for school-based assessments [1, 56]. This form of assessment is one of the most widely adopted and features in many of the internationally recognized test batteries such as Alpha-Fit, ASSO-FTB, and EuroFit. The assessment consists of adjusting the grip span to suit the hand size of the participant. The participant is then asked to squeeze the dynamometer continuously as hard as possible for 3 s with the elbow in full extension down by the side of the body [57, 58]. This method of assessing hand grip strength is deemed the most reliable protocol to assess hand grip strength in adolescents and is also used among younger children to assess grip strength [57]. While it is acknowledged that hand grip strength is influenced by age, sex, hand size, grip span, posture, the position of the elbow, forearm and wrist orientation, the arm-by-the-side method provides the most appropriate protocol to account for such differences and accounts for differences in brand of dynamometer [57, 58].

In recent years, the sophistication of the literature surrounding handgrip strength has grown. Various cut points for different assessments have been created to align further the relationship between strength and health, including the development of bone health-related grip strength cut points for youth [59]. This may allow for tracking healthy bone development in community settings and, indeed, school settings. Such developments in muscular fitness assessments open the possibility and opportunity for teachers to develop meaningful health-related fitness data related to muscular fitness.

While the three methods of assessing muscular fitness covered are deemed relatively simple and suitable for the school environment, the degree to which PE teachers use such protocols is not understood. Furthermore, no existing literature studies whether teachers use such measures to monitor students and inform muscular fitness activity program design. Where research has been conducted, it is often reported that the teachers are not fully confident or competent in conducting and interpreting such assessments [19, 60].

15.4 Developing Muscular Fitness

Adolescence and childhood are key periods for developing muscular fitness activity competency. Effective promotion of muscular strength, endurance, and power, enabling children and adolescents to perform bodily movements more efficiently and effectively, will ensure muscular fitness is developed [61]. With the growing body of evidence surrounding the benefits of muscular fitness, there are concerns regarding the misuse of the terms "strength training" and "resistance training," with much of the current literature on youth overlooking the principles of specificity and the subsequent adaptation in muscular fitness (i.e., strength and power) [17, 34, 62]. The development of muscular fitness is dependent on the type, frequency, intensity (load), and volume (amount) of muscular fitness activity conducted [14]. Traditionally, the prescription of muscular fitness activity is aligned to a "repetition continuum," which recommends a volume and intensity scale to elicit a specific adaptation [63, 64]. The general concept of the "repetition continuum" is that higher volume and low-intensity muscular fitness activity will induce endurance adaptations, with low volume and high intensity more aligned to power adaptations. However, this continuum has been recently challenged [65] and much of the work conducted to date involves young men and is not generalizable to children and adolescents.

Regarding muscular fitness delivery in youth guidance for prescription is provided in the form of an international position statement [66], adapted from the original UK Strength and Conditioning (UKSCA) position stand. Since the inception of the international position stand, there have been very few changes. The international position stand brings together leaders in pediatric exercise science, pediatric medicine, physical education, strength and conditioning, and sports medicine to provide guidance around an area of PA that has been largely overlooked [66]. More recently, this position has been adopted by the American Academy of Pediatrics to provide further guidance on the appropriate prescription of muscular fitness activity in youth [67]. The following training variables are provided for consideration when developing structured muscular fitness programs in youth and consider the major position stands that provide muscular fitness activity guidance:

15.4.1 Exercise Selection

Similar to existing literature surrounding adult muscular fitness exercise selection [14, 68, 69], there is an emphasis on the suitability principles and familiarity of equipment and movements carried out. It is suggested that when youth are competent in moving their bodies (i.e., lunging, squatting, press-ups, and pulling movements) and can respond to coaching cues, traditional forms of muscular fitness activity (i.e., weightlifting, free weights, and plyometrics) can be introduced [66]. To develop competency in movement and to support the development of youth with minimal muscular fitness activity experience (termed a low training age), it is suggested that motor skill competency is assessed and developed prior to conducting more complex muscular fitness activity movements such as weightlifting (i.e., snatch and clean and jerk) [66]. For youth with previous muscular fitness activity experience (high training age), it is suggested to select exercises that possess dynamic qualities and can be enhanced through multi-joint exercises that are velocity-specific and typically come in the form of weightlifting and plyometric type movements [70, 71]. It is acknowledged that while exercise selection is necessary to elicit specific adaptations [72], supervision of exercises can result in improved movement quality and muscular fitness [73–75]. Furthermore, the supervision of muscular fitness activity in a controlled environment may ensure the safety of movements conducted and increase the efficacy of muscular fitness activity [76].

15.4.2 Training Volume and Intensity

Successful muscular fitness outcomes are dependent on the manipulation of volume (total number of repetitions) and intensity (the weight being moved) [66]. The dose-response relationship between muscular fitness activity intensity and improvements in motor performance, such as running, jumping, and throwing, in young people has been reported in previous literature [77]. Furthermore, the relationship between intensity and volume prescription is inverse, whereby increased load (intensity) requires lower volume (number of repetitions), and both variables must be considered together to avoid injury [78–81]. To prescribe volume and intensity, teachers and youth sports coaches must assess one repetition maximum (1rm) and assign a load based on a percentage [82–84]. However, while maximal strength assessments in youth are deemed safe and appropriate, some PE teachers may be put off conducting such assessments due to their perceived complexity and lack of muscular fitness activity knowledge [13]. However, simple field-based measures of muscular fitness, such as those described in the section earlier, can provide an assessment to inform muscular fitness activity prescription by monitoring muscular fitness progression. Previous literature suggests that vertical jump and hand grip strength are correlated to 1rm strength values in youth [44, 85]. While not as accurate as 1rm, this approach may serve as an appropriate measure of muscular fitness to inform prescription and monitor progression in school and recreational settings.

15.4.3 Progression of Volume and Intensity

The starting volume and intensity for youth depend on training age and technical competency [13]. However, it is generally accepted that all youth start at a low intensity and volume irrespective of training age until the PE teacher or coach can verify their technical competency to progress [82–84]. Low volume (1–2 sets of 1–3 repetitions) and low intensity (under 60% of 1rm) are recommended to start multi-joint movements such as squatting [66]. Once movement competence is achieved, the individual can progress to 2 to 4 sets of 6 to 12 repetitions with a low to moderate training intensity (under 80% 1 rm). Advanced youth can finally progress to lower volume and higher intensity, provided the individual is competent in the movement. It is generally accepted that intensity increases of 5–10% are reasonable, provided that the individual can comfortably carry out 15 repetitions at the previous weight. Once the intensity has been increased, the volume drops back down and gradually progresses until meeting 15 competent repetitions and once again increasing intensity.

To assist teachers and youth sport coaches in the development of youth muscular fitness activity prescription, the resistance training skills competency (RTSC) framework (Fig. 15.2) and an associated checklist have been developed [72]. The RTSC framework provides recommendations based on each participant's resistance training skill competency and muscular strength. Additionally, the supporting checklist can assess exercise performance and communicate the specific actions and behaviors required for this exercise. While it is evident that the tools to assist teachers and youth sports coaches exist in the literature, it is not fully understood if and how these tools are applied and the extent of the ability and knowledge of the same

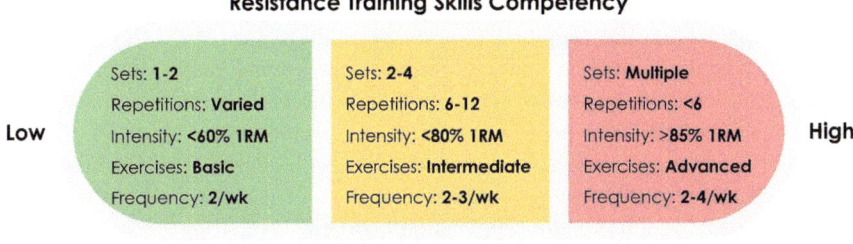

Fig. 15.2 Resistance training skills competency framework. 1RM, one repetition maximum [72]. (Source: Faigenbaum and McFarland [72]. Copyright © 2016 American College of Sports Medicine. Used with permission)

practitioners to prescribe muscular fitness activity safely and effectively. Further research is required to provide insight into the current knowledge levels of PE teachers to highlight areas of development in the delivery of muscular fitness activity.

15.5 Muscular Fitness Benefits and Risks

Understanding specific muscular fitness outcomes and their association with health indicators is paramount for informing future program design and delivery. For example, it has been reported that strength (the ability to produce force against an external resistance) may reduce levels of disability and cardiovascular disease in later life if appropriately developed during adolescence [86]. Additionally, power (the ability to accomplish muscular work per unit of time) is fundamental in combatting physical declines associated with sarcopenia and maintaining mobility and performance for everyday life in older adults [87, 88]. However, as we age, muscular power declines at a faster rate than muscular strength, directly impacting health and quality of life and further supporting the need to investigate specific muscular fitness outcomes and their association with indicators of health [89, 90].

Throughout childhood and adolescence, it is recognized that the development of muscular fitness is not homogenous, with muscle morphology, androgen levels, growth, and maturation all contributing to the development of strength and power throughout the development process [66, 83]. The associations between strength and power and health indicators are yet to be fully investigated in youth due to the inherent muscular fitness development heterogeneity associated with the growth and maturation process. Improvements in muscular fitness have been associated with improvements in cardiorespiratory fitness (CRF) [91, 92], metabolic function and efficiency (i.e., glucose transport capacity and lipid oxidation) [3, 24, 93], and bone health [94] in youth.

Muscular fitness activity has recently been associated with long-term health benefits when exposure to a training stimulus occurs during childhood and adolescence as part of organized PA [2]. Some of the health benefits include reductions in fat mass, increased bone density, and improvements in psychological health [95, 96]. Much of the existing PA literature focuses on traditional aerobic MVPA (such as ambulatory activities such as walking, running, playground games, invasion game sports, etc.), which is associated with health benefits such as decreased adiposity, reductions in metabolic syndrome, and type 2 diabetes later in life [56, 97–99]. Although evidence acknowledges muscular fitness interventions for enhancing health and PA, recent research expresses a need to investigate further the role of resistance-based exercise and its application to youth [100, 101].

Although the health benefits of muscular fitness are well supported within the literature, concerns regarding the safety and efficacy of muscular fitness activity still exist in schools [6, 19]. These concerns may prevent muscular fitness activity from being conducted in schools and further exacerbate declines in muscular fitness witnessed in children and adolescents [1, 6–8]. A concern often reported is that of injury. However, injury rates for children and adolescents participating in structured muscular fitness activity are typically lower than those occurring in many sports and, interestingly, than those occurring during school play [67, 102]. Additionally, concerns remain regarding the stunting of growth among children and adolescents who engage in muscular fitness activity. These concerns lack any scientific foundation and are largely based on myths and assumptions [83].

15.5.1 Psychosocial Health and Muscular Fitness Activity

Psychosocial health has been shown to be positively impacted when engaging in structured PA [103]. Improved self-efficacy, reductions in anxiety and depression, and improvements in self-esteem and PA enjoyment are all indicative of PA participation [95, 100]. PA is also associated with increased academic performance, increased self-efficacy and lower depression, and behavioral issues [104]. Furthermore, improving muscular fitness is associated with positive psychological health, including improved confidence and self-efficacy, and reduced anxiety [96, 105, 106]. Engaging in muscular fitness activity has also been shown to benefit cognitive function, academic performance, and on-task behaviors in school-aged youth [107]. Although some research shows positive responses in psychological health following muscular fitness interventions, data is still limited and warrants further investigation [40]. In the available literature, positive changes in psychological health have been reported following muscular fitness interventions and include increased confidence and self-efficacy [108, 109].

It has been suggested that long-term compliance with PA must focus on what individuals *like to do* and less on what they *have to do,* leading to intrinsically motivated participation in PA. Given the reported inclination of adolescent boys to participate in muscular fitness activity, it would be prudent to explore this relationship further and make conscious efforts to provide structured exposure in the school setting [110]. Additionally, adolescent girls have also expressed a desire to engage in more fitness-based activities as part of their PE curriculum, including a focus on muscular fitness activity [111]. As the literature surrounding muscular fitness activity advances, practitioners and researchers alike should remain cognizant of the potential gender bias cultivated from preconceived ideologies of masculine identities associated with muscular fitness activity [112]. Universal characteristics of hegemonic masculinities in PE are related to strength and speed, and are often influenced by social factors and are not necessarily the representative of participants views and experiences [112]. Furthermore, the glorification of masculinity in PE may have a negative influence on participation as a result of gendered pressures that may exacerbate insecurities and negatively affect participation across both sexes [113]. While there is merit in conducting research with specific sexes to account for physiological differences, the translation of knowledge into practice should avoid gendered habitus based on historical views of gender that may be detrimental to PA and PE participation across both sexes. Historically, PE has remained gendered in its delivery and may reserve muscular fitness activities for young boys, which may exacerbate the growing PA dropout rates in youth [111, 114, 115]. It should be acknowledged that muscular fitness activity is a popular form of PA that is conducted globally by both genders, often in the same commercial environments.

Formal PE may be an individual's only exposure to PA [116] and, therefore, must seek to elicit a positive psychological response if PA is to become habitual. If students are positively engaged in PA by enhancing enjoyment, engagement, and performance through PE, PA increases. Furthermore, insufficient PA remains a contributing factor to obesity and its associated health problems. Therefore, it is important to develop PA interventions that will enhance the self-perceptions of children and adolescents already disengaged, overweight, and with poor experiences in relation to PA. Many obese and disengaged individuals avoid PA as most current activities delivered in schools are aerobic in nature, thus excluding those individuals who possess a higher fat mass [117]. There is a growing body of literature that indicates youth with a higher fat mass are also subject to a higher fat-free mass, in turn placing them in a favorable position compared to their leaner peers with regards to muscular fitness activity by virtue of absolute strength [118, 119]. By combining the physiological adaptations of muscular fitness such as increased limb control and kinesthetic awareness, with improved self-perceptions in competency, this may encourage individuals who perceive themselves proficient in muscular fitness to actively pursue different types of MVPA [93, 108]. While it is postulated that muscular fitness activity may be an attractive form of exercise for overweight and obese children and adolescents, the role of self-determination theory in muscular fitness activity is overlooked in young people [40]. It has been suggested that muscular fitness activity may provide an opportunity for a form of PA that is aligned with what young people *want to do* while also providing an inclusive form of PA that accommodates overweight and obese adolescents [40, 120–122]. Collectively, the greater involvement, intent, and ability to conduct muscular fitness activity competently alongside peers may allow for elements of self-determination theory (SDT) to be satisfied.

Self-determination theory (SDT [123]) is a framework commonly utilized to examine the relationship between motivation and PA [124]. The need to cater to what individuals *like to do* is further supported by the notion that the development of positive self-perceptions, leading to increased enjoyment, may contribute to increases in habitual life-long PA (LLPA) [125, 126]. SDT is made up of three components: competence, relatedness, and autonomy. By satisfying all of these basic psychological needs, an individual can secure optimal psychological health and functioning [127]. Competence is how one feels toward the task when reflecting upon the level of mastery. A sense of mastery may be present in young people with a higher fat mass when taking part in muscular fitness due to their higher fat-free mass, allowing them to outperform their leaner peers [128]. Furthermore, potential improvements in kinesthetic awareness, limb control, and muscular fitness may increase competence in PA and catalyze future PA participation in overweight, obese, and previously sedentary children and young people [93].

The second element of SDT is that of autonomy, which is the level of perceived control for the individual. Exercise involving load being added as the individual improves their level of competence can expect to see loads of up to 5–10% added once the individual can comfortably perform 15 repetitions of a given movement while maintaining correct form [72, 129]. This method of adding load to progress the intensity of the muscular fitness allows for greater perceived autonomy while ensuring loads are not increased dramatically, allowing for safe progressions. The perceived control that the child or adolescent has over their load increases allows for an approach that places a degree of autonomy on the individual. This method of increasing load may be conducive to supporting autonomy with regard to exercise progression; allowing individuals to regulate the PA outcome themselves may enhance the intrinsic appeal. By allowing for an amount of autonomy within the curriculum and, ultimately, the expression of PA, it supports the participants in the decision-making process, allowing them to make the choices they want.

The final element of SDT is relatedness. Muscular fitness activity may allow the participant to feel part of the process alongside their peers, which may increase PA participation [130, 131]. Relatedness refers to the feeling of closeness and belonging to a social group. Muscular fitness activity may catalyze positive feedback from peers when considering that previously disengaged and overweight youth may outperform some of their leaner peers, allowing them to feel part of the social group [80]. This connection and feeling of acceptance from peers, whether it be through increases in motor control or by virtue of a higher fat-free mass, may support the promotion of PA in youth [128]. However, while it is hypothesized that overweight youth may benefit from being provided with the opportunity to outperform their leaner peers, PE and PA participation should remain balanced. The balance of providing opportunities for all children and adolescents, irrespective of body type, can be achieved by providing a varied curriculum and moving away from the current overemphasis on team sports and aerobic MVPA [121]. Furthermore, while such social comparisons are not to be encouraged in schools and PE, they are an unavoidable aspect of school life [132]. Indeed, given the current lack of focus on muscular fitness in schools, there may be a chance for young people to develop muscular fitness together and build competence in an activity where previous exposure has been limited [133]. Given the incompleteness of the current evidence base surrounding muscular fitness activity and psychological correlates and determinants, it would be beneficial to contextualize them using a socioecological model. Socioecological models provide a framework to understand the various personal, social, and environmental factors that facilitate and restrict PA [134–136]. These factors are represented in the youth PA promotion model (YPAPM) [136]. The YPAPM socioecological approach provides a framework that goes beyond investigating individual factors associated with PA, allowing for the social and built environment to be considered and inform future intervention design. Applying the YPAPM to future muscular fitness lesson design may improve understanding of factors that may predispose, reinforce, or enable participation in muscular fitness activity.

15.5.2 Muscular Fitness and Motor Skill

It is understood that motor skill is a correlate of PA, with youth possessing high levels of motor skill engaging in more PA than their less able counterparts [137, 138]. Failing to develop adequate motor skills during a child's development may result in poor fundamental movement skills and a lack of confidence and motivation to engage in PA [138]. Motor skill developed through muscular fitness activity may help support further participation in various forms of PA and engage youth and emerging young adults in ongoing PA [3]. The development of muscular fitness provides both functional (changes in motor unit coordination) and structural (muscle hypertrophy) changes that impact motor skills [77] and develop motor skills and fundamental movement skills such as jumping, throwing, and balancing [139]. Such adaptations have resulted in improvement in jumping, running, and throwing following structured muscular fitness activity [77]. It is suggested that if muscular fitness activity is not conducted during youth development, there is a potential for motor skill competence to decrease further over time. To allow children and adolescents to participate in all expressions of PA, there is a need to develop motor skills and movement confidence in the first instance, allowing for the development of prerequisite skills that are indicative to participating in varying forms of PA later in life [82]. Involving young people in muscular fitness activity may help suppress the inverse relationship between motor skill performance and the prevalence of overweight and obesity through reductions in PA [118, 140, 141].

15.5.3 Life-Long Physical Activity

LLPA is defined as activities that carry over from childhood into adulthood, require minimal equipment, and are generally reserved for one or two people [142]. Schools play a key role in catalyzing successful LLPA outcomes [100]. It has been suggested that the school environment and PE in particular are well placed to enhance young people's knowledge of lifelong health [143]. Therefore, exposure and teaching specific to PA guidelines designed to support health may cultivate an awareness of healthy behaviors as adolescents transition into adulthood. Ensuring acquisition of knowledge regarding muscular fitness activity may support lifelong engagement in a popular mode of adult PA and work toward reducing the lack of PA knowledge evidenced in adults [144]. Indeed, teachers and specialist PE teachers recognize the benefits of muscular fitness activity across a range of age groups and the contribution such activity has in developing overall fitness in preparation for lifelong PA engagement [19, 145–147].

Although team sports are enjoyed by many, competitive team sports may fail to engage the least active and skilled youth [148]. Team sports, although integral to PE, generally lack significant carry-over into adult life, and the opportunity to take part in organized sports drops off significantly post-formal education [149].

Fairclough et al. [150] raised concerns over the contribution of PE to the promotion of LLPA in northwest secondary schools in England. Fairclough et al. went on to suggest that PE should develop LLPA as part of the curriculum to increase exposure to activities that youth may face in adult life. Furthermore, Hills et al. [151] highlighted the potential schools have to develop the necessary skills and knowledge to sustain an active life beyond formal education.

Whitehead [152] defines physical literacy as "the motivation, confidence, physical competence, knowledge and understanding to value and take responsibility for engagement in PAs for life." Thus, by addressing the potential positive impact schools have on developing LLPA, there is an opportunity to develop physically literate pupils, enhancing lifelong engagement in PA. Activities such as yoga, cycling, and muscular fitness have been highlighted by adolescents as an expression of PA that they would like to explore, yet the curriculum lacks diversity in PA, favoring aerobic-based MVPA and team sports [153].

Muscular fitness activity fulfils the criteria associated with LLPA, yet few studies have assessed longitudinal outcomes regarding the impact of muscular fitness activity in formal PE and their tracking into adult life [154]. However, the work of Kjonniksen [149] displayed positive associations between youth exposure to PA when provided with a choice of activity in a formal setting and their positive tracking into adulthood, supporting the notion that varying modalities of PA should be utilized to elicit an impact on LLPA. By exploring varied forms of PA that young people may encounter after formal PE, a curriculum that promotes individual success and ultimately enjoyment may provide young people with the skills and confidence to participate in other forms of PA later in life [128, 139].

15.5.4 Muscular Fitness Activity and Disadvantaged Youth

Socioeconomic status (SES) measured using adolescent-based (pocket money and academic performance) and family-based (housing tenure, parents education, family affluence) indicators are closely related to health behaviors [155]. Previous research has found family affluence is positively associated with PA [156, 157]. Furthermore, low SES is associated with lower fitness levels and less intention to pursue an active lifestyle [158, 159]. Additionally, unfit young people are more likely to be deprived, with qualitative data suggesting cost and access to facilities are barriers to PA [160]. Policy makers and school stakeholders should consider SES and interventions that support deprived population groups that may be at increased risk of not meeting PA recommendations indictive of good health. It has been suggested that schools may provide such a safe and accessible environment that allows for PA participation independent of socioeconomic status [18, 161, 162].

When it comes to muscular fitness activity and gym-based PA, it may only be possible in the school setting for those individuals from disadvantaged backgrounds due to increasing charges to use public and commercial sports facilities [110, 163]. The lack of access to public sports and recreation facilities have been found to promote health inequalities [164, 165], yet few studies have addressed how individuals from disadvantaged communities may benefit from muscular fitness activity interventions in the schools. Schools may provide an opportunity to reach the majority of children irrespective of background characteristics and socioeconomic status [18]. Engaging children in PA at school may support a life-long willingness to continue engaging in PA following formal education. When considering the possible lack of access to facilities that may help develop muscular fitness, it is apparent schools may have a central role in addressing this inequality [158].

15.6 School-Based Muscular Fitness

Schools have the facilities and the curricula to promote and support health promotion including fitness programs independent of a pupils' sociodemographic profile [18, 166]. As such, schools are suitable settings to promote and support muscular fitness activity [17, 32, 40, 66, 72, 167]. In England, the National Curriculum for PE (NCPE) (DfE, 2014) outlines four aims for the subject as follows: (1) develop competence to excel in a broad range of PAs; (2) ensure students are physically active for sustained periods of time; (3) engage in competitive sports and activities; and (4) lead healthy active lives. Current recommendations from the UK government highlight the development of strength as a mandated element of PE for children and young people aged 7–16 [168]. The development of strength resides within the healthy active lives aspect of the PE curriculum and contributes to improving muscular fitness. Despite the broad aims of PE, with aims 2 and 4 specifically focused on PA and health, the curriculum is typically dominated by traditional team sports [148, 169]. This may be due to a lack of specific guidance on how to appropriately develop healthy lives, which would include the development of muscular fitness [4]. Similar recommendations are echoed in America [170] and Australia [171]. Indeed, if carried out correctly, muscular fitness activity can contribute to and support the aims of PE and form part of a health-related PE pedagogy [148, 172, 173]. The integration of muscular fitness activity into the curriculum, with specific guidance on the methods and approaches to facilitate the delivery of muscular fitness activity, can ensure that all curriculum aims are met for respective PE curriculums.

Despite schools being recognized as suitable settings, much of the research is conducted with high school athletes [167]. However, schools do provide a unique setting that allows for periodized models of exposure to muscular fitness activity at regular points throughout the academic year, which supports the development of muscular fitness [174]. One of the unique benefits of schools is that term time muscular fitness activity delivered during PE can be appropriately periodized and can extend beyond the recommended minimum of 23 weeks of consistent exposure suggested to muscular fitness in youth [175]. The use of term-time structure has been theoretically applied in a high school in New Zealand [167]. The 35 to 40-week structure of a term was deemed sufficient to stimulate meaningful adaptations for strength, power, speed, and aerobic capacity in both children and adolescents [167].

Furthermore, it is acknowledged that doing muscular fitness twice a week is enough to increase muscle muscular fitness [83, 176]. Therefore, a curriculum that includes two periods a week, on alternate days, would adequately develop muscular fitness [83, 176]. However, the success of muscular fitness activity delivery is still dependent upon the skill and knowledge levels of the individual delivering the activity to manipulate training variables to elicit a desired adaptation [60]. It is suggested that if muscular fitness activity is to be implemented in schools, the delivering staff must be suitably qualified [60, 72, 176].

In addition to the testing considerations necessary for the implementation of muscular fitness interventions, the timing and period of delivery is equally as important [177, 178]. The school environment lends itself well to the development of macrocycles that cover an academic year [167]. Furthermore, the structure of terms within the academic year could provide a way to develop detailed planning lasting between 2 and 6 weeks in the form of a mesocycle [63]. Consideration to time constraints placed upon the school should be taken into consideration when developing muscular fitness interventions. Typically, exposure to PA is conducted within PE sessions lasting 45–60 min [179], allowing for a suitable amount of time to conduct effective muscular fitness activity in the school setting [66]. Overall, methods of constructing long term planning are not only pragmatically appropriate to the school environment, but also widely recognized within muscular fitness literature, in both youth and adults [14]. Teachers should consider the potential for the academic year to act as a construct for periodization, while adhering to recognized protocols for program design to enhance specific muscular fitness adaptations. Muscular fitness activity in schools should be approached with an informed appreciation for the nuances involved in program design, delivery, and a clear objective of the muscular fitness adaptation required. For delivery success at a larger scale, training must be provided to teachers and school coaches to deliver muscular fitness activity confidently and effectively.

While the school environment is unique in providing a largely mandatory setting to a broad range of youth [180], it should seek to make the most of every opportunity to incorporate PA. School policy makers and teachers may benefit from exploring enhanced, extended, and expanded opportunities (TEO) for youth PA and muscular fitness development in conjunction with complex behavioral theories [180] and avoid repeating the shortcomings evidenced in school-based aerobic MVPA intervention design. TEO allows for a pragmatic approach to intervention design, expanding on PA opportunity by adding to the current PA opportunities, extending PA by adding additional time to current PA opportunities, and enhancing PA by augmenting existing PA opportunities [180]. Addressing both TEO and motivational psychological constructs may enhance the quality of the PA experience and positively impact intervention outcomes [180]. Particular attention may be well placed for those young people in the latter years of their formal education, providing an opportunity to participate in muscular fitness activity may fulfil both a desire [153] and a need to explore a mode of PA that supports LLPA [181]. School stake holders and policy makers should utilize TEO to allow both teachers and students to become familiar with the prescription of muscular fitness activity through the addition of its use within a school setting. This may help dispel some of the myths surrounding implementation (i.e., the need for specialist equipment and muscular fitness activity in injurious) [182] and cultivate positive intervention design in schools.

15.6.1 Teachers Delivery of Muscular Fitness

Unfortunately, it has been reported that some PE teachers avoid implementing muscular fitness activity as part of health-based PE and PA promotion due to perceived barriers, including a lack of facilities, teacher confidence, and time [183–185]. Such perceived barriers can be overcome through continued professional development (CPD) and support to improve foundational knowledge [17]. Knowledge of muscular fitness activity has been assessed among PE teachers in America and suggested that current competence levels to deliver muscular fitness activity in a school setting require improvement [60]. Although the literature surrounding muscular fitness activity delivery in schools is limited, evidence of successful interventions to improve knowledge of muscular fitness activity delivery has emerged from Australia [186, 187]. Kennedy and colleagues conducted one-day in-person workshops with teachers from 16 secondary schools to equip them with the necessary theoretical and practical knowledge to deliver muscular fitness activity. While the research in Australia is promising, other countries, such as the UK, lack research into the provision of PE teacher CPD, specifically in muscular fitness.

Despite levels of muscular fitness declining among some school-aged youth [1, 7, 8], there is little investigation into how to support teachers in the delivery of this health-enhancing activity [188]. Current CPD opportunities focus on team sports, games, and dance [189]. To support teachers in delivering muscular fitness activity as part of health-based PE, foundational knowledge and ongoing professional development opportunities are required to ensure safe and developmentally appropriate practice [60]. Within CPD provision, muscular fitness is aligned to developing health-based pedagogy. Currently, teachers and CPD providers are unsure about developing health-based PE content, making it challenging to develop CPD for health pedagogies such as muscular fitness activity [189, 191].

Research into PE teacher CPD is relatively new [190] and there is still a lack of clarity on what constitutes PE CPD, how it is accessed and what subjects should be covered [192]. However, the quality and content of PE CPD have received increased attention in recent years, with teachers expected to take a more research-informed approach to their lesson planning and delivery [193, 194]. CPD in the context of PE refers to a wide variety of specialized training, formal or informal education, or advanced professional learning intended to help teachers improve their professional knowledge, competence, skills, tools, and effectiveness in the delivery of quality PE [195]. Research suggests that current CPD opportunities for PE teachers lack relevance and require more thought to ensure it meets the requirements of the PE teacher [196, 197]. Additionally, there are concerns that some teachers are not aware of their existing knowledge gaps and, therefore, do not seek out suitable CPD that could enhance or inform their teaching, especially in health pedagogies such as muscular fitness activity [198]. The lack of knowledge reported in health-based PE can be attributable to a lack of focus during initial teacher training [188, 198] and limited opportunity to engage in related CPD. If PE is to remain a key component in tackling physical inactivity and promoting health in young people, appropriate CPD that enhances the knowledge and competence of teachers needs to be developed and disseminated [199].

Some teachers have reported difficulty accessing CPD, constrained by time and financial requirements of traditional face-to-face training opportunities [200]. Additionally, insufficient provision and limited accessibility contribute to low levels of CPD [199, 201]. In recent years, a move to online CPD has provided an opportunity to overcome time and financial costs barriers [202]. However, online CPD provision is in the early stages of use, and much work is needed to understand the feasibility and suitability of delivery to teachers [196]. Despite online CPD being in the early stages, recent qualitative research has suggested teachers require CPD to be: (1) evidence-based; (2) provide pedagogical content knowledge and not just content knowledge; (3) be informed by teachers and translatable to practice; (4) facilitate communities of practice; (5) be interactive; (6) be simple to navigate; and (7) be highly visual [196]. Recent work has taken the needs and requirements of PE teachers to develop online CPD that improved knowledge regarding the delivery of muscular fitness activity in schools.

15.6.2 Pedagogical Considerations

Session delivery and pedagogical considerations are of paramount importance to ensure engagement and inclusivity. Over the last two decades there has been a surge in pedagogical approaches to the delivery of PE, both structured and opportunistic throughout the school day [203]. Two approaches lend themselves well to muscular fitness delivery in the school environment when taking into consideration the approaches to muscular fitness session delivery discussed earlier in this chapter.

When considering muscular fitness pedagogy, a non-linear pedagogical constraints-led approach may be beneficial. This would allow for manipulation of environmental, task, and individual factors to enhance delivery [204] and such approaches may work well with muscular fitness delivery. Environmental constraints encompass the physical and social elements that influence the acquisition of movement skills, playing a crucial role in fostering a motivational atmosphere that engages students. Students' enjoyment of PAs is deeply influenced by their perceptions of the motivational climate around them [205]. A study of 4397 year 9 Finnish students found that environments that focus on task orientation, relatedness, and autonomy lead to greater enjoyment in physical education classes [205]. Furthermore, there may be advantages of allowing students to choose their own training variables, which may result in enhanced motivation and performance [206].

Research involving 128 high school athletes showed that those in a supportive and task-oriented climate within their strength and conditioning programs exhibited higher levels of effort, enjoyment, competence, intrinsic motivation, and commitment, highlighting the importance of a positive training atmosphere [207]. The study also suggested methods to foster such an environment, including acknowledging students' efforts and progress, encouraging teamwork, viewing mistakes as learning opportunities, emphasizing the importance of each student's role in the team, and fostering respectful interactions. An intervention lasting a year showed that moving the motivational climate toward task involvement and away from ego orientation has a beneficial effect on students' attitudes toward exercise and sports, which may subsequently improve relationships with exercise and PA [208]. These insights reveal that the environment plays a crucial and modifiable role in the effectiveness of muscular fitness training programs. Qualified teachers and coaches can adjust activities to suit various contexts, ages, and abilities allowing for an inclusive environment. By implementing task constraints, teachers can prompt students to discover and address movement challenges. For example, having a band around the knees during a squat to ensure knees do not collapse in, balancing an object on the head to maintain an upright posture, and seeking peer feedback. While individual constraints such as the learner's physical, physiological, cognitive, and emotional characteristics are mostly fixed, teachers need to consider these factors to adapt delivery effectively. For example, an individual's squat stance may be influenced by their leg length. Although physical attributes are often genetically determined, coaches can impact physiological factors like strength, power, and movement skills through well-planned training programs.

Another approach to muscular fitness delivery would be to take a health-based model approach. This approach to delivery focuses on the health of individual students, encouraging them to take ownership and understand the implications that engaging in PA has on their health and well-being [209, 210]. The model underscores the importance of students recognizing the value of leading a physically active lifestyle, equipped with the knowledge to select suitable PAs that enhance their health and well-being now and in the future [209]. It impacts areas related to personal growth, social development, and emotional well-being. A health-based model fulfilled through muscular fitness or strength training should integrate various components aimed at improving students' physical health, fitness levels, and overall well-being. This approach evolves from traditional skill-cantered models to health-centered models emphasizing MVPA or sport-focused engagement. While in the context of muscular fitness or strength specific delivery, moderate to vigorous activity may seem redundant, the integration of strength and skill-based training, for instance, has demonstrated improvements in aerobic capacity, muscular fitness, and fundamental movement skills, which are crucial for sustained participation in MVPA [211]. Such programs typically involve a circuit of strength and skill-based exercises, leading to significant health and fitness benefits without reported injuries. To help inform a well-rounded approach to overall physical development, the youth physical development model provides a systematic approach to developing physical performance in young athletes, emphasizing the importance of muscular strength alongside CRF and other fitness qualities [212]. This evidence-based approach highlights the role of muscular fitness in preventing chronic diseases, enhancing performance, and supporting overall health.

References

1. Dooley FL, Kaster T, Fitzgerald JS, Walch TJ, Annandale M, Ferrar K, et al. A systematic analysis of temporal trends in the handgrip strength of 2,216,320 children and adolescents between 1967 and 2017. Sports Med. 2020;50(6):1129–44.
2. García-Hermoso A, Ramírez-Campillo R, Izquierdo M. Is muscular fitness associated with future health benefits in children and adolescents? A systematic review and meta-analysis of longitudinal studies. Sports Med. 2019;49(7):1079–94.
3. Smith JJ, Eather N, Morgan PJ, Plotnikoff RC, Faigenbaum AD, Lubans DR. The health benefits of muscular fitness for children and adolescents: a systematic review and meta-analysis. Sports Med. 2014;44(9):1209–23.
4. Chalkley A. Muscle and bone strengthening activities for children and young people (5 to 18 years): a rapid evidence review. Public Health England; 2021. p. 1–42.
5. Villa-González E, Barranco-Ruiz Y, García-Hermoso A, Faigenbaum AD. Efficacy of school-based interventions for improving muscular fitness outcomes in children: a systematic review and meta-analysis. Eur J Sport Sci. 2023;23(3):444–59.
6. Cohen D, Voss C, Taylor M, Delextrat A, Ogunleye A, Sandercock G. Ten-year secular changes in muscular fitness in English children. Acta Paediatr. 2011;100(10):e175–7.
7. Kaster T, Dooley FL, Fitzgerald JS, Walch TJ, Annandale M, Ferrar K, et al. Temporal trends in the sit-ups performance of 9,939,289 children and adolescents between 1964 and 2017. J Sports Sci. 2020;38:1913–23.
8. Sandercock GRH, Cohen DD. Temporal trends in muscular fitness of English 10-year-olds 1998–2014: an allometric approach. J Sci Med Sport. 2019;22(2):201–5.
9. Tomkinson GR, Kaster T, Dooley FL, Fitzgerald JS, Annandale M, Ferrar K, et al. Temporal trends in the standing broad jump performance of 10,940,801 children and adolescents between 1960 and 2017. Sports Med. 2021;51(3):531–48.
10. Đurić S, Sember V, Starc G, Sorić M, Kovač M, Jurak G. Secular trends in muscular fitness from 1983 to 2014 among Slovenian children and adolescents. Scand J Med Sci Sports. 2021;31(9):1853–61.
11. Pate RR, Daniels S. Institute of medicine report on fitness measures and health outcomes in youth. JAMA Pediatr. 2013;167(3):221–2.
12. Corbin CB, Janz KF, Baptista F. Good health: the power of power. J Phys Educ Recreat Dance. 2017;88(9):28–35.
13. Welk G, Janz K, Laurson K, Mahar M, Zhu W, Pavlovic A. Development of criterion-referenced standards for musculoskeletal fitness in youth: considerations and approaches by the FitnessGram Scientific Advisory Board. Meas Phys Educ Exerc Sci [Internet]. 2022 [cited 2022 May 12]. Available from: https://www.tandfonline.com/doi/abs/10.1080/1091367X.2021.2014331.
14. Suchomel TJ, Nimphius S, Bellon CR, Stone MH. The importance of muscular strength: training considerations. Sports Med. 2018;48(4):765–85.
15. Gamble P. Implications and applications of training specificity for coaches and athletes. Strength Cond J. 2006;28(3):54–8.
16. Cassar S, Salmon J, Timperio A, Naylor PJ, Van Nassau F, Contardo Ayala AM, et al. Adoption, implementation and sustainability of school-based physical activity and sedentary behaviour interventions in real-world settings: a systematic review. Int J Behav Nutr Phys Act. 2019;16(1):1–13.

17. Cox A, Fairclough SJ, Kosteli MC, Noonan RJ. Efficacy of school-based interventions for improving muscular fitness outcomes in adolescent boys: a systematic review and meta-analysis. Sports Med. 2020;50(3):543–60.
18. Love R, Adams J, van Sluijs EMF. Are school-based physical activity interventions effective and equitable? A meta-analysis of cluster randomized controlled trials with accelerometer-assessed activity. Obes Rev. 2019;20(6):859–70.
19. Cox A, Noonan RJ, Fairclough SJ. PE teachers' perceived expertise and professional development requirements in the delivery of muscular fitness activity: PE Teacher EmPOWERment Survey. Eur Phys Educ Rev. 2022;29:251–67. https://doi.org/10.1177/1356336X221134067.
20. Faigenbaum AD, Best TM, MacDonald J, Myer GD, Stracciolini A. Top 10 research questions related to exercise deficit disorder (EDD) in youth. Res Q Exerc Sport. 2014;85(3):297–307.
21. Faigenbaum AD, Rebullido TR, MacDonald JP. Pediatric inactivity triad: a risky PIT. Curr Sports Med Rep. 2018;17(2):45–7. https://doi.org/10.1249/JSR.0000000000000450.
22. Eliakim A, Falk B, Armstrong N, Baptista F, Behm DG, Dror N, et al. Aerobic exercise and training during youth. Pediatr Exerc Sci. 2019;31(11):2577–605.
23. Clark BC, Manini TM. What is dynapenia? Nutrition. 2012;28(5):495–503.
24. Meinhardt U, Witassek F, Petrò R, Fritz C, Eiholzer U. Strength training and physical activity in boys: a randomized trial. Pediatrics. 2013;132(6):1105–11.
25. Eiholzer U, Meinhardt U, Petrò R, Witassek F, Gutzwiller F, Gasser T. High-intensity training increases spontaneous physical activity in children: a randomized controlled study. J Pediatr. 2010;156(2):242–6.
26. Lubans DR, Cliff DP. Muscular fitness, body composition and physical self-perception in adolescents. J Sci Med Sport. 2011;14(3):216–21.
27. Lubans DR, Smith JJ, Plotnikoff RC, Dally KA, Okely AD, Salmon J, et al. Assessing the sustained impact of a school-based obesity prevention program for adolescent boys: the ATLAS cluster randomized controlled trial. Int J Behav Nutr Phys Act. 2016;13(1):92.
28. Detter F, Nilsson JA, Karlsson C, Dencker M, Rosengren BE, Karlsson MK. A 3-year school-based exercise intervention improves muscle strength – a prospective controlled population-based study in 223 children. BMC Musculoskelet Disord [Internet]. 2014;15(1). Available from: https://www.scopus.com/inward/record.uri?eid=2-s2.0-84932189108&doi=10.1186%2f1471-2474-15-353&partnerID=40&md5=eefdfd968322602c9542ca2e449ce832.
29. De Ste Croix MBA. Isokinetic assessment and interpretation in paediatric populations: why do we know relatively little? Isokinet Exerc Sci. 2012;20(4):275–91.
30. Keating X, Liu X, Stephenson R, Guan J, Hodges M. Student health-related fitness testing in school-based physical education: strategies for student self-testing using technology. Eur Phys Educ Rev. 2020;26(2):552–70.
31. Yager Z, Alfrey L, Young L. The psychological impact of fitness testing in physical education: a pilot experimental study among Australian adolescents. J Teach Phys Educ. 2021;1(aop):1–9.
32. Cohen DD, Voss C, Sandercock GRH. Fitness testing for children: let's mount the zebra! J Phys Act Health. 2015;12(5):597–603.
33. Lloyd RS, Oliver JL, Faigenbaum AD, Myer GD, De Ste Croix MBA. Chronological age vs. biological maturation: implications for exercise programming in youth. J Strength Cond Res. 2014;28(5):1454–64.
34. Moran J, Sandercock GRH, Ramírez-Campillo R, Meylan C, Collison J, Parry DA. A meta-analysis of maturation-related variation in adolescent boy athletes' adaptations to short-term resistance training. J Sports Sci. 2017;35(11):1041–51.
35. Moran J, Sandercock G, Ramirez-Campillo R, Clark CCT, Fernandes JFT, Drury B. A meta-analysis of resistance training in female youth: its effect on muscular strength, and shortcomings in the literature. Sports Med. 2018;48(7):1661–71.
36. Radnor JM, Oliver JL, Waugh CM, Myer GD, Lloyd RS. The influence of maturity status on muscle architecture in school-aged boys. Pediatr Exerc Sci. 2020;32:89–96.

37. Carvalho HM, Coelho-e-Silva M, Valente-dos-Santos J, Gonçalves RS, Philippaerts R, Malina R. Scaling lower-limb isokinetic strength for biological maturation and body size in adolescent basketball players. Eur J Appl Physiol. 2012;112(8):2881–9.
38. Cohen R, Mitchell C, Dotan R, Gabriel D, Klentrou P, Falk B. Do neuromuscular adaptations occur in endurance-trained boys and men? Appl Physiol Nutr Metab. 2010;35(4):471–9.
39. Dotan R, Mitchell C, Cohen R, Klentrou P, Gabriel D, Falk B. Child-adult differences in muscle activation-a review. Pediatr Exerc Sci. 2012;24(1):2–21.
40. Ten Hoor GA, Plasqui G, Ruiter RAC, Kremers SPJ, Rutten GM, Schols AMWJ, et al. A new direction in psychology and health: resistance exercise training for obese children and adolescents. Psychol Health. 2016;31(1):1–8.
41. Tomlinson DJ, Erskine RM, Morse CI, Winwood K, Onambélé-Pearson G. The impact of obesity on skeletal muscle strength and structure through adolescence to old age. Biogerontology. 2016;17(3):467–83.
42. Gomez-Bruton A, Gabel L, Nettlefold L, Macdonald H, Race D, McKay H. Estimation of peak muscle power from a countermovement vertical jump in children and adolescents [Internet]. J Strength Cond Res. 2019;33:390–8. Available from: www.nsca.com.
43. Nuzzo JL, Cavill MJ, Triplett NT, Mcbride JM. A descriptive study of lower-body strength and power in overweight adolescents. Pediatr Exerc Sci. 2009;21:34–46.
44. Castro-Piñero J, Ortega FB, Artero EG, Girela-Rejón MJ, Mora J, Sjöström M, et al. Assessing muscular strength in youth: usefulness of standing long jump as a general index of muscular fitness. J Strength Cond Res. 2010;24(7):1810–7.
45. Moya-Ramón M, Juan-Recio C, Lopez-Plaza D, Vera-Garcia FJ. Dynamic trunk muscle endurance profile in adolescents aged 14–18: normative values for age and gender differences. J Back Musculoskelet Rehabil. 2018;31(1):155–62.
46. Brotons-Gil E, García-Vaquero MP, Peco-González N, Vera-Garcia FJ. Flexion-rotation trunk test to assess abdominal muscle endurance: reliability, learning effect, and sex differences. J Strength Cond Res. 2013;27(6):1602–8.
47. Knudson D, Johnston D. Validity and reliability of a bench trunk-curl test of abdominal endurance. J Strength Cond Res. 1995;9(3):165–9.
48. Knudson D, Johnston D. Analysis of three test durations of the bench trunk-curl. J Strength Cond Res. 1998;12(3):150–1.
49. Sidney K, Jetté M. The partial curl-up to assess abdominal endurance: age and sex standards. Sports Med Train Rehabil. 1990;2(1):47–56.
50. Moreland J, Finch E, Stratford P, Balsor B, Gill C. Interrater reliability of six tests of trunk muscle function and endurance. J Orthop Sports Phys Ther. 1997;26(4):200–8.
51. Evans K, Refshauge KM, Adams R. Trunk muscle endurance tests: reliability, and gender differences in athletes. J Sci Med Sport. 2007;10(6):447–55.
52. Ito T, Shirado O, Suzuki H, Takahashi M, Kaneda K, Strax TE. Lumbar trunk muscle endurance testing: an inexpensive alternative to a machine for evaluation. Arch Phys Med Rehabil. 1996;77(1):75–9.
53. McGill SM, Childs A, Liebenson C. Endurance times for low back stabilization exercises: clinical targets for testing and training from a normal database. Arch Phys Med Rehabil. 1999;80(8):941–4.
54. FitnessGram Administration Manual [Internet]. Human Kinetics. 2017 [cited 2022 Sep 6]. Available from: https://www.human-kinetics.co.uk/9781450470469/fitnessgram-administration-manual.
55. Knaggs HE. Essentials of exercise physiology. 2nd ed. McArdle WD, Katch FL, Katch VL. Biochem Mol Biol Educ. 2002;30(6):433–4.
56. Ruiz JR, Castro-Piñero J, España-Romero V, Artero EG, Ortega FB, Cuenca MM, et al. Field-based fitness assessment in young people: the ALPHA health-related fitness test battery for children and adolescents. Br J Sports Med. 2011;45(6):518–24.

57. España-Romero V, Ortega FB, Vicente-Rodríguez G, Artero EG, Rey JP, Ruiz JR. Elbow position affects handgrip strength in adolescents: validity and reliability of Jamar, DynEx, and TKK Dynamometers. J Strength Cond Res. 2010;24(1):272–7.
58. Roberts HC, Denison HJ, Martin HJ, Patel HP, Syddall H, Cooper C, et al. A review of the measurement of grip strength in clinical and epidemiological studies: towards a standardised approach. Age Ageing. 2011;40(4):423–9.
59. Saint-Maurice PF, Laurson K, Welk GJ, Eisenmann J, Gracia-Marco L, Artero EG, et al. Grip strength cutpoints for youth based on a clinically relevant bone health outcome. Arch Osteoporos. 2018;13(1):92.
60. McGladrey BW, Hannon JC, Faigenbaum AD, Shultz BB, Shaw JM. High school physical educators' and sport coaches' knowledge of resistance training principles and methods. J Strength Cond Res. 2014;28(5):1433–42.
61. Stricker PR, Faigenbaum AD, McCambridge TM. Resistance training for children and adolescents. Pediatrics [Internet]. 2020 [cited 2021 Nov 2];145(6). Available from: https://pediatrics.aappublications.org/content/145/6/e20201011.
62. Gamble P. Periodization of training for volleyball. Strength Cond J. 2006;28(5):56–66.
63. Haff GG. Program design for resistance training. In: Haff GG, Triplett NT, editors. Essent Strength Train Cond. 2016, p. 439–70.
64. Coffey TH. Delorme method of restoration of muscle power by heavy resistance exercises. Treat Serv Bull Can Dep Veterans Aff. 1946;1(2):8–11.
65. Schoenfeld BJ, Grgic J, Van Every DW, Plotkin DL. Loading recommendations for muscle strength, hypertrophy, and local endurance: a re-examination of the repetition continuum. Sports. 2021;9(2):1–25.
66. Lloyd RS, Faigenbaum AD, Stone MH, Oliver JL, Jeffreys I, Moody JA, et al. Position statement on youth resistance training: the 2014 International Consensus. Br J Sports Med. 2014;48(7):498–505.
67. Stricker PR, Faigenbaum AD, McCambridge TM; FITNESS COSMA. Resistance training for children and adolescents. Pediatrics [Internet]. 2020 [cited 2021 Oct 28];145(6). Available from: https://pediatrics.aappublications.org/content/145/6/e20201011.
68. Suchomel TJ, Nimphius S, Stone MH. The importance of muscular strength in athletic performance. Sports Med. 2016;46(10):1419–49.
69. Suchomel TJ, Wagle JP, Douglas J, Taber CB, Harden M, Gregory Haff G, et al. Implementing eccentric resistance training—part 1: a brief review of existing methods. J Funct Morphol Kinesiol. 2019;4(2):38.
70. Faigenbaum AD, McFarland JE, Keiper FB, Tevlin W, Ratamess NA, Kang J, et al. Effects of a short-term plyometric and resistance training program on fitness performance in boys age 12 to 15 years. J Sports Sci Med. 2007;6(4):519–25.
71. Lloyd RS, Oliver JL, Hughes MG, Williams CA. The effects of 4-weeks of plyometric training on reactive strength index and leg stiffness in male youths. J Strength Cond Res. 2012;26(10):2812–9.
72. Faigenbaum AD, McFarland JE. Resistance training for kids: right from the start. ACSMs Health Fit J. 2016;20(5):16–22. https://doi.org/10.1249/FIT.0000000000000236.
73. Coutts AJ, Murphy AJ, Dascombe BJ. Effect of direct supervision of a strength coach on measures of muscular strength and power in young rugby league players. J Strength Cond Res. 2004;18(2):316–23.
74. Klusemann MJ, Pyne DB, Fay TS, Drinkwater EJ. Online video-based resistance training improves the physical capacity of junior basketball athletes. J Strength Cond Res. 2012;26(10):2677–84.
75. Smart DJ, Gill ND. Effects of an off-season conditioning program on the physical characteristics of adolescent rugby union players. J Strength Cond Res. 2013;27(3):708–17.
76. Peitz M, Behringer M, Granacher U. A systematic review on the effects of resistance and plyometric training on physical fitness in youth- what do comparative studies tell us? PLoS One. 2018;13(10):e0205525.

77. Behringer M, Vom Heede A, Matthews M, Mester J. Effects of strength training on motor performance skills in children and adolescents: a meta-analysis. Pediatr Exerc Sci. 2011;23:186–206.
78. Behm DG, Faigenbaum AD, Falk B, Klentrou P. Canadian Society for Exercise Physiology position paper: resistance training in children and adolescents. Appl Physiol Nutr Metab. 2008;33(3):547–61.
79. Carpinelli RN. Critical commentary: the NSCA position statement on youth resistance training. Med Sport Med Sport. 2012;16(1):46–50.
80. Faigenbaum AD, Lloyd RS, MacDonald J, Myer GD. Citius, Altius, Fortius: beneficial effects of resistance training for young athletes: narrative review. Br J Sports Med. 2016;50(1):3–7.
81. Grgic J, Schoenfeld BJ, Davies TB, Lazinica B, Krieger JW, Pedisic Z. Effect of resistance training frequency on gains in muscular strength: a systematic review and meta-analysis. Sports Med. 2018;48(5):1207–20.
82. Faigenbaum AD, Lloyd RS, Myer GD. Youth resistance training: past practices, new perspectives, and future directions. Pediatr Exerc Sci. 2013;25:591–604.
83. Myers AM, Beam NW, Fakhoury JD. Resistance training for children and adolescents. Transl Pediatr. 2017;6(3):137–43.
84. Radnor JM, Oliver JL, Waugh CM, Myer GD, Moore IS, Lloyd RS. The influence of growth and maturation on stretch-shortening cycle function in youth. Sports Med. 2018;48(1):57–71.
85. Milliken LA, Faigenbaum AD, Loud RL, Westcott WL. Correlates of upper and lower body muscular strength in children. J Strength Cond Res. 2008;22(4):1339–46.
86. Henriksson H, Henriksson P, Tynelius P, Ortega FB. Muscular weakness in adolescence is associated with disability 30 years later: a population-based cohort study of 1.2 million men. Br J Sports Med. 2018;0(10):1–11.
87. Quinlan JI, Maganaris CN, Franchi MV, Smith K, Atherton PJ, Szewczyk NJ, et al. Muscle and tendon contributions to reduced rate of torque development in healthy older males. J Gerontol – Ser Biol Sci Med Sci. 2018;73(4):539–45.
88. Fielding RA, Vellas B, Evans WJ, Bhasin S, Morley JE, Newman AB, et al. Sarcopenia: an undiagnosed condition in older adults. Current consensus definition: prevalence, etiology, and consequences. International Working Group on Sarcopenia. J Am Med Dir Assoc. 2011;12(4):249–56.
89. Alcazar J, Guadalupe-Grau A, García-García FJ, Ara I, Alegre LM. Skeletal muscle power measurement in older people: a systematic review of testing protocols and adverse events. J Gerontol – Ser Biol Sci Med Sci. 2018;73(7):914–24.
90. Cadore EL, Izquierdo M. Muscle power training: a hallmark for muscle function retaining in frail clinical setting. J Am Med Dir Assoc. 2018;19(3):190–2.
91. Alberga AS, Prud D, Sigal RJ, Goldfield GS, Hadjiyannakis S, Phillips P, et al. ARTICLE Effects of aerobic training, resistance training, or both on cardiorespiratory and musculoskeletal fitness in adolescents with obesity: the HEARTY trial. Child Appl Physiol Nutr Metab. 2016;41:255–65.
92. Chung-Wah YC, Mary McManus A, So HK, Chook P, Au CT, Martin Li A, et al. Effects of resistance training on cardiovascular health in non-obese active adolescents. World J Clin Pediatr. 2016;5(3):293–300.
93. Bea JW, Blew RM, Howe C, Hetherington-Rauth M, Going SB. Resistance training effects on metabolic function among youth: a systematic review. Pediatr Exerc Sci [Internet]. 2017;29. Available from: https://doi.org/10.1123/pes.2016-0143.
94. Torres-Costoso A, López-Muñoz P, Martínez-Vizcaíno V, Álvarez-Bueno C, Cavero-Redondo I. Association between muscular strength and bone health from children to young adults: a systematic review and meta-analysis. Sports Med. 2020;50(6):1163–90.
95. Fedewa AL, Candelaria A, Erwin HE, Clark TP. Incorporating physical activity into the schools using a 3-tiered approach. J Sch Health. 2013;83(4):290–7.

96. Collins H, Booth JN, Duncan A, Fawkner S, Niven A. The effect of resistance training interventions on 'the self' in youth: a systematic review and meta-analysis. Sports Med – Open. 2019;5(1):29.
97. Mintjens S, Menting MD, Daams JG, Van Poppel MNM, Roseboom TJ, Gemke RJBJ, et al. Cardiorespiratory fitness in childhood and adolescence affects future cardiovascular risk factors: a systematic review of longitudinal studies key points. Sports Med. 2018;48:2577–605.
98. Ruiz JR, Castro-Piñero J, Artero EG, Ortega FB, Sjöström M, Suni J, et al. Predictive validity of health-related fitness in youth: a systematic review. Br J Sports Med. 2009;43:909–23.
99. Joan Poitras V, Ellen Gray C, Borghese MM, Carson V, Chaput JP, Janssen I, et al. Systematic review of the relationships between objectively measured physical activity and health indicators in school-aged children and youth 1. 2016 [cited 2019 Feb 9]. Available from: http://nrcresearchpress.com/doi/suppl/10.1139/apnm-2015-0663.
100. Kennedy SG, Smith JJ, Morgan PJ, Peralta LR, Hilland TA, Eather N, et al. Implementing resistance training in secondary schools. Med Sci Sports Exerc. 2018;50(1):62–72.
101. Smith JJ, Morgan PJ, Plotnikoff RC, Stodden DF, Lubans DR. Mediating effects of resistance training skill competency on health-related fitness and physical activity: the ATLAS cluster randomised controlled trial. J Sports Sci. 2016;34(8):772–9.
102. Eisenberg ME, Wall M, Neumark-Sztainer D. Muscle-enhancing behaviors among adolescent girls and boys. Pediatrics. 2012;130(6):1019.
103. Morgan PJ, Saunders KL, Lubans DR. Improving physical self-perception in adolescent boys from disadvantaged schools: psychological outcomes from the Physical Activity Leaders randomized controlled trial. Pediatr Obes. 2012;7(3):e27–32.
104. Spruit A, Assink M, van Vugt E, van der Put C, Stams GJ. The effects of physical activity interventions on psychosocial outcomes in adolescents: a meta-analytic review. Clin Psychol Rev. 2016;45:56–71.
105. Faigenbaum AD, Myer GD. Resistance training among young athletes: safety, efficacy and injury prevention effects. Br J Sports Med. 2010;44(1):56–63.
106. Padilla-Moledo C, Ruiz JR, Ortega FB, Mora J, Castro-Piñero J. Associations of muscular fitness with psychological positive health, health complaints, and health risk behaviors in Spanish children and adolescents. J Strength Cond Res. 2012;26(1):167–73.
107. Robinson K, Riley N, Owen K, Drew R, Mavilidi MF, Hillman CH, et al. Effects of resistance training on academic outcomes in school-aged youth: a systematic review and meta-analysis. Sports Med. 2023;53(11):2095–109.
108. Schranz N, Tomkinson G, Olds T. What is the effect of resistance training on the strength, body composition and psychosocial status of overweight and obese children and adolescents? A systematic review and meta-analysis. Sports Med. 2013;43(9):893–907.
109. Velez A, Golem DL, Arent SM. The impact of a 12-week resistance training program on strength, body composition, and self-concept of hispanic adolescents. J Strength Cond Res. 2010;24(4):1065–73.
110. Cox A, Fairclough SJ, Noonan RJ. "It's just not something we do at school". Adolescent boys' understanding, perceptions and experiences of muscular fitness activity. Int J Environ Res Public Health. 2021;18(9):4923.
111. Cowley ES, Watson PM, Foweather L, Belton S, Thompson A, Thijssen D, et al. "Girls aren't meant to exercise": perceived influences on physical activity among adolescent girls—the HERizon project. Children [Internet]. 2021 [cited 2021 Oct 4];8(1). Available from: https://pubmed.ncbi.nlm.nih.gov/33430413/.
112. Lagestad P, Ropo E, Bratbakk T. Boys' experience of physical education when their gender is in a strong minority. Front Psychol [Internet]. 2021 [cited 2022 Dec 7];12. Available from: https://www.frontiersin.org/articles/10.3389/fpsyg.2021.573528.
113. Metcalfe S. Adolescent constructions of gendered identities: the role of sport and (physical) education. Sport Educ Soc. 2018;23(7):681–93.
114. Coen SE, Rosenberg MW, Davidson J. 'It's gym, like g-y-m not J-i-m': exploring the role of place in the gendering of physical activity. Soc Sci Med (1982). 2018;196:29–36.

115. Corr M, McSharry J, Murtagh EM. Adolescent girls' perceptions of physical activity: a systematic review of qualitative studies. Am J Health Promot. 2019;33(5):806–19.
116. Sutherland R, Campbell E, Nathan N, Wolfenden L, Lubans DR, Morgan PJ, et al. A cluster randomised trial of an intervention to increase the implementation of physical activity practices in secondary schools: study protocol for scaling up the Physical Activity 4 Everyone (PA4E1) program. BMC Public Health. 2019;19(1):883.
117. Mcmanus AM, Mellecker RR. Physical activity and obese children. J Sport Health Sci. 2012;1:141–8.
118. Colella D, Morano M, Robazza C, Bortoli L. Body image, perceived physical ability, and motor performance in nonoverweight and overweight Italian children. Percept Mot Skills. 2009;108(1):209–18.
119. Riddiford-Harland DL, Steele JR, Baur LA. Upper and lower limb functionality: are these compromised in obese children? Int J Pediatr Obes. 2006;1(1):42–9.
120. Hoor GAT, Kok G, Rutten GM, Ruiter RAC, Kremers SPJ, Schols AMJW, et al. The Dutch 'Focus on Strength' intervention study protocol: programme design and production, implementation and evaluation plan. 2016;16:496.
121. ten Hoor GA, Kok G, Peters GJY, Frissen T, Schols AMWJ, Plasqui G. The psychological effects of strength exercises in people who are overweight or obese: a systematic review. Sports Med. 2017;47(10):2069–81.
122. Ten Hoor GA, Rutten GM, Van Breukelen GJP, Kok G, Ruiter RAC, Meijer K, et al. Strength exercises during physical education classes in secondary schools improve body composition: a cluster randomized controlled trial. Int J Behav Nutr Phys Act [Internet]. 2018;15(1). Available from: https://doi.org/10.1186/s12966-018-0727-8.
123. Deci EL, Ryan RM. The general causality orientations scale: self-determination in personality. J Res Pers. 1985;19(2):109–34.
124. Owen KB, Smith J, Lubans DR, Ng JYY, Lonsdale C. Self-determined motivation and physical activity in children and adolescents: a systematic review and meta-analysis. Prev Med. 2014;67:270–9.
125. Weiss JW, Liu I, Sussman S, Palmer P, Unger JB, Cen S, et al. After-school supervision, psychosocial impact, and adolescent smoking and alcohol use in China. J Child Fam Stud. 2006;15(4):445–62.
126. Wagnsson S, Lindwall M, Gustafsson H. Participation in organized sport and self-esteem across adolescence: the mediating role of perceived sport competence. J Sport Exerc Psychol. 2014;36(6):584–94.
127. Ryan RM, Deci EL. Self-determination theory and the facilitation of intrinsic motivation, social development, and well-being. Am Psychol. 2000;55(1):68–78.
128. Babic MJ, Morgan PJ, Plotnikoff RC, Lonsdale C, White RL, Lubans DR. Physical activity and physical self-concept in youth: systematic review and meta-analysis. Sports Med. 2014;44(11):1589–601.
129. Dahab KS, McCambridge TM. Strength training in children and adolescents: raising the bar for young athletes? Sports Health. 2009;1(3):223–6.
130. Cuevas R, García-López LM, Serra-Olivares J. Sport education model and self-determination theory: an intervention in secondary school children. Kinesiology. 2016;48(1):10.26582/k.48.1.15.
131. Standage M, Duda JL, Ntoumanis N. A test of self-determination theory in school physical education. Br J Educ Psychol. 2005;75(3):411–33.
132. O'Keefe PA, Ben-Eliyahu A, Linnenbrink-Garcia L. Shaping achievement goal orientations in a mastery-structured environment and concomitant changes in related contingencies of self-worth. Motiv Emot. 2013;37(1):50–64.
133. Ten Hoor GA, Rutten GM, Van Breukelen GJP, Kok G, Ruiter RAC, Meijer K, et al. Strength exercises during physical education classes in secondary schools improve body composition: a cluster randomized controlled trial. Int J Behav Nutr Phys Act. 2018;15(1):92.

134. Sallis JF, Cervero RB, Ascher W, Henderson KA, Kraft MK, Kerr J. An ecological approach to creating active living communities. Annu Rev Public Health. 2006;27:297–322.
135. Abdelghaffar EA, Hicham EK, Siham B, Samira EF, Youness EA. Perspectives of adolescents, parents, and teachers on barriers and facilitators of physical activity among school-age adolescents: a qualitative analysis. Environ Health Prev Med. 2019;24(1):21.
136. Welk GJ. The youth physical activity promotion model: a conceptual bridge between theory and practice. Quest. 1999;51(1):5–23. https://doi.org/10.1080/00336297.1999.10484297.
137. Barnett LM, Stodden D, Cohen KE, Smith JJ, Lubans DR, Lenoir M, et al. Fundamental movement skills: an important focus. J Teach Phys Educ. 2016;35(3). https://doi.org/10.1123/jtpe.2014-0209.
138. De Meester A, Stodden D, Goodway J, True L, Brian A, Ferkel R, et al. Identifying a motor proficiency barrier for meeting physical activity guidelines in children. J Sci Med Sport. 2018;21(1):58–62.
139. Lubans DR, Morgan PJ, Cliff DP, Barnett LM, Okely AD. Fundamental movement skills in children and adolescents. Sports Med. 2010;40(12):1019–35.
140. Barros WMA, da Silva KG, Silva RKP, da Silva Souza AP, da Silva ABJ, Silva MRM, de Sousa Fernandes MS, de Souza SL, de Oliveira Nogueira Souza V. Effects of overweight/obesity on motor performance in children: a systematic review. Front Endocrinol [Internet]. 2022 [cited 2024 Feb 16];12. Available from: https://www.frontiersin.org/journals/endocrinology/articles/10.3389/fendo.2021.759165.
141. Lopes VP, Rodrigues LP, Maia JAR, Malina RM. Motor coordination as predictor of physical activity in childhood. Scand J Med Sci Sports. 2011;21(5):663–9.
142. Ross JG, Dotson CO, Gilbert GG, Katz SJ. What are kids doing in school physical education? J Phys Educ Recreat Dance. 1985;56(1):73–6.
143. Penney D, Jess M. Physical education and physically active lives: a lifelong approach to curriculum development. Sport Educ Soc. 2004;9(2):269–87.
144. Knox ECL, Musson H, Adams EJ. Knowledge of physical activity recommendations in adults employed in England: associations with individual and workplace-related predictors. Int J Behav Nutr Phys Act. 2015;12(1):69.
145. Daly RM, Ducher G, Hill B, Telford RM, Eser P, Naughton G, et al. Effects of a specialist-led, school physical education program on bone mass, structure, and strength in primary school children: a 4-year cluster randomized controlled trial. J Bone Miner Res Off J Am Soc Bone Miner Res. 2016;31(2):289–98.
146. McGladrey BW, Hannon J, Faigenbaum A, Shultz B, Shaw J. High school physical educators' and sport coaches' knowledge of resistance training principles and methods. J Strength Cond Res [Internet]. 2014 [cited 2024 Feb 16];28. Available from: https://consensus.app/papers/school-physical-educators-sport-coaches-knowledge-mcgladrey/7b3ecc1ed3ea575aaae098da2b3620dc/.
147. Lanier KV, Killian CM, Burnett R. Integrating strength and conditioning into a high school physical education curriculum: a case example. J Phys Educ Recreat Dance. 2021;92:18–26.
148. Green K. Mission impossible? Reflecting upon the relationship between physical education, youth sport and lifelong participation. Sport Educ Soc [Internet]. 2014 [cited 2017 Sep 30];19. Available from: http://www.tandfonline.com/action/journalInformation?journalCode=cses20.
149. Kjønniksen L, Torsheim T, Wold B. Tracking of leisure-time physical activity during adolescence and young adulthood: a 10-year longitudinal study. Int J Behav Nutr Phys Act. 2008;5:69.
150. Fairclough S, Stratton G, Baldwin G. The contribution of secondary school physical education to lifetime physical activity. Eur Phys Educ Rev. 2002;8(1):69–84.
151. Hills AP, Dengel DR, Lubans DR. Supporting public health priorities: recommendations for physical education and physical activity promotion in schools. Prog Cardiovasc Dis. 2015;57(1873-1740 (Electronic)):368–74.
152. Whitehead M. Physical literacy: throughout the lifecourse. Abingdon, Oxford: Routledge; 2010.

153. Corder K, Atkin AJ, Ekelund U, van Sluijs EM. What do adolescents want in order to become more active? BMC Public Health. 2013;13(1):718.
154. Smith JJ, DeMarco M, Kennedy SG, Kelson M, Barnett LM, Faigenbaum AD, et al. Prevalence and correlates of resistance training skill competence in adolescents. J Sports Sci. 2018;36(11):1241–9.
155. Moor I, Kuipers MAG, Lorant V, Pförtner TK, Kinnunen JM, Rathmann K, et al. Inequalities in adolescent self-rated health and smoking in Europe: comparing different indicators of socioeconomic status. J Epidemiol Community Health. 2019;73(10):963–70.
156. Foster HME, Celis-Morales CA, Nicholl BI, Petermann-Rocha F, Pell JP, Gill JMR, et al. The effect of socioeconomic deprivation on the association between an extended measurement of unhealthy lifestyle factors and health outcomes: a prospective analysis of the UK Biobank cohort. Lancet Public Health. 2018;3(12):e576–85.
157. Borraccino A, Lemma P, Iannotti RJ, Zambon A, Dalmasso P, Lazzeri G, et al. Socioeconomic effects on meeting physical activity guidelines: comparisons among 32 countries. Med Sci Sports Exerc. 2009;41(4):749–56.
158. Wolfe AM, Lee JA, Laurson KR. Socioeconomic status and physical fitness in youth: findings from the NHANES National Youth Fitness Survey. J Sports Sci. 2020;38(5):534–41.
159. Shrewsbury VA, Foley BC, Flood VM, Bonnefin A, Hardy LL, Venchiarutti RL, et al. School-level socioeconomic status influences adolescents' health-related lifestyle behaviors and intentions. J Sch Health. 2018;88(8):583–9.
160. Charlton R, Gravenor MB, Rees A, Knox G, Hill R, Rahman MA, et al. Factors associated with low fitness in adolescents – a mixed methods study. BMC Public Health. 2014;14(1):764.
161. Mura G, Rocha NBF, Helmich I, Budde H, Machado S, Wegner M, et al. Physical activity interventions in schools for improving lifestyle in European countries. Clin Pract Epidemiol Ment Health. 2015;11(Suppl 1 M5):77–101.
162. van Sluijs EMF, Ekelund U, Crochemore-Silva I, Guthold R, Ha A, Lubans D, et al. Physical activity behaviours in adolescence: current evidence and opportunities for intervention. Lancet. 2021;398(10298):429–42.
163. Ramchandani G, Shibli S, Kung SP. The performance of local authority sports facilities in England during a period of recession and austerity. Int J Sport Policy Politics. 2018;10(1):1–17.
164. Parnell M, Gee I, Foweather L, Whyte G, Knowles Z. Children of smoking and non-smoking households' perceptions of physical activity, cardiorespiratory fitness, and exercise. Children. 2021;8(7):552.
165. Higgerson J, Halliday E, Ortiz-Nunez A, Brown R, Barr B. Impact of free access to leisure facilities and community outreach on inequalities in physical activity: a quasi-experimental study. J Epidemiol Community Health. 2018;72(3):252–8.
166. CDC. Comprehensive school physical activity programs [Internet]. Comprehensive School Physical Activity Programs. 2012 [cited 2020 Oct 26]. Available from: http://www.shapeamerica.org/cspap/index.cfm.
167. Pichardo AW, Oliver JL, Harrison CB, Maulder PS, Lloyd RS. Integrating resistance training into high school curriculum. Strength Cond J. 2019;41(1):39–50.
168. Foster D, Roberts N. Physical education, physical activity and sport in schools. Res Brief [Internet]. 2022 [cited 2022 Jul 18]. Available from: https://commonslibrary.parliament.uk/research-briefings/sn06836/.
169. Green K. Lifelong participation, physical education and the work of Ken Roberts. Sport Educ Soc. 2002;7(2):167–82.
170. Logan K, Cuff S, LaBella CR, Brooks MA, Canty G, Council on Sports Medicine and Fitness, et al. Organized sports for children, preadolescents, and adolescents. Pediatrics. 2019;143(6):e20190997.
171. The Australian Physical Literacy Framework.
172. Andermo S, Hallgren M, Nguyen TTD, Jonsson S, Petersen S, Friberg M, et al. School-related physical activity interventions and mental health among children: a systematic review and meta-analysis. Sports Med – Open [Internet]. 2020 [cited 2022 Jul 19];6(1). Available from: https://doi.org/10.1186/s40798-020-00254-x.

173. Lubans DR, Smith JJ, Peralta LR, Plotnikoff RC, Okely AD, Salmon J, et al. A school-based intervention incorporating smartphone technology to improve health-related fitness among adolescents: rationale and study protocol for the NEAT and ATLAS 2.0 cluster randomised controlled trial and dissemination study. BMJ Open [Internet]. 2016 [cited 2018 Jul 19];6. Available from: https://doi.org/10.1136/bmjopen-2015-010448.
174. Faigenbaum A, Meadors L. A coach's dozen: an update on building healthy, strong, and resilient young athletes. Strength Cond J. 2017;39:27–33.
175. Lesinski M, Prieske O, Granacher U. Effects and dose–response relationships of resistance training on physical performance in youth athletes: a systematic review and meta-analysis. Br J Sports Med. 2016;50(13):781.
176. dos Santos Duarte Junior MA, López-Gil JF, Caporal GC, Mello JB. Benefits, risks and possibilities of strength training in school Physical Education: a brief review. Sport Sci Health. 2022;18(1):11–20.
177. Drenowatz C, Greier K. Resistance training in youth – benefits and characteristics. J Biomed. 2018;3. https://doi.org/10.7150/jbm.25035.
178. Faigenbaum AD, Kraemer WJ, Blimkie CJR, Jeffreys I, Micheli LJ, Nitka M, et al. Youth resistance training: updated position statement paper from the national strength and conditioning association. J Strength Cond Res. 2009;23(5 Suppl):S60–79.
179. Duehring MD, Feldmann CR, Ebben WP. Strength and conditioning practices of United States high school strength and conditioning coaches. J Strength Cond Res. 2009;23(8):2188–203.
180. Beets MW, Okely A, Glenn Weaver R, Webster C, Lubans D, Brusseau T, et al. The theory of expanded, extended, and enhanced opportunities for youth physical activity promotion. Int J Behav Nutr Phys Act. 2016;13(1):120.
181. Hulteen RM, Smith JJ, Morgan PJ, Barnett LM, Hallal PC, Colyvas K, et al. Global participation in sport and leisure-time physical activities: a systematic review and meta-analysis. Prev Med. 2016;95:14–25.
182. Steele J, Fisher J, Skivington M, Dunn C, Arnold J, Tew G, et al. A higher effort-based paradigm in physical activity and exercise for public health: making the case for a greater emphasis on resistance training. BMC Public Health. 2017;17(1):300.
183. Kennedy SG, Smith JJ, Estabrooks PA, Nathan N, Noetel M, Morgan PJ, et al. Evaluating the reach, effectiveness, adoption, implementation and maintenance of the Resistance Training for Teens program. Int J Behav Nutr Phys Act. 2021;18(1):1–18.
184. Naylor PJ, Nettlefold L, Race D, Hoy C, Ashe MC, Wharf Higgins J, et al. Implementation of school based physical activity interventions: a systematic review. Prev Med. 2015;72:95–115.
185. Nathan N, Elton B, Babic M, McCarthy N, Sutherland R, Presseau J, et al. Barriers and facilitators to the implementation of physical activity policies in schools: a systematic review. Prev Med. 2018;107:45–53.
186. Kennedy SG, Smith JJ, Hansen V, Lindhout MIC, Morgan PJ, Lubans DR. Implementing resistance training in secondary schools: an exploration of teachers' perceptions [Internet]. 2018. Available from: http://www.acsm-tj.org.
187. Kennedy SG, Peralta LR, Lubans DR, Foweather L, Smith JJ. Implementing a school-based physical activity program: process evaluation and impact on teachers' confidence, perceived barriers and self-perceptions. Phys Educ Sport Pedagogy. 2019;24(3):233–48.
188. Cale L, Harris J, Duncombe R. Promoting physical activity in secondary schools: growing expectations, 'same old' issues? Eur Phys Educ Rev. 2016;22(4):526–44.
189. Armour KM, Makopoulou K. Great expectations: teacher learning in a national professional development programme. Teach Teach Educ. 2012;28(3):336–46.
190. Ennis CD. Routledge handbook of physical education pedagogies [Internet]. In: Ennis CD, editor. Routledge handbook of physical education pedagogies. Routledge; 2016 [cited 2022 Jul 6]. Available from: https://www.taylorfrancis.com/books/9781317589518.
191. Pühse U, Barker D, Brettschneider WD, Feldmeth A, Gerlach E, McCuaig L, et al. International approaches to health-oriented physical education – local health debates and differing conceptions of health. Int J Phys Educ. 2011;3:2–14.

192. Tannehill D, Demirhan G, Čaplová P, Avsar Z. Continuing professional development for physical education teachers in Europe. Eur Phys Educ Rev. 2021;27(1):150–67.
193. Osmond-Johnson P, Campbell C, Faubert B. Supporting professional learning: the work of Canadian teachers' organizations. 2018;45(1):17–32. https://doi.org/101080/1941525720181486877.
194. Beni S, Fletcher T, Chróinín DN. Teachers' engagement with professional development to support implementation of meaningful physical education. J Teach Phys Educ. 2021;1(aop):1–10.
195. Lander N, Lewis S, Nahavandi D, Amsbury K, Barnett LM. Teacher perspectives of online continuing professional development in physical education. Sport Educ Soc. 2022;27(4):434–48.
196. Lander N, Lewis S, Nahavandi D, Amsbury K, Barnett LM. Teacher perspectives of online continuing professional development in physical education. [Internet]. 2020 [cited 2021 Oct 20]. https://doi.org/10.1080/1357332220201862785. Available from: https://www.tandfonline.com/doi/abs/10.1080/13573322.2020.1862785.
197. Makopoulou K. An investigation into the complex process of facilitating effective professional learning: CPD tutors' practices under the microscope. 2017;23(3):250–66. https://doi.org/10.1080/1740898920171406463.
198. Alfrey L, Webb L, Cale L. Physical education teachers' continuing professional development in health-related exercise: a figurational analysis. 2012;18(3):361–79. http://doi.org/101177/1356336X12450797.
199. Armour K, Harris J. Making the case for developing new PE-for-health pedagogies. Quest. 2013;65(2):201–19.
200. Sato T, Haegele JA, Foot R. In-service physical educators' experiences of online adapted physical education endorsement courses. Adapt Phys Act Q. 2017;34(2):162–78.
201. Ward P, van der Mars H. Confronting the challenge of continuous professional development for physical education teacher educators. J Phys Educ Recreat Dance. 2020;91(1):7–13.
202. Lantz-Andersson A, Lundin M, Selwyn N. Twenty years of online teacher communities: a systematic review of formally-organized and informally-developed professional learning groups. Teach Teach Educ. 2018;75:302–15.
203. Arufe-Giráldez V, Sanmiguel-Rodríguez A, Ramos-Álvarez O, Navarro-Patón R. News of the pedagogical models in physical education—a quick review. Int J Environ Res Public Health. 2023;20(3):2586.
204. Renshaw I, Chow JY. A constraint-led approach to sport and physical education pedagogy. Phys Educ Sport Pedagogy. 2019;24(2):103–16.
205. Jaakkola T, Wang CKJ, Soini M, Liukkonen J. Students' perceptions of motivational climate and enjoyment in Finnish physical education: a latent profile analysis. J Sports Sci Med. 2015;14(3):477–83.
206. Halperin I, Wulf G, Vigotsky AD, Schoenfeld BJ, Behm DG. Autonomy: a missing ingredient of a successful program? Strength Cond J. 2018;40(4):18–25.
207. Chamberlin JM, Fry MD, Iwasaki S. High school athletes' perceptions of the motivational climate in their off-season training programs. J Strength Cond Res. 2017;31(3):736–42.
208. Christodoulidis T, Papaioannou A, Digelidis N. Motivational climate and attitudes towards exercise in Greek senior high school: a year-long intervention. Eur J Sport Sci. 2001;1(4):1–12.
209. Haerens L, Cardon G, De Bourdeaudhuij I, Kirk D. Toward the development of a pedagogical model for health-based physical education. Quest. 2011;63(3):321–38.
210. McEvilly N, Verheul M, Atencio M, Jess M. Physical education for health and wellbeing: a discourse analysis of Scottish physical education curricular documentation. Discourse Stud Cult Polit Educ. 2014;35(2):278–93.
211. Faigenbaum AD, Bush JA, Mcloone RP, Kreckel MC, Farrell A, Ratamess NA, et al. Benefits of strength and skill-based training during primary school physical education. J Strength Cond Res. 2015;29(5):1255–62.
212. Lloyd RS, Oliver JL. The youth physical development model: a new approach to long-term athletic development. Strength Cond J. 2012;34(3):61–72.

Chapter 16
Inclusive Physical Activity Practices for Disabled Children and Adolescents

Thi Nancy Huynh, Justin Haegele, Maeghan E. James, and Kelly P. Arbour-Nicitopoulos

16.1 Introduction

The interdisciplinary field of adapted physical activity (PA) focuses on the promotion of active lifestyles and sport participation among disabled people, including disabled students within schools. Given the interdisciplinary nature of the field, educators and practitioners (e.g., therapists) in adapted PA, such as those promoting or providing PA opportunities to disabled children and adolescents in schools, are influenced by a variety of practical, philosophical, and social considerations when making decisions about how to provide services, what services to provide, and reasons why to provide them. In this chapter, we review a collection of considerations that may help to inform educators and practitioners on the *whats, whys, and hows* of providing PA opportunities for disabled students. These considerations begin with conversations about disability, ableism, inclusion, and school settings, before moving into overviews on the importance of PA for disabled students, promising practices for supporting school-based PA for disabled students, and practical applications and measurement for implementing and evaluating school-based PA.

Prior to engaging in conversations about PA and disability, we first must disclose our use of language about disability within this chapter. We recognize that the

---

T. N. Huynh · K. P. Arbour-Nicitopoulos (✉)
Faculty of Kinesiology and Physical Education, University of Toronto, Toronto, ON, Canada
e-mail: kelly.arbour@utoronto.ca

J. Haegele
Department of Human Movement Sciences, Old Dominion University, Norfolk, VA, USA

M. E. James
Healthy Active Living and Obesity Research Group, Children's Hospital of Eastern Ontario Research Institute, Ottawa, ON, Canada

Department of Pediatrics, Faculty of Medicine, University of Ottawa, Ottawa, ON, Canada

language that we use to describe disabled people reflects our beliefs about disability, impairment, and disabled people. We also recognize that person-first language (e.g., person with disabilities), which is intended to prioritize a person as a human first and that impairment is just one of many attributes, is a commonly accepted disability related language to use. However, for the purposes of this chapter, we use identity-first language (i.e., disabled person), which is aligned with the social model of disability discourse (more on that below) and recognizes that individuals who are oppressed by social barriers are disabled by society. We would be remiss here, though, not to note, as Spencer and colleagues [1] have, that we have a responsibility to represent participants and communities using the words and descriptions they choose, and therefore, service providers should be receptive to unique and individualized language preferences of the disabled people they interact with while engaging in activities.

16.2 What Is a Disability?

Understandings of what disability is or means have changed over time. These changes are largely influenced by who is considered the cognitive authority, or the professional organization or collection of people who have social capital to establish definitions and act as key gatekeepers, in specific fields [2].

Today, there are a variety of frameworks for understanding disability that influence how society, including service providers within schools, interact with and think about those with disabilities. For example, a service provider's orientation toward disability might influence (a) their expectations for disabled students, (b) the type and quality of instructions they provide, (c) the language they use when discussing disability, and (d) what is considered "competent" within PA environments [3–5]. In this section, we briefly describe two dominant conceptualizations of disability discourse, the medical model and social model, as well as a newer understanding of disability through the social relational model. With that, it is important for readers to understand that we are not endorsing the adoption of any of these models specifically, but rather attempting to provide some thoughts and comments on models for readers to shape their thinking toward disability.

16.2.1 Medical Model

The medical model of disability discourse emerged when doctors and scientists replaced religious leaders as cognitive authority within societies [2]. Because members of the medical community most often work from a biological perspective, they conceptualize disability as largely a biological product that resides within the individual as a defect, or failure, of a body system that is abnormal or pathological [6]. Within this lens, disability is an individual phenomenon that results in limited functioning that is viewed as a problem [6] and can include structural or functional deficiencies caused by physical, sensory, affective, or cognitive disorders [4]. As such, disability is viewed as being inherently negative and is therefore something that society should help to remediate or "fix" using interventions [7]. Historically, medical model thinking has underpinned many aspects of research and practice within adapted PA and in the promotion of PA for disabled children and adolescents. For example, the types and goals of interventions and research, which are often focused on achieving normative status [8], are largely influenced by medical understandings of disability. Similarly, the medical model is characterized by a heavy reliance on medical professionals as being important gatekeepers who can restrict or provide resources and benefits. That is, in some contexts (e.g., the United States), adapted PA services within schools are only offered and available to those who present a medical diagnosis, therefore centering the role of the medical professional as gatekeepers to service.

16.2.2 Social Model

The social model of disability discourse, often presented as a juxtaposition to the medical model, has gained popularity among adapted PA scholars and practitioners. With the social model, medical professionals are supplanted by academics and disabled advocates, as well as non-disabled allies, as the cognitive authority. According to the social model, limitations associated with disability are not thought of as being a product of impairment but are rather associated with limitations imposed on people with impairments by society [9]. It is important to note, here, that social model thinkers consider impairment to be an abnormality of the body (e.g., restriction or malfunction of a limb), whereas disability is considered to be the disadvantages that are caused by social institutions that do not take disabled people into account and therefore exclude them from major social life [10]. The distinction between disability as a product of impairment as opposed to limitations placed on disabled people within society, is important to keep in mind, as advocates for the social model contest that there is nothing inherently disabling about having an impairment. Rather, advocates indicate that disability is imposed, in addition to impairments, by the way individuals with impairments are excluded from fully participating in their community.

According to social model advocates, impairment should be considered a form of diversity, like gender, sexual orientation, or racial diversity, that offers a unique perspective and should be celebrated and valued [11]. Interventions should therefore not be directed toward "fixing" disability or attempting to capture normalized performance values [8] but rather focus on social change. Social model thinkers and advocates claim that with social change, having an impairment would not substantially reduce one's well-being, and that many problems typically associated with disability may disappear if people's attitudes toward disabled individuals would change. The overarching message of the social model is a call to move society from one which discriminates against those with impairments.

16.2.3 Social Relational Model

While the medical and social models of disability discourse have gained considerable attention, there are many other models that influence thinking about disability internationally. For example, one model that has emerged from criticisms of both the medical and social models is the social relational model of disability discourse [12]. According to the social relational model, impairments are thought to have direct effects on experiences that can simultaneously occur with socially engendered structural or attitudinal restrictions [13]. That is, disability is something that is imposed on top of restrictions that exist because of one's impairment [13, 14]. Importantly, and unlike the medical and social models, the social relational model stresses the effects of both one's impairment as well as the social or structural limitations brought on by society. According to the social relational model, disability can be experienced in a number of social contexts or experiences, which may include the immediate everyday physical and social influences of impairment, negative experiences with attitudes toward disability, or structural disability (e.g., being physically excluded from environments, opportunities, etc.) [13]. For those interested in the social relational model, we would encourage further reading of the work of Solveig Mangus Reindal [13, 14].

16.2.4 Ableism

Ableism, like sexism, racism, or heterosexism, is a form of prejudice and discrimination that is inherent to legal, educational, and ethical practices. Ableism classifies an entire group, disabled people, as "less than" or abnormal, whereas non-disabled people are viewed as superior or "normal" [15]. An ableist society treats nondisabled people as the standard (or, "normal"), which results in public spaces (such as schools) that are built to serve standard people, inherently excluding disabled people and, in educational contexts, disabled students. Some have connected ableism to the medical model, because disabled people are viewed as needing to be changed in order to fit within existing, ableist spaces.

Ableism can come in a number of different forms. Direct ableism, for example, is both conscious and oppressive in nature, where nondisabled people purposely dehumanize disabled people. Some examples of direct ableism may include (a) nondisabled people complaining that disabled people receive too many benefits or special privileges (like, disabled parking spots), (b) suspecting disabled people are "faking it" or do not need resources provided for them, or (c) overprotecting or sheltering disabled people in fear that activities are too "risky" for them. The third example here might have particular relevance in sport or PA spaces, where disabled children and adolescents are often prevented from opportunities because adults believe active play, exercise, or sport may be too risky, which takes away options for risk and devalues their human dignity [16]. A second type of ableism, indirect ableism, is unconscious behavior that is not intended to cause harm but does. This may take the form of using verbal expressions that communicate an insult or slight in relation to a disability, such as phrases like "you're acting bi-polar" or "why are you so OCD about this?" Finally, systemic or institutional ableism is ableism that is deeply rooted into our social structures as a result of centuries of active discrimination against disabled people. This type of ableism is often unnoticed and unquestioned among nondisabled people, since it is deeply rooted in their understandings of how the world exists. But, it can include things like physical barriers to access, limited opportunities, restricted freedom to move around settings or spaces, and ongoing failures to address these issues.

16.3   Inclusion in Schools

Within the field of adapted PA, the term *inclusion* is used in a variety of different ways, often without clear definitions or conceptualizations [17]. This is problematic, as without providing explicit definitions when using the term, *inclusion* can be used in a variety of different forms, which can ultimately affect the decisions made by practitioners. For example, one definition of inclusion that is commonly used is to describe a placement or setting in which disabled students and nondisabled students are educated together [18]. In this definition, all contexts in which disabled and nondisabled students are together would be considered inclusive, regardless of the curriculum, pedagogies, or practices that occur within those spaces [17, 19]. This definition has some shortcomings, though, as materially based definitions, which only take into consideration the physical space an individual is located, do not consider how people experience those spaces [19]. With this in mind, we will use the term "integrated" or "regular" throughout the rest of the chapter, to describe a physical space or place that has disabled and nondisabled people together, but does not assume "inclusiveness."

In recent years, conceptualizations of inclusion have begun to extend beyond materiality and center on the feelings and experiences of disabled people themselves. For example, Haegele and Maher [19] conceptualize inclusion as an intersubjective experience, which fosters feelings of belonging, acceptance, and value. This conceptualization is well aligned with the "nothing about us, without us" movement that emphasizes the importance of empowering disabled people through centering their voices when constructing experiences [20] as well as social justice pedagogical practices (more on that below).

Within this experiential conceptualization, inclusion extends beyond just an individual's physical existence within a space or activity and considers an individual's experience within those spaces. There are a number of important implications for practitioners regarding inclusion being conceptualized as an intersubjective experience. First, and foremost, existing within an integrated space does not guarantee experiences of inclusion. Rather, service providers must ask disabled students to share their feelings and experiences, by actively communicating with them about their time within the space or activity. Relatedly, since inclusion is thought of as a feeling, observational methods, such as inclusion checklists, would not be able to capture or evaluate the inclusiveness of a program and inclusive strategies would not necessarily support inclusion. Rather, to reiterate again, service providers can only understand the inclusiveness of their programs by speaking directly with those experiencing the program.

16.4 Physical Activity, Schools, and Disabled Students

It is well documented that PA for children and adolescents improves cognition, muscle tone, and overall well-being [21], including for disabled children and adolescents [22, 23]. Yet, we know that disabled children and adolescents tend not to meet established international PA guidelines of an average of at least 60 min of moderate-to-vigorous intensity aerobic activity each day [24–26] and therefore may be missing out on some of these psychological and physiological benefits. To help promote PA opportunities for disabled children and adolescents, we must understand what factors might enable or prevent their participation. To date, many barriers have been identified that may restrict disabled students from being physically active outside of schools [27–29]. These barriers include environmental constraints (e.g., accessibility, transportation), lack of appropriate programs, and available opportunities [28]. Less research has been done to explore factors that help enable PA participation; however, it is logical to suggest that the removal of some of the aforementioned barriers could help to enhance the likelihood of disabled children and adolescents engaging in activity, and therefore, reaping the associated health benefits.

Schools have been identified as a context that can inherently reduce barriers to PA for disabled children and adolescents and promote PA. Physical activity can take place in several different contexts within schools, including extracurricular or intramural sport activities, recess, and physical education (PE) classes. Physical education classes, specifically, have been identified as a context which has the potential to provide opportunities for all students, regardless of ability, to participate in PA. Notably, disabled students are often reliant on school-based programming, such as PE classes, to obtain their daily PA [30]. School-based PE can also take different forms, depending on the culture and context of the schools as well as legislative requirements of the country, including integrated or general PE settings (i.e., where disabled and nondisabled students are educated together), self-contained settings (i.e., where disabled students are educated together as a group), or other unique settings, such as reverse mainstreamed settings (i.e., larger groups of disabled students with small numbers of nondisabled students).

16.5 Promising Practices for Supporting School-Based Physical Activity

To support and bring in the lived experiences of disabled students into the classroom, a call to action for social justice approaches are needed in school-based PA [31] and PE spaces [32]. For social justice approaches to be implemented, practitioners and educators must be open to reflexivity as well as alleviation of power. Aligning with the writings of Paulo Freire [33] in the *Pedagogy of the Oppressed*, liberation should be a mutual process, in which both disabled students, educators, and practitioners work together to create opportunities for school-based PA. Freire's [33] notions are also related to global disability activists in the field, such as James Charlton [20] who asserts, "Nothing about us without us," and Sandy Ho who stated in Alice Wong's edited series of essays in *Disability Visibility* [34], "Taking up space as a disabled person is always revolutionary." Furthermore, practitioners and educators must view teaching as a fluid process and design their programming with a focus on empowering the voices of disabled children and adolescents. Practitioners and educators must also critically analyze how their biases affect their teaching strategies in ways that both create (e.g., differentiated assessment) and take away power (e.g., standardized testing) from disabled students. Educators and practitioners are also challenged to think about creative ways that they can meaningfully engage disabled students in the work that they do (e.g., co-creation of lesson plans and assessments).

To explore how reflexivity and meaningful engagement can be achieved, the next section will discuss strategies for practitioners and educators within school-based settings to actively engage disabled students. It is crucial to acknowledge that there is no one-size-fits-all strategy, and educators and practitioners should adapt these practices as best as they can to their context. What this means, is that the strategies we discuss in this chapter are only suggestions, and that practitioners and educators must work together with disabled students to see what works best for them. Educational practices have historically centered on school-based PE contexts, and largely within integrated spaces, however we will attempt to speak broadly about these practices across school-based spaces and places.

16.5.1 Strategies for Supporting School-Based Physical Activity for Disabled Students

16.5.1.1 Supporting Belonging, Acceptance, and Value Through Community Engagement

In many adapted PA texts, readers will find a host of best practices or "inclusive strategies" geared toward educating disabled students within school-based PE contexts. However, many of these practices or strategies are based on material definitions of inclusion and do not take into consideration the opinions or voices of disabled people themselves [19].

> Community engagement is a health promotion concept that empowers marginalized populations by facilitating power-sharing, mutual learning from all involved parties, and conducting needs assessments for specific groups [35].

With this point in mind, a critical strategy for those supporting PA for disabled students within school-based contexts, particularly when conceptualizing inclusion as an intersubjective experience, is to center the voices of disabled students in their decision-making process through community engagement. Community engagement provides an opportunity to empower disabled people to advocate and improve self-efficacy [35]. For example, community engagement would include having educators or other power holders actively communicating with disabled students about their experiences within school contexts (e.g., PE) and with activities regularly to ensure that they are having meaningful experiences that support feelings of acceptance, belonging, and value. Furthermore, community engagement could include engaging the school community such as disabled students, teachers, administrators, educational assistants, caregivers, and professionals (such as occupational therapists) in creating individualized PA goals and lessons for disabled students.

Community engagement has provided opportunities for professionals to think about disabled individuals more holistically and allow for reflections on how practitioners can address the needs of disabled students and their families [36]. While considering inclusion as intersubjective experiences, we must also recognize the challenges with community engagement, including differing priorities and values amongst groups, feelings of tokenism, and burdening the disabled population. Ways to counteract these challenges as an educator or practitioner are to ensure that disabled students share what they value in their learning, what outcomes they would like to gain from school PA programs, what level of time and commitment they are comfortable with to assist in the co-creation process of lessons, as well as meaningful compensation for their time (e.g., community service hours, reference letters, work experience).

> **Questions to practitioners and educators:**
> - What are some ways that you may be promoting normative standards and values in your classes?
> - What are ways to move away from those practices?

16.5.1.2 Preservice Training and Continual Learning

Common barriers to PA participation in schools for disabled students are educator and practitioner knowledge and attitudes [37, 38]. While we recognize that there are many systemic barriers (e.g., preservice and in-service training in teaching disabled students, funding, time, and shared values amongst educators and administrators) that may reproduce lack of knowledge and poor attitudes toward disabled students, we encourage practitioners and educators to make small changes in their classroom spaces. For instance, practitioners and educators can work to learn more about disabled populations and be reflexive in their teaching attitudes and practices. Practitioners and educators can also improve their knowledge by taking professional development courses and other opportunities related to adapted PA, depending on the country or region they are working within. Moreover, educators and practitioners can speak to colleagues in different departments or reach out to their networks who work with disabled students outside of the school settings, perhaps coaches or camp coordinators to discuss teaching strategies. Aligning with the Freire's [33] notion of alleviation of power, practitioners and educators must also challenge their own knowledge, be comfortable with being uncomfortable, and be driven to improve their teaching pedagogies.

16.5.1.3 Quality Participation: A Framework to Support School-Based Physical Activity

Quality participation is one way to promote school-based PA and aligns closely with conversations surrounding the intersubjectivity of inclusion [19], as well as the process of liberation [33]. First conceptualized by Martin Ginis and colleagues [39] and then contextualized to disability sport by Evans and colleagues [40], quality participation is an evidence-based framework that centers around their being constant exposure to one or more of six experiential aspects of participation. These experiential aspects are referred within the Quality Participation framework as building blocks –which can promote quality experiences in sport settings that can consequently lead to quality participation (i.e., feeling satisfied, having fun, and achieving personally meaningful goals). These building blocks include autonomy (e.g., choice), belongingness (e.g., acceptance), challenge (e.g., appropriately tested), engagement (e.g., being in flow or in-the-moment), mastery (e.g., a sense of achievement), and meaning (e.g., personal or social roles). We recognize that the definition of belongingness and acceptance are combined within the quality participation framework, but also must note that they too can be conceptually distinct. The quality participation framework was developed using a rigorous and systematic process involving a consensus-building process with disabled paraathletes, caregivers of disabled adolescent athletes, disability sport coaches and researchers and has been further supported through qualitative and quantitative studies [40]. The quality

Table 16.1 Strategies to promote the building blocks of quality participation

Building block	Definition	Building block specific strategies to implement in school-based physical activity
Autonomy	Having independence, choice, and control	Variety of equipment including adaptive equipment and games. Students can choose schedule and activities (e.g., Free Fridays). Activity stations [31]
Belongingness	Feeling part of a group, included, accepted, and/or respected by others	Co-operative games. Ice breakers. Group activities
Challenge	Feeling appropriately tested	Establishing the goals for each student and individualizing challenges based on those goals
Engagement	Feeling focused, in-the-moment, and absorbed; experiencing flow	Understanding what students enjoy and implementing it into lessons. Rapport building to understand what students need to be engaged
Mastery	Experiencing achievement, competence; having sense of accomplishment	Providing constructive feedback that assists students in working toward achieving goals
Meaning	Contributing toward obtaining a personal or socially meaningful goal; feeling a sense of responsibility to others	Challenging students to think about their "why" and purpose in PE contexts and make sure that is represented in what they are doing

participation framework also includes supporting strategies that can be used to promote quality participation in PA in school spaces through gaining a conceptual understanding of how students perceive each of the building blocks and ensuring these experiences are applied within PA school settings.

Table 16.1 illustrates some strategies, based on research by Evans et al. [40] as well as some of the authors' research on this framework in school settings [41] to promote the building blocks of quality participation. These strategies are a starting point, and therefore, we recommend educators and practitioners to collaborate with their disabled students on how they can apply these strategies within their school spaces. For instance, by meeting with students and asking them what makes them feel autonomous in PA settings (perhaps having choice in the equipment to be used), educators and practitioners can implement those requests within their lessons. For more information on the quality participation framework, we refer readers to Evans et al.'s [40] research as well as the practical guides for Building Quality Participation in Sport that are available on the Canadian Disability Participation Project website (https://cdpp.ca/resources-and-publications/blueprint-building-quality-participation-sport-children-youth-and-adults).

16.6 Practical Applications and Measurement for the Implementation and Evaluation of School-Based Physical Activity in Disabled Students

Now that we have discussed some strategies that can be used to support school-based PA for disabled students; in this third and final section of the chapter, we focus on more detailed considerations of implementing those strategies to promoting and evaluating PA of disabled students, with a particular focus on overall PA and fitness levels of disabled students.

16.6.1 Practical Considerations of Promoting Overall Physical Activity in Disabled Students

Schools are part of a "whole systems approach" for ensuring all students, including disabled students, can be afforded with the opportunity to engage in PA for optimal health [42]. As such, practitioners and educators have a responsibility of ensuring that PA is implemented and evaluated in ways that consider the needs and full capabilities of disabled students. Below are some considerations to do so.

16.6.1.1 Physical Activity Guidelines and School-Based Physical Activity

The promotion of PA in school-aged children and adolescents has traditionally been directed toward participation in moderate to vigorous intensity physical activity (MVPA) [42]. As mentioned earlier in the chapter, international PA guidelines recommend that children and adolescents spend, on average, at least 60 min each day in MVPA, with emphasis on aerobic-type activity [42]. This recommendation is associated with many health outcomes for children and adolescents, including better cardiorespiratory and muscular fitness, cardiometabolic health, academic achievement, emotion regulation, and quality of life [43, 44]. However, within the research that has informed this PA guideline, minimal evidence exists from studies of disabled children and adolescents [45]. Of the studies that have been included, most have focused on children with attention deficit and hyperactivity disorder, autism and intellectual disability, have samples of disabled children and adolescents with more mild impairment severity and who are ambulatory [46]. The lack of diversity in the study samples brings into question the appropriateness of using conventional PA guidelines when working with disabled students.

In 2021, disability-specific PA guidelines were put forth in the United Kingdom based on scientific evidence of the health benefits from PA done outside of clinical settings specifically for disabled children and young people (aged 2–17 years) [47]. Complementing this research was co-production work done through a knowledge user panel of disabled children and adolescents, and caregivers to create a knowledge tool for communicating the guidelines to disabled children and adolescents [47]. The disability-specific guideline noted that adolescents (aged 2–17 years) were encouraged to participate in 120–180 min of aerobic MVPA each week. Of particular interest is that the evidence informing this disability-specific guideline encourages choice in how the total volume of PA is accumulated over the week (e.g., 20 min per day, 3 times per week) rather than the one-size-for-all approach that is taken within the more conventional PA guideline for children and adolescents [47]. From the co-production process, the panel emphasized how activity intensity is often "an unnecessary, irrelevant, and confusing" message to communicate to disabled children and young people [47]. The panel emphasized the value of asking about intensity when discussing PA with disabled children and young people, and the need to start gradually with those who are more novice to PA while encouraging them to be physically active in ways they find enjoyable and that make them feel good [47].

Within schools, practitioners and educators have an important role in facilitating the PA participation of their students. For disabled students, there are often limited opportunities outside of school-time for engaging in meaningful PA. For instance, access to accessible PA spaces and knowledgeable program leaders are key barriers to PA for disabled students [28, 48]. Applying an individualized approach that is guided by students' interests and needs (as previously discussed), rather than conventional guidelines, is one way that educators and practitioners can better support the PA of disabled students. The intensity of the PA may be less of a priority for some disabled students than having the opportunity to be physically active (and thus a greater focusing on participation-related goals). Meanwhile, activity intensity may matter for disabled students who are aiming to work toward performance-related goals (e.g., beating a personal best time for the 400 m swim). Being open to facilitating quality participation experiences through the use of the quality participation framework [39, 40], and not solely focusing on PA guidelines, can allow for exploration, enjoyment, and ultimately continued participation in PA among disabled students.

16.6.1.2 School Sports Participation in Disabled Students

Sports within schools are a cornerstone experience for many students, whether it be through playing organized sports and active games during PE class or recess time, or on a school sports team. Students' participation in sport should consider not only their performance (e.g., points scored per game, skills, attendance) but also their experiences while participating (e.g., feeling engaged or part of the team). Too often is there a greater emphasis being placed on students' performance in sports and PE rather than equal (if not greater) prioritization of whether students are taking part in sports that make them feel satisfied, having fun in the activities, and feeling that they are achieving meaningful outcomes from their involvement in the activities (i.e., quality sport experience) [40].

Encouraging and supporting students' participation in sport, and more broadly PA, should also focus on their physical literacy. As defined by Whitehead [49], physical literacy is an embodied human experience that involves the "motivation, confidence, physical competence, and knowledge and understanding to value and take responsibility for engaging in physical activities for life" [49]. Educators and practitioners who adopt a physical literacy approach consider the relationships and interactive effects of the various domains of physical literacy (e.g., physical competence, motivation, enjoyment), rather than their isolated effects, and how they contribute to a student's individualized physical literacy journey [24, 49, 50].

Quality sport participation and physical literacy are approaches that align with the United Nations' Promoting Quality PE Policy of the United Nations Educational, Scientific and Cultural Organization [50]. Quality PE focuses on aspects related to "frequency, variety, inclusivity, and value content (e.g., fair play respect, friendship) to ensure that the right to access PE is realized by all students" [51]. Quality PE is distinct from PE as it promotes the use of a balanced instructional approach to PE through the integration of physical, mental, and social-emotional learning to enhance educational and employment outcomes [51]. Quality PE requires educators to be open to flexibility with rules and curricula and ensuring that the physical, social, and activity environments are welcoming, safe, and inclusive to disabled students as well as other equity-deserving students [51].

16.6.1.3 Practical Considerations for Promoting Fitness in Disabled Students

Many educators and practitioners may find themselves in a position of having to assess the fitness levels of their students. Fitness assessments most often consider one of the following categories: cardiorespiratory fitness, muscular strength and endurance, body composition, balance and, to a lesser extent in children, flexibility [52, 53]. The reasons for conducting school-based fitness assessments vary and may include, but are not limited to, there being a focus on fitness within the curriculum or that the educator or practitioner requires knowledge on students' baseline fitness levels to guide focus on individualized goals or adaptations of activities.

When considering the diverse needs and abilities of disabled students, educators and practitioners may feel challenged, at times, with how they incorporate fitness assessments into their teaching that allows for students to demonstrate their full capabilities. At the core of most fitness assessments are comparisons to criterion-referenced standards such as age or biological sex (e.g., male, female). In most instances, fitness assessments require educators and practitioners to compare their students to standards that have been validated in samples of nondisabled children and adolescents, and have been understudied, in terms of their reliability and validity, in disabled students [54, 55]. In line with our earlier discussion on ableism [15], fitness assessments based on criterion-referenced standards dictate the norm for being "physically fit" from a medicalized, health-related perspective. When compared to referenced values, disabled students most often score below cut-off values on fitness testing such as the shuttle run test, overarm throwing, standing long jump, and sit-ups, which has resulted in a narrative of disabled students being less physically fit than age- or sex-matched peers without disabilities [55, 56]. The standardized administration and scoring (e.g., same tasks and materials, set order of completion, limited verbal instruction) of fitness assessments, while argued necessary to make comparisons among groups and across settings, pose challenges when assessing the fitness levels of disabled students. Modifications that account for each student's preferences and learning and communication styles, such as being afforded with additional guidance to perform tasks correctly (e.g., verbal explanation and demonstrations, using a pacer or balance support from an instructor or peer while performing the task), addition of a familiarization period of the testing environment, rest periods, and practice trials can assist in students' understanding, motivation and confidence, and overall task performance [55, 57]. Rather than focusing on standardized scores or cut-offs, educators and practitioners are encouraged to consider how the fitness assessments they use within their teaching practices allow for monitoring of students' individualized progress toward goals over time that are meaningful to student success.

16.7 Pragmatic Measures and Practices for Evaluating School-Based Physical Activity Among Disabled Students

Understanding disabled students' PA participation and fitness levels is critical to quality PE. This understanding allows for educators and practitioners to meet students where they are currently at and identify areas for improvement at the individual, instructor, and school level. The school setting can provide unique opportunities as well as challenges to PA assessments for disabled students. The main priority when conducting assessments in school settings is that all students have a quality experience. Not all students will have the same physical, cognitive, and social abilities, and therefore, modifications to assessments may be needed to ensure quality participation. This section highlights three common types of assessment tools and discusses the opportunities and barriers associated with each type. This section also explores ways to modify assessment tools so that they are more appropriate and feasible to use with disabled students.

16.7.1 Common Assessment Types

There are three main types of assessments used to measure aspects related to PA and fitness. The first type is device-based measures, which refer to using a device (e.g., a Fitbit) to measure students' PA. Devices such as accelerometers, pedometers,

Fitbits, and Apple Watches allow for the collection of various types of PA data including steps per day, minutes of PA, and in some cases, calories burned, heart rate, and sleep.

Another common assessment tool used in PE is standardized observational assessment. Standardized assessments include fitness assessments (e.g., the shuttle run) and motor skill assessments (e.g., Test of Gross Motor Skill Development) [58]. Conducting standardized assessments in PE can provide valuable information to educators and practitioners regarding the fitness and skill levels as well as overall participation of students. With the information gained from fitness and motor skills assessments, PE lessons can be tailored to target areas that students are needing to improve within, as well as activities and/or teaching practices that can be modified using the supporting strategies discussed in Table 16.1 to improve participation levels as well as performance indicators in PE class.

The third type of assessment we will discuss in this section are student and proxy-reported questionnaires. Questionnaires provide an opportunity to gather information about students' PA participation in a relatively feasible and cost-effective way. Questionnaires can be completed using traditional pen and paper methods or they can be administered using online survey platforms like Google Forms. Questionnaires can be completed by students themselves (i.e., self-report) or by parents or educators (e.g., proxy report). Many questionnaires exist that capture participation in PA that include PA type (e.g., PE class, organized sport), time (e.g., duration spent being active), and intensity (e.g., light, moderate, vigorous intensity). Some questionnaires have also been developed that capture motor skill development and physical literacy (e.g., the Physical Literacy Assessment Youth-Self) [59] and quality participation in PA such as the Measure of Experiential Aspects of Participation developed by Caron and colleagues [60].

Table 16.2 presents an overview and examples of measurement tools for each type of assessment, along with considerations that must be made by educators and practitioners when administering these three different types of assessments with disabled students.

16.8 Using Assessment Tools in Physical Education Settings

When using PA and fitness assessments in school settings, it is important that disabled students are included and provided with equitable opportunities to complete the assessments to the best of their abilities. This practice aligns with the concept of community engagement, whereby disabled students are given the opportunity to have voice in what assessment is most meaningful to them. Moreover, it is critical that PA and fitness assessments are conducted in a way that promote quality participation for all students. Similar approaches that can be used to adapt school-based PAs (discussed earlier in the chapter) can also be used to adapt PA and fitness assessments. A helpful tool educators and practitioners can consider using for modifying PA assessments to meet the needs, interests, and abilities of disabled students

Table 16.2 A summary of the three types of assessments commonly used in physical activity and fitness evaluations and considerations when working with disabled students

Assessment type	Descriptions	Examples	Opportunities	Challenges
Devices	A common approach to measuring physical activity participation and aspects of fitness is through the use of physical activity and fitness trackers or devices.	Fitbits, Garmin watch, Apple watch, ActiGraph accelerometers, pedometers	Measuring physical activity using a device provides a mostly un-biased measurement of activity. Accelerometers are considered the "gold standard" for physical activity measurement. Physical activity and fitness trackers are becoming more commonly used and therefore students may already have these devices. Wearing a device can be fun and interesting for students.	Devices for measuring physical activity were created for nondisabled individuals and therefore, challenges remain with the accuracy of the data from these devices for disabled people. Physical activity and fitness trackers are expensive and are not a readily accessible tool for most educators and practitioners. Some students, especially those with sensory processing difficulties, may find wearing a device uncomfortable.
Standardized tests	Standardized tests are one way to assess students' fitness and motor skills. Typically, these assessments have strict protocols for how to administer the test to ensure consistency across all students. These tests are administered and scored by the educator or practitioner	*Health and fitness* Shuttle run, push-ups test, sit, and reach. *Motor skills* Test of Gross Motor Development (TGMD), Brockport Physical Fitness Test (BPFT), Bruininks-Oseretsky Test of Motor Proficiency-2 (BOT-2). *Physical Literacy* Physical Literacy Assessment for Youth (PLAY-Fun)	Standardized assessments provide a systematic way to observe students' skills and abilities. Scores on standardized assessments can be used to compare a student's skills and abilities over time. Standardized assessments provide insight into the skill levels and abilities in a physical education class or on a sports team.	Normative values that accompany standardized tests are usually based on nondisabled students and can be ableist in nature. Some activities included in a standardize test may not be appropriate for all students. For example, an assessment item measuring how fast a student runs would not be appropriate for a student using a wheelchair modifications to this item would be necessary.

Questionnaires/ surveys	Questionnaires/ surveys can be used as a tool to collect information about physical activity, fitness, and physical literacy. Questionnaires and surveys can be completed by the student themselves, by a educator, or by a caregiver	International Physical Activity Questionnaire for Adolescents (IPAQ-A), Physical Literacy Assessment for Youth-Self (PLAY-Self)	Questionnaires and surveys provide a relatively convenient way to assess aspects of physical activity and fitness. Questionnaires and surveys can be completed online and from anywhere.	Some questions may be difficult to understand and may require an adult's assistance completing the questions to ensure understanding. Completing a questionnaire using the pen/paper method may not be feasible for students who have visual impairments or who have significant upper limb impairments. Not all online questionnaire platforms are accessible and can be used with a screen reader.

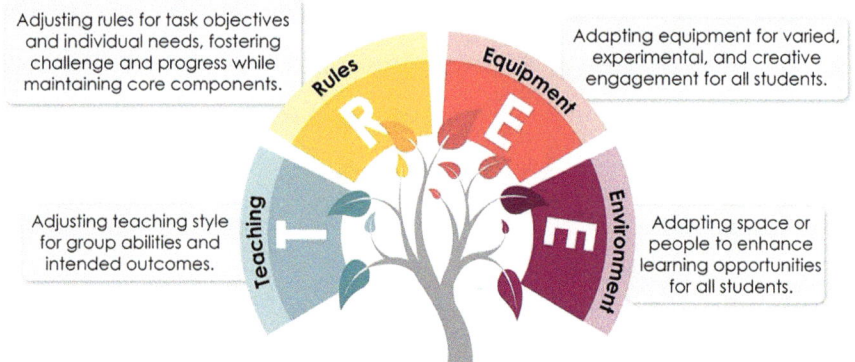

Fig. 16.1 The TREE framework and examples

is the TREE framework, with the acronym focusing on four areas to consider around modifying activities and assessments: Teaching, Rules, Equipment, and Environment [61]. The TREE framework (Fig. 16.1) functions as a mental map for educators and practitioners to ensure that they are prepared to facilitate PA and fitness assessments that will best capture the abilities and skills of all students as appropriately as possible.

16.8.1 Using the TREE Framework to Modify Physical Activity and Fitness Assessments

The following section will discuss two scenarios where educators are looking to assess the fitness and PA levels of their disabled and nondisabled students. For each scenario, we provide a discussion on the steps taken to choose the best-fitting assessment tool and how the TREE framework can be used as a guide for educators and practitioners to modify the assessment in an effort to ensure all students are included and have a quality experience.

> **Scenario #1**
> Mr. Jansen teaches a grade five PE class and is looking for a standardized test that can be used to measure students' PE skills. He teaches 20 students, including a student named Jessica who has cerebral palsy. Jessica is ambulatory, but often uses a walker to assist them when moving around. Dale is another student in Mr. Jansen's class. Dale has difficulty staying on tasks and often disengages during PE. Mr. Jansen is looking for assessment tools that will capture the PE skills of all students in his class and can foster a fun and meaningful PA experience for his students.

In Scenario 1, Mr. Jansen is looking to assess aspects of fitness among the students in his class. These assessments will be used to inform a portion of their grade for PE. Given that there is a student in Mr. Jansen's class who has a physical disability and there are also students who have difficulty staying on task, Mr. Jansen needs to select assessment tools that will best capture the diverse abilities of each of his 20 students.

The biggest challenge associated with using standardized assessments to measure the fitness and physical skill levels of disabled students is that these assessments were not designed for disabled students (as previously discussed in the chapter). These assessments often come with strict procedures for administering the test to ensure standardization, which often prevents equitable participation from disabled students. For example, testing procedures may only include verbal instructions, which may be difficult for some students to understand (e.g., students with cognitive impairments). Therefore, the results from the test may not reflect a student's actual ability but rather a student's ability (or inability) to understand instructions that are only provided using spoken communication.

Standardized assessments are often associated with "criterion-referenced values" (sometimes referred to as "normative values") that categorize students into different levels of ability. As discussed earlier, these normative values are often ableist in nature as they were developed using data from nondisabled individuals. This is important to keep in mind if using the results of a standardized assessment (and how students rank relative to such normative values) as a performance indicator. We must note that standardized assessment is not a practice that we ascribed to but recognize that others (e.g., administrators, researchers) may suggest educators and practitioners do so. In Mr. Jansen's case, it would be beneficial to speak to all of his students and understand what their individualized goals are, and from there, he can conduct the assessments multiple times throughout the year. This will allow Mr. Jansen to focus on individual-level improvement on the tasks instead of comparing students' results to "normative" values to determine their skill level.

An assessment tool that may be useful in this scenario is the Test of Gross Motor Development-3rd Edition (TGMD-3) [58], which is a commonly used motor skill assessment in school settings. Given that the TGMD-3 was designed for nondisabled students, and Mr. Jansen's class includes a student with cerebral palsy and another student who has difficulty staying on task, comparing students' performance on the TGMD-3 to the normative values associated with the test would not be appropriate. Modifying some of the TGMD-3 procedures and scoring are needed to ensure all students have an opportunity to participate fully and to the best of their abilities.

Using the TREE framework as a guide, we can modify the TGMD-3 such that it meets the needs of the students in Mr. Jansen's class and provides him with results that best represents students' actual capabilities, and therefore more appropriate information to include within his reporting on the students' evaluation. For example, Mr. Jansen can add visual instructions (*Teaching*) for the TGMD-3 that students can refer to throughout the lesson. This may be helpful for the student who has difficulty staying on task but will also be beneficial to other students in his class. The

Rules for the TGMD-3 could be modified to allow for greater participation from students who need physical supports. For example, instead of having students perform the kicking and throwing skills with their dominant hand (a rule that is outlined in the TGMD-3 manual), Mr. Jansen could give all of his students a choice for which side to use, which could account for some students who need higher physical supports and may experience physical impairments on one side of the body. Modifying the *Equipment* could also be helpful in creating an equitable experience for all of Mr. Jansen's students. For example, he could provide various sizes of balls for the throwing and kicking activities to account for a range of abilities. Finally, Mr. Jansen can choose to conduct the assessments in an *Environment* that has minimal distractions, has a flat and uniform surface to promote balance, and is familiar and comfortable for the students.

> **Scenario #2**
> Ms. Fletcher coaches the junior boys' basketball team as East Gate Highschool. There is one student on the basketball team who has Down syndrome and another student who experiences sight loss. She has never coached a team that had disabled students and wants to measure how engaged the students on her team are. To do this, Ms. Fletcher is looking for a measurement tool to assess students' physical activity participation on the basketball team.

In Scenario 2, Ms. Fletcher is a coach for her school's junior boys' basketball team. She is interested in measuring the PA levels of the students on the team to understand the PA participation levels of all team members. Two members of the basketball team have a diagnosed disability: Down syndrome and sight loss. Given this, Ms. Fletcher wants to ensure that the assessment tool chosen to assess PA will accurately reflect the participation levels of all the students on the team.

Device-based assessments provide an opportunity to measure PA levels without relying on self-reported data which helps to reduce biases and has been shown to be feasible to use with disabled children and adolescents [62]. However, the use of devices can be quite costly and are often not accessible to educators and practitioners in a school setting. That said, PA trackers are becoming more mainstream, and it is possible that students already own one of these devices. If this is the case, there may be opportunity to utilize the information provided by a student's activity tracker into PA assessments and a strategy moving forward on how to monitor their activity levels.

A more feasible option may be the use of pedometers, which are small devices that track step counts. If using monitoring devices as an assessment tool, it is important to keep in mind that most devices were developed for nondisabled individuals and similar to standardized fitness tests, data from these devices are often analyzed based on normative values developed through research with nondisabled children and adolescents. Studies examining the accuracy of device-based PA assessment tools, such as accelerometers, have demonstrated that estimates of PA among disabled children are often inaccurate [63, 64].

Ms. Fletcher explores the possibility of using devices to measure PA but realizes this will not be feasible to use with her team. She decides to use a questionnaire instead to capture the students' participation in PA. There are several validated questionnaires that have been developed by researchers to measure PA. Some questionnaires are designed for coaches, educators, or caregivers to complete based on their observations of the child (referred to as proxy reported questionnaires), and others are designed for children and adolescents to complete themselves (i.e., self-reported questionnaires). Ms. Fletcher decides to use the adolescent version of the *International Physical Activity Questionnaire* (IPAQ), which is meant for students to complete on their own [65]. Despite questionnaires being feasible to assess PA within this particular scenario, there are challenges that should be addressed. First, questionnaires rely on an individual's ability to recall events and, in the case of PA, specific details such as minutes spent in a particular intensity of PA. Therefore, using questionnaires introduce bias to the data being collected. In addition, it is extremely important that when administering questionnaires with students, efforts are made to ensure students understand the questions being asked.

Ms. Fletcher can use the TREE framework as a guide to modify how she administers the questionnaire so that it is inclusive to all students on the basketball team. With regard to *Teaching* modifications, Ms. Fletcher can ensure that clear instructions are provided to the students and have additional coaches or volunteers present to provide one-on-one assistance with completing the questionnaire. For disabled students, this may require one-on-one assistance with completing the questionnaire or rephrasing questions such that they are at a reading level appropriate for the student. Ms. Fletcher may also decide to change the *Rules* associated with the questionnaire. Typically, standardized questionnaires require the questions to be administered as is, without changing the wording and order of any of the questions. Ms. Fletcher knows from conversations with other educators that the student on the team with Down syndrome requires more reading support than other students on the team. Therefore, Ms. Fletcher could provide alternative phrasing on the questionnaire that will allow for all students to read, understand, and participate to the best of their ability. Printing the questionnaires is determined to be most feasible as this way Ms. Fletcher can bring physical copies of the questionnaire to the basketball practice thus reducing concerns around students not having access to a computer to complete the questionnaire online. However, Ms. Fletcher recognizes paper administration of the questionnaire will not be accessible for the blind student on her team. Therefore, Ms. Fletcher can change the *Equipment* used to deliver the questionnaire to accommodate all students on the team. She knows from speaking with the blind student that they typically use an iPad with a screen reader function in class. Knowing this, Ms. Fletcher creates an online version of the questionnaire using a survey platform (i.e., Google Forms) and confirms that the survey platform is compatible for use with a screen reader. To avoid potentially singling out the one blind student on the team, which could make him uncomfortable, Ms. Fletcher decides to give all students on the team a choice to complete the questionnaire at the basketball practice or using a computer at home. Finally, the *Environment* where the questionnaire is administered is important. Having somewhere for the students to complete the questionnaire away from distractions would help to keep students focused and which could help students recall their previous PA behaviors. Having coaches and volunteers available will help to foster a supportive and inclusive environment while the students complete the questionnaire.

16.9 Conclusion

Educators and practitioners must consider that there is no one-size-fits-all solution to promoting, implementing, and evaluating school-based PA for disabled students. What is important in this work is that educators and practitioners seek out the voices of disabled students in the PA spaces that directly involve and affect them. In this chapter, we have outlined various approaches for facilitating engagement with disabled students in school-based PA; for example, educators and practitioners can actively seek the perspectives of disabled students on their subjective experiences of inclusion and the quality participation building blocks that can be targeted within their teaching practices. Additionally, collaboration among educators and practitioners, as well as the broader school community (including disabled students, caregivers, educational assistants, administration, and therapists), is critical in developing individualized PA plans that align with the meaningful goals of disabled students in PE. This community engagement can also offer the opportunity for a critical review of necessary assessment tools to be used for disabled students as well, with a larger focus on individual improvement over time versus a one-time assessment period. As emphasized throughout the chapter, we encourage practitioners and educators to challenge dominant discourses of thought within school spaces by liberating themselves through learning from and about disabled students and improving their pedagogical practice. It is in this process of mutual liberation [33], that we all can move the needle in the direction of supporting quality PA opportunities for disabled students.

References

1. Spencer NL, Peers D, Eales L. Disability language in adapted physical education: what is the story? In: Routledge handbook of adapted physical education. Abingdon, Oxon: Routledge; 2020. p. 131–44.
2. Humpage L. Models of disability, work and welfare in Australia. Soc Policy Adm. 2007;41(3):215–31. https://doi.org/10.1111/j.1467-9515.2007.00549.x.
3. Barton L. Disability, physical education and sport: some critical observations and questions. In: Fitzgerald H, editor. Disability and youth sport. London: Routledge; 2009. p. 39–50.
4. Haegele JA, Hodge S. Disability discourse: overview and critiques of the medical and social models. Quest [Internet]. 2016;68(2):193–206. Available from: https://doi.org/10.1080/00336297.2016.1143849.

5. Haslett D, Smith B. Viewpoints toward disability: conceptualizing disability in adapted physical education. In: Haegele JA, Hodge SR, Shapiro DR, editors. Routledge handbook of adapted physical education. Abingdon, Oxon: Routledge; 2020. p. 48–64.
6. Goodley D. Disability studies: an interdisciplinary introduction. Disabil Stud. 2016:1–296.
7. Mitra S. The capability approach and disability. J Disabil Policy Stud. 2006;16(4):236–47. Available from: https://doi.org/10.1177/10442073060160040501.
8. Giese M, Haegele JA, Maher AJ. The ableist underpinning of normative motor assessments in adapted physical education. J Teach Phys Educ. 2023;1(aop):1–7.
9. Palmer M, Harley D. Models and measurement in disability: an international review. Health Policy Plan. 2012;27(5):357–64.
10. Goodley D. 'Learning difficulties', the social model of disability and impairment: challenging epistemologies. Disabil Soc. 2001;16(2):207–31.
11. Roush SE, Sharby N. Disability reconsidered: the paradox of physical therapy. Phys Ther. 2011;91(12):1715–27.
12. Robertson S. Sociologies of disability and illness: Contested ideas in disability studies and medical sociology. Sociol Health Illn. 2007;29(7):1108–9.
13. Reindal SM. Disability, capability, and special education: towards a capability-based theory. Eur J Spec Needs Educ. 2009;24(2):155–68.
14. Reindal SM. A social relational model of disability: a theoretical framework for special needs education? Eur J Spec Needs Educ. 2008;23(2):135–46.
15. Smith B, Mallick K, Monforte J, Foster C. Disability, the communication of physical activity and sedentary behaviour, and ableism: a call for inclusive messages. Br J Sports Med. 2021;55(20):1121–2.
16. Ball L, Lieberman LJ, Haibach-Beach P. Dignity of risk in physical education for students with visual impairments. EC Ophthalmol. 2021;12(3):12–7.
17. Haegele JA. Inclusion illusion: questioning the inclusiveness of integrated physical education. Quest. 2019;71(4):387–97. https://doi.org/10.1080/00336297.2019.1602547.
18. Haegele JA, Wilson WJ. 10 things I hate about 'inclusion' in physical education. In: Goodwin DL, Connolly M, editors. Reflexivity & change in adaptive physical activity: overcoming hubris. Routledge; 2023.
19. Haegele JA, Maher AJ. Toward a conceptual understanding of inclusion as intersubjective experiences. Educ Res. 2023;52(6):385–93.
20. Charlton JI. Nothing about us without us: disability oppression and empowerment. Univ of California Press; 1998.
21. Sibley BA, Etnier JL. The relationship between physical activity and cognition in children: a meta-analysis. Pediatr Exerc Sci. 2003;15(3):243–56.
22. Aitchison B, Rushton AB, Martin P, Barr M, Soundy A, Heneghan NR. The experiences and perceived health benefits of individuals with a disability participating in sport: a systematic review and narrative synthesis. Disabil Health J. 2022;15(1):101164.
23. Martin JJ. Benefits and barriers to physical activity for individuals with disabilities: a social-relational model of disability perspective. Disabil Rehabil. 2013;35(24):2030–7.
24. Arbour-Nicitopoulos KP, Kuzik N, Vanderloo LM, Martin Ginis KA, James ME, Bassett-Gunter RL, et al. Expert appraisal of the 2022 Canadian Para Report Card on physical activity for children and adolescents with disabilities. Adapt Phys Activ Q. 2023;40(3):465–74.
25. Ng K, Sit C, Arbour-Nicitopoulos K, Aubert S, Stanish H, Hutzler Y, Silva DA, Kang MG, López-Gil JF, Lee EY, Asunta P. Global Matrix of Para Report Cards on physical activity of children and adolescents with disabilities. Adapt Phys Act Q. 2023;1(aop):1–22.
26. Stanish H, Ross SM, Lai B, Haegele JA, Yun J, Healy S. US Physical Activity Para Report Card for children and adolescents with disabilities. Adapt Phys Act Q. 2023;1(aop):1–8.
27. Shields N, Synnot AJ. An exploratory study of how sports and recreation industry personnel perceive the barriers and facilitators of physical activity in children with disability. Disabil Rehabil. 2014;36(24):2080–4.

28. Shields N, Synnot AJ, Barr M. Perceived barriers and facilitators to physical activity for children with disability: a systematic review. Br J Sports Med. 2012;46(14):989–97.
29. Stanish H, Curtin C, Must A, Phillips S, Maslin M, Bandini L. Enjoyment, barriers, and beliefs about physical activity in adolescents with and without autism spectrum disorder. Adapt Phys Act Q. 2015;32(4):302–17.
30. Case L, Ross S, Yun J. Physical activity guideline compliance among a national sample of children with various developmental disabilities. Disabil Health J. 2020;13(2):100881.
31. Block ME, Fines A. Examining physical activity for individuals with disabilities through a social justice lens. Kinesiol Rev. 2021;11(1):80–7.
32. Hodge SR, Jordan RD, Smith KJ. Intersectionality, disability, justice, and critical pedagogy. In: Reflexivity and change in adaptive physical activity. Routledge; 2022. p. 123–35.
33. Freire P. Pedagogy of the oppressed. New York Continuum. 1970;72:43–70.
34. Wong A, editor. Disability visibility: first-person stories from the twenty-first century. New York: Vintage; 2020.
35. Cyril S, Smith BJ, Possamai-Inesedy A, Renzaho AM. Exploring the role of community engagement in improving the health of disadvantaged populations: a systematic review. Glob Health Action. 2015;8(1):29842.
36. Vargas CM, Arauza C, Folsom K, Luna MD, Gutiérrez L, Frerking PO, Shelton K, Foreman C, Waffle D, Reynolds R, Cooper PJ. A community engagement process for families with children with disabilities: lessons in leadership and policy. Matern Child Health J. 2012;16:21–30.
37. Tarantino G, Makopoulou K, Neville RD. Inclusion of children with special educational needs and disabilities in physical education: a systematic review and meta-analysis of teachers' attitudes. Educ Res Rev. 2022;36:100456.
38. Tanure Alves ML, Storch JA, Harnisch G, Strapasson AM, da Cunha P, Furtado OL, Lieberman L, et al. Physical education classes and inclusion of children with disability: Brazilian teachers' perspectives. Movimento. 2017;23(4):1229–44.
39. Ginis KA, Evans MB, Mortenson WB, Noreau L. Broadening the conceptualization of participation of persons with physical disabilities: a configurative review and recommendations. Arch Phys Med Rehabil. 2017;98(2):395–402.
40. Evans MB, Shirazipour CH, Allan V, Zanhour M, Sweet SN, Ginis KA, Latimer-Cheung AE. Integrating insights from the parasport community to understand optimal experiences: the Quality Parasport Participation Framework. Psychol Sport Exerc. 2018;37:79–90.
41. Huynh N, Bassett-Gunter R, Atkinson M, Arbour-Nicitopoulos K. Exploring perspectives of youth with and without intellectual and developmental disabilities and varying intersectional identities towards a mixed abilities physical education program and quality participation experiences. J Exerc Mov Sport (SCAPPS refereed abstracts repository). 2023;54(1). https://www.scapps.org/jems/index.php/1/article/view/3058.
42. World Health Organization. Global action plan on physical activity 2018–2030: more active people for a healthier world. World Health Organization; 2019.
43. Carson V, Chaput JP, Janssen I, Tremblay MS. Health associations with meeting new 24-hour movement guidelines for Canadian children and youth. Prev Med. 2017;95:7–13.
44. Wu XY, Han LH, Zhang JH, Luo S, Hu JW, Sun K. The influence of physical activity, sedentary behavior on health-related quality of life among the general population of children and adolescents: a systematic review. PLoS One [Internet]. 2017 [cited 2021 Jul 8];12(11):e0187668. Available from: https://journals.plos.org/plosone/article?id=10.1371/journal.pone.0187668.
45. Martin Ginis KA, van der Ploeg HP, Foster C, Lai B, McBride CB, Ng K, Pratt M, Shirazipour CH, Smith B, Vásquez PM, Heath GW. Participation of people living with disabilities in physical activity: a global perspective. Lancet. 2021;398(10298):443–55.
46. Bull FC, Al-Ansari SS, Biddle S, Borodulin K, Buman MP, Cardon G, Carty C, Chaput J-P, Chastin S, Chou R, Dempsey PC, DiPietro L, Ekelund U, Firth J, Friedenreich CM, Garcia L, Gichu M, Jago R, Katzmarzyk PT, et al. World Health Organization 2020 guidelines on physical activity and sedentary behaviour. Br J Sports Med. 2020;54(24):1451–62. https://doi.org/10.1136/bjsports-2020-102955.

47. Smith B, Rigby B, Netherway J, Wang W, Dodd-Reynolds C, Oliver E, Bone L, Foster C. Physical activity for general health in disabled children and disabled young people: summary of a rapid evidence review for the UK Chief Medical Officers' update of the physical activity guidelines. London: Department of Health and Social Care; 2022.
48. Martin Ginis KA, Ma JK, Latimer-Cheung AE, Rimmer JH. A systematic review of review articles addressing factors related to physical activity participation among children and adults with physical disabilities. Health Psychol Rev. 2016;10(4):478–94.
49. Whitehead M. Definition of physical literacy: developments and issues. In: Physical literacy across the world. Abingdon, Oxon: Routledge; 2019. p. 8–18.
50. Cairney J, Dudley D, Kwan M, Bulten R, Kriellaars D. Physical literacy, physical activity and health: toward an evidence-informed conceptual model. Sports Med. 2019;49:371–83.
51. Promoting quality physical education policy. Unesco.org. 2022 [cited 2023 Dec 3]. Available from: https://www.unesco.org/en/quality-physical-education.
52. Pescatello LS, editor. ACSM's guidelines for exercise testing and prescription. Lippincott Williams & Wilkins; 2014.
53. National Center for Health Physical Activity and Disability (NCHPAD). Fitness assessments for individuals who use a wheelchair: toolkit for the fitness professional [cited 2023 Dec 3]. Available from: https://www.nchpad.org/fppics/NCHPAD_Fitness%20Assessments_revised.pdf.
54. Balemans AC, Fragala-Pinkham MA, Lennon N, Thorpe D, Boyd RN, O'Neil ME, Bjornson K, Becher JG, Dallmeijer AJ. Systematic review of the clinimetric properties of laboratory-and field-based aerobic and anaerobic fitness measures in children with cerebral palsy. Arch Phys Med Rehabil. 2013;94(2):287–301.
55. Wouters M, Evenhuis HM, Hilgenkamp TI. Systematic review of field-based physical fitness tests for children and adolescents with intellectual disabilities. Res Dev Disabil. 2017;61:77–94.
56. Wouters M, Evenhuis HM, Hilgenkamp TI. Physical fitness of children and adolescents with moderate to severe intellectual disabilities. Disabil Rehabil. 2020;42(18):2542–52.
57. Verschuren O, Ketelaar M, Keefer D, Wright V, Butler J, Ada L, Maher C, Reid S, Wright M, Dalziel B, Wiart L. Identification of a core set of exercise tests for children and adolescents with cerebral palsy: a Delphi survey of researchers and clinicians. Dev Med Child Neurol. 2011;53(5):449–56.
58. Ulrich DA. The test of gross motor development-3 (TGMD-3): administration, scoring, and international norms. Spor Bilim Derg. 2013;24(2):27–33.
59. Sport for Life. PLAYself Workbook. Canada: Sport for Life; 2016. Available from: https://sportforlife.ca/wp-content/uploads/2016/12/PLAYself_Workbook.pdf [Accessed 24 July 2024].
60. Caron JG, Martin Ginis KA, Rocchi M, Sweet SN. Development of the measure of experiential aspects of participation for people with physical disabilities. Arch Phys Med Rehabil. 2019;100(1):67–77.
61. The Inclusion Club. Introduction to the TREE framework. 2017 [cited 2023 Dec 30]. Available from: http://theinclusionclub.com/e12-introduction-to-the-tree-framework/.
62. Bremer E, Arbour-Nicitopoulos KP, Tsui B, Ginis KA, Moore SA, Best KL, Voss C. Feasibility and utility of a Fitbit tracker among ambulatory children and youth with disabilities. Pediatr Exerc Sci. 2023;1(aop):1–9.
63. McGarty AM, Penpraze V, Melville CA. Calibration and cross-validation of the ActiGraph wGT3X+ accelerometer for the estimation of physical activity intensity in children with intellectual disabilities. PLoS One. 2016;11(10):e0164928.
64. Leung W, Siebert EA, Yun J. Measuring physical activity with accelerometers for individuals with intellectual disability: a systematic review. Res Dev Disabil. 2017;67:60–70.
65. Hagströmer M, Bergman P, De Bourdeaudhuij I, Ortega FB, Ruiz JR, Manios Y, Rey-López JP, Phillipp K, Von Berlepsch J, Sjöström M. Concurrent validity of a modified version of the International Physical Activity Questionnaire (IPAQ-A) in European adolescents: the HELENA Study. Int J Obes. 2008;32(5):S42.

Index

A

Academic performance, 5, 47, 174–177, 182, 183, 215, 223, 224, 233, 234, 238, 241, 245, 275, 276, 337, 341
Accelerometers, 75, 94, 96–100, 102, 103, 214, 215, 270, 274, 372, 374, 379
Accessibility, 57, 101, 313, 345, 364
Active breaks, 233–247
Active School Flag (ASF), 254, 255, 286
Active travel, 193–206
Activity guidelines, 20–23, 29–31, 369–370
Activity leaders, 286
Activity zones, 221, 222
Adolescence, 3–32, 56, 59, 108, 121, 133–137, 154, 169, 170, 176, 233, 280, 286, 330, 333, 336
Adolescents, 9–12, 15–20, 23–26, 31, 32, 41, 42, 44, 45, 49, 50, 55, 56, 59, 68, 69, 74–81, 83, 90–93, 96–99, 103, 104, 108, 135, 143, 148, 150, 151, 153, 154, 168–174, 178, 179, 181, 193–196, 198–202, 204, 206, 217, 220, 222, 224, 233, 234, 251, 252, 257, 258, 260–262, 269–272, 275–278, 280, 285, 294, 305–311, 314–316, 320, 321, 329–333, 336–341, 343, 359, 361, 363–365, 367, 369–371, 375, 378, 379

B

Before-school, 269, 289
Body mass index (BMI), 4, 13, 44, 81, 110, 114–116, 171, 173, 179, 216, 217, 223, 243, 244, 253, 308

C

Cardiorespiratory fitness (CRF), 9, 13, 81, 108, 109, 111, 112, 115, 119, 121–123, 173, 174, 200, 201, 206, 234, 242, 244, 275, 307, 319, 336, 347, 371
Child, 7, 23, 29–31, 49, 51, 54, 55, 73, 83, 93, 96, 99, 116, 134, 138–145, 148, 153–155, 178, 179, 182, 194, 213, 215, 216, 224, 253, 257, 259, 260, 287, 297, 339, 340, 379
Child development, 6, 42
Childhood, 3–32, 42, 50, 52, 56, 59, 72–74, 83, 108, 110, 111, 118, 124, 133–138, 142, 150, 154, 168, 169, 178, 179, 193, 198, 200, 216, 221, 233, 245, 252, 259, 290, 314, 333, 336, 340
Children, 4, 41, 68, 90, 108, 133, 169, 193, 213, 233, 251, 269, 285, 305, 327, 359
Classroom-based physical activity, 234–237, 245–247
Cognition, 8, 43, 109, 175–177, 183, 215–216, 234, 235, 245, 275, 280, 364
Community partners, 254, 258–260, 294, 296
Commuting to schools, 193–199, 201, 286
Comprehensive School Physical Activity Program (CSPAP), 182, 183, 255, 256, 259, 260, 287, 296
Creating Active Schools (CAS), 254, 256

D

Diaries, 94, 101, 102, 270
Disabilities, 17, 47, 50, 108, 134, 138, 140, 142, 144, 146–152, 154, 155, 307, 310, 336, 359–363, 365, 367–369, 372, 377, 378

E

Effectiveness, 58, 72, 92, 96, 134, 142, 148, 153, 172–175, 200, 218–221, 245, 269, 273–276, 279, 280, 288, 289, 303, 306, 312, 313, 315, 316, 344, 346
Exercises, 3, 7–12, 16, 18, 19, 21, 22, 24, 44, 47, 72, 89, 98, 109, 169, 173–175, 177, 180, 206, 238, 242, 244–247, 260, 273, 276, 289, 303–308, 311, 313–320, 328, 329, 333–336, 338, 339, 346, 363

F

Fitness, 14, 43, 80, 97, 108, 133, 171, 201, 217, 237, 275, 288, 303, 327, 369
Fitness assessments, 107–124, 330, 332, 371–373, 376–380

G

Game equipment, 218–220
Geolocation systems, 94

H

Hand strength, 112
Health outcomes, 3, 14, 16, 41, 43, 50, 55, 60, 81, 133, 170, 180, 199, 274, 275, 304, 306, 310, 311, 316, 320, 327, 369
Health promotion, 21, 42, 109, 117, 181, 303–306, 315, 342
Healthy lifestyles, 10, 12, 53, 58, 59, 168, 169, 240
Healthy Schools, 223
High-intensity interval training (HIIT), 242, 245, 303–321

I

Implementation, 17, 54, 57–59, 68, 103, 108, 118–122, 135, 137, 142, 151, 174, 181, 217, 222–224, 237–238, 240–246, 253–256, 258, 261, 262, 269, 271–273, 276–280, 286, 289, 296, 311, 314–317, 343, 344, 369–372

Inclusion, 57, 103, 174, 175, 178, 182, 219, 239, 240, 256, 274, 279, 310, 359, 363–364, 366, 367, 380
Infants, 4–6, 12–14, 18, 23, 26, 31, 45, 48, 50–52, 138–140
Interventions, 4, 42, 81, 90, 117, 134, 171, 198, 214, 234, 251, 273, 288, 306, 328, 361
Interviews, 51, 74, 91, 94, 100–102, 293

K

Knowledge and understandings, 68, 70–72, 75–79, 81, 83, 341, 371

L

Lifestyles, 5, 9, 10, 14–16, 19, 58, 59, 72, 80, 93, 100, 104, 167–170, 178, 183, 193, 197, 216, 257, 259, 286, 291, 341, 346, 359
Lifetime engagement, 70, 72, 76–79

M

Mental health, 4–8, 10, 12–16, 43, 44, 55, 90, 108, 168, 169, 174, 180, 198, 214, 306, 310, 311, 327
Morning, 202, 213, 215, 220, 270, 272, 274, 276, 277
Motivation and confidence, 72, 75, 76, 81, 317, 372
Motor assessments, 133–155
Motor delays, 133, 134, 142, 144, 145
Motor development, 133–137, 140–142, 154, 294, 374
Movement behaviors, 41–60, 103, 170, 197–199
Muscle-strength, 7, 13, 23, 201, 242, 244, 285, 327, 329
Muscle-strengthening activities, 20, 327–347

O

Out of school time, 259, 312

P

Pedometers, 75, 76, 94, 95, 98, 99, 372, 374, 378
Physical active lessons, 237–239
Physical activity (PA), 3, 41, 67, 89, 107, 133, 167, 193, 213, 233, 251, 269, 285, 304, 327, 359

Index

Physical competence, 68, 70–79, 81, 83, 170, 171, 313, 317, 341, 371
Physical education (PE), 56, 57, 67–70, 73, 74, 93, 121, 143, 148, 150–152, 167–184, 203–205, 214, 223, 237, 246, 253–261, 272, 279, 286–288, 293, 295, 306, 307, 311–314, 317, 318, 320, 329, 330, 333–345, 364–366, 368, 370–380
Physical endurance, 175
Physical fitness, 3, 12, 23, 67, 75, 107–124, 146, 169–176, 180–183, 213, 216, 236, 237, 243, 245, 257, 309, 317, 320, 374
Physical literacies, 67–83, 180, 203, 311, 313–314, 321, 329, 341, 371, 373–375
Preschoolers, 4–6, 12–14, 18, 20, 26–30, 41–45, 48, 51, 53, 54, 56, 58, 108, 115–117, 119, 121–123, 219–222
Public health, 4, 17, 19, 25, 44, 50, 53, 56, 58, 67, 69, 70, 90, 99, 107, 110, 122, 168, 170, 175, 178, 180, 183, 184, 193, 206, 251, 252, 256, 304, 313

Q

Questionnaires, 75, 76, 79, 91–94, 99–102, 140, 373, 375, 379, 380

R

Recommendations, 12, 16–32, 44–47, 49–51, 53–55, 59, 90, 92, 96, 115, 120, 169, 171, 179, 180, 182, 183, 198, 199, 214, 223, 224, 233, 234, 237, 240, 246, 269, 277–280, 296, 304, 306, 317–320, 328, 335, 341, 342, 369

S

School break, 213, 220, 224
School guidelines, 287–288
School programs, 260, 277, 287, 290, 297

School promotion, 327–347
Schools, 11, 42, 73, 92, 108, 133, 167, 193, 213, 233, 252, 269, 286, 304, 328, 359
Schools on the Move, 254, 286
School systems, 108, 117, 251–254, 256–260, 262, 270
Sedentary behaviors (SB), 3–32, 41–43, 46, 48–51, 53–56, 58, 81, 89, 93, 96, 109, 169, 170, 172, 197–199, 221, 233, 272, 293
Sleep durations, 13, 41, 42, 46, 47, 50, 53–55, 58, 59, 96, 199
Smartphones, 25, 97, 98, 100, 101, 104, 204
Social ecological model, 252
Stakeholders, 44, 52, 69, 70, 120, 121, 221, 224, 240, 244, 262, 269, 271, 272, 276–280, 316, 341
Standing long jump (SLJ), 113, 116, 308, 327, 331, 372
Structure games, 6, 68, 69

T

Teacher trainings, 173, 256, 258, 345
Teaching strategies, 176, 365, 367
Toddlers, 4–6, 12–14, 18, 21, 23, 26–31, 43, 45, 48, 51–54, 138–140
Transport, 28, 31, 97, 98, 109, 195, 196, 201–206, 269–271, 277–279, 297, 336

W

Waist circumference, 44, 81, 114, 173, 223, 308, 309
Whole-of-school physical activity, 254–261

Y

Youth, 11, 41, 90, 108, 133, 167, 194, 214, 252, 271, 285, 304, 327
Youth fitness, 117, 215, 217